PESTICIDE RESIDUES IN FOOD

TECHNOLOGIES FOR DETECTION

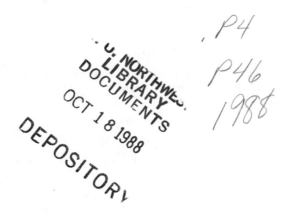
CONGRESS OF THE UNITED STATES   OFFICE OF TECHNOLOGY ASSESSMENT

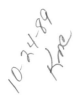

Recommended Citation:

U.S. Congress, Office of Technology Assessment, *Pesticide Residues in Food: Technologies for Detection,* OTA-F-398 (Washington, DC: U.S. Government Printing Office, October 1988).

Library of Congress Catalog Card Number 88-600566

For sale by the Superintendent of Documents
U.S. Government Printing Office, Washington, DC 20402-9325
(order form can be found in the back of this report)

Foreword

Pesticides are an integral part of agriculture today, but their use can lead to residues in agricultural products. Because of their potential adverse human health effects, the Federal Government sets limits on allowable levels of pesticide residues in food and animal feed and monitors these products to enforce those levels.

Federal monitoring and enforcement action is dependent on technical capability to detect pesticides. A major concern is that Federal regulatory agencies cannot practically monitor food for all pesticides of health concern. OTA was asked to assess whether existing and emerging technologies could improve Federal monitoring of pesticide residues in food. In addition, OTA examined the Federal research programs dedicated to improving Federal analytical capabilities for the detection of pesticides in food.

This study was requested by the House Committee on Energy and Commerce Subcommittee on Oversight and Investigations; the House Committee on Agriculture; and its Subcommittee on Domestic Marketing, Consumer Relations, and Nutrition. The Senate Committee on Agriculture, Nutrition, and Forestry and the House Agriculture Subcommittee on Department Operations, Research, and Foreign Agriculture endorsed the request.

OTA appreciates the valuable assistance of the study's workshop participants and observers, authors of commissioned technical papers, and the many other individuals from the public and private sectors who provided information throughout the course of this assessment and reviewed a draft of the report. As with all OTA studies, the content of this report is the sole responsibility of OTA.

JOHN H. GIBBONS
Director

OTA Workshop Participants:
Technologies To Detect Pesticide Residues in Food, Mar. 14-16, 1988

Henry Conacher
Food Research Division
Health and Welfare Canada
Ottawa, Canada

John Cowell
Environmental Sciences Department
Monsanto Co.
St. Louis, MO

William Cusick
Chemistry Laboratory Services
Department of Food and Agriculture
Sacramento, CA

Richard Ellis
Chemistry Division
Food Safety and Inspection Service
U.S. Department of Agriculture
Washington, DC

Silvia Canseco Gonzalez
Plant and Animal Health Office
Agriculture Department
Cozoacan, Mexico City

Kenneth Hill
Environmental Chemistry Laboratory
Agricultural Research Service
U.S. Department of Agriculture
Beltsville, MD

Kenneth Hunter
Westinghouse Bio-Analytic Systems Corp.
Rockville, MD

Lyle Johnson
Analytical Bio-Chemistry Laboratories, Inc.
Columbia, MO

Bruce Kropscott
Analytical and Environmental Chemistry
Dow Chemical Co./USA
Midland, MI

Harry Lento
Corporate Analytical Chemistry
Campbell Soup Co.
Camden, NJ

Julius Menn
Plant Science Institute
Agricultural Research Service
U.S. Department of Agriculture
Beltsville, MD

Ralph Mumma
Pesticide Research Laboratory
Pennsylvania State University
University Park, PA

W. Harvey Newsome
Pesticide Section
Food Research Division
Health and Welfare Canada
Ottawa, Canada

Cynthia Peck
Analytical and Environmental Chemistry
Dow Chemical Co./USA
Midland, MI

Jack Plimmer
Environmental Chemistry Laboratory
Agricultural Research Service
U.S. Department of Agriculture
Beltsville, MD

Leon Sawyer
Center for Food Safety and Applied Nutrition
Food and Drug Administration
U.S. Department of Health and Human Services
Washington, DC

Jim Seiber
Department of Environmental Toxicology
University of California
Davis, CA

Sarah Taylor
Congressional Research Service
The Library of Congress
Washington, DC

Charles Trichilo
Residue Chemistry Branch
Office of Pesticides and Toxic Substances
Environmental Protection Agency
Washington, DC

NOTE: OTA appreciates and is grateful for the valuable assistance and thoughtful critiques provided by the workshop participants. The workshop participants do not, however, necessarily approve, disapprove, or endorse this report. OTA assumes full responsibility for the report and the accuracy of its contents.

OTA Project Staff
Pesticide Residues in Foods: Technologies and Methodologies for Detection

Roger C. Herdman, *Assistant Director, OTA*
Health and Life Sciences Division

Walter E. Parham, *Food and Renewable Resources Program Manager*

Susan Shen, *Project Director*

Contractors

H. Anson Moye, *University of Florida*

Allen Ruby, *In-House Contractor*

Lisa Olson, *Editor*

Administrative Staff

Ellis Lewis, *Administrative Assistant*

Nellie Hammond, *Secretary*

Carolyn Swann, *Secretary*

Abbreviations and Acronyms

ADI —Acceptable Daily Intake
AFID —alkali flame ionization detector
AOAC —Association of Official Analytical Chemists
CCPR —Codex Alimentarius Committee on Pesticide Residues
CDFA —California Department of Food and Agriculture
CES —compound evaluation system
CFSAN —Center for Food Safety and Applied Nutrition (of FDA)
DDT —dichlorodiphenyl trichloroethane
ECD —electron capture detector
EDB —ethylene dibromide
ELISA —enzyme-linked immunosorbent assay
EPA —Environmental Protection Agency
FDA —Food and Drug Administration
FFDCA —Federal Food, Drug, and Cosmetic Act
FIA —Federal Insecticide Act
FIFRA —Federal Insecticide, Fungicide, and Rodenticide Act
FMIA —Federal Meat Inspection Act
FOI —Freedom of Information
FPD —flame photometric detector
FR —Federal Register
FSIS —Food Safety and Inspection Service
FTE —full-time equivalents
GC —gas chromatography
GLC —gas liquid chromatography
GPC —gel permeation chromatograpy
HECD —Hall microelectrolytic conductivity detector
HPLC —high performance liquid chromatography
IR —infrared (detector)
ITD —ion trap detector
IUPAC —International Union of Pure and Applied Chemistry

LC —liquid chromatography
LIMS —Laboratory Information Management Systems
LOQ —limits of quantitation
LUO —laboratory unit operations
MOG —Mills, Onley, and Gaither
MOU —memorandum of understanding
MRP —multiresidue procedure
MRL —maximum residue limits
MRM —multiresidue method
MS —mass spectrometry
MSD —mass selective detector
NBS —National Bureau of Standards
NOEL —No Observable Effect Level
NPD —nitrogen-phosphorus detector
NRP —National Residue Program
NTIS —National Technical Information Service
OMA —*Official Methods of Analysis*
PAM —*Pesticide Analytical Manual*
PC —paper chromatography
PCB —polychlorinated biphenyls
PICRC —Pesticide and Industrial Chemicals Research Center (of FDA)
RRT —relative retention time
SF —supercritical fluid
SFC —supercritical fluid chromatography
SFE —supercritical fluid extraction
SI —Surveillance Index
SIM —single ion monitoring
SPE —solid phase extraction
SRM —single residue method
TDRC —Total Diet Research Center (of FDA)
TDS —Total Diet Study
TLC —thin layer chromatography
UAR —unidentified analytical response
USDA/ARS—United States Department of Agriculture/Agricultural Research Service
UV/VIS —ultraviolet-visible (light detector)

Contents

Page

Abbreviations and Acronyms vii

Chapter 1: Introduction 3

Chapter 2: Federal Pesticide Residues in Food Monitoring Programs 7

Chapter 3: Contemporary Analytical Techniques for Pesticide Residues
    in Food 21

Chapter 4: Immunoassay: An Emerging Technology......................... 37

Chapter 5: Automation in Today's Pesticide Laboratory 49

Chapter 6: Pesticide Analytical Methods................................. 59

Chapter 7: Federal Methods Development Programs for Detecting Pesticides
    in Food 75

Chapter 8: Summary and Options 87

Appendix A: OTA Workshop Participants and Observers 109

Appendix B: OTA Workshop Papers 112

Appendix C: Glossary of Terms 230

Chapter 1
Introduction

CONTENTS

Page

Introduction 3
Chapter 1 References 4

Chapter 1
Introduction

Pesticides, in general, are chemicals used worldwide in agricultural production to destroy or control weeds, insects, fungi, and other pests. Some of those pesticides remain on food as residues. When pesticides are applied improperly, resulting residues can pose significant health risks to consumers. To protect U.S. consumer health, Federal and State programs have been established to monitor levels of pesticide residues present in domestic and imported food and fodder and to prevent the marketing of food containing residues that either exceed specific levels (known as tolerances) set by the Environmental Protection Agency or for which no tolerances have been established for that food.

Public concern over pesticide residues in food has been increasing during the last decade. For example, a recent 1988 national survey by the Food Marketing Institute showed that approximately 75 percent of consumers are very concerned about pesticides in their food; that percentage is higher than that of consumers worried about cholesterol, fats, salt, additives, or any other components (2). Contributing to such concerns have been the discovery of hazardous effects from certain pesticides once deemed safe, e.g., ethylene dibromide (EDB) and chlordane, and publicized acute food poisonings from improperly used pesticides, e.g., the aldicarb contamination of watermelon in the Western United States and Canada in 1985. Finally, the high level of uncertainty concerning the health effects of pesticide residues has heightened consumer concern.

One factor in this uncertainty is the technical capability of Federal and State programs to analyze food for all pesticides. These programs are faced with an enormous number of pesticide/food combinations to test, and the difficulty of the task is compounded by a lack of information on what pesticides actually have been used on specific crops (especially for imports). Analyzing for all pesticides on all types of food products is currently impossible because of limitations in testing methods as well as time and resource constraints. Although the number of pesticide/food combinations to address can be narrowed by focusing on the potentially moderate to high health hazard combinations, current analytical methods are not adequate to identify and quantify all residues of these pesticide/food combinations within available resources.

Although Federal data show that only a small percentage of food samples tested violate established tolerances, a gray area exists for those pesticides and pesticide/food combinations that are not being analyzed because of the cost or time of analysis or that cannot be detected by existing analytical methods. Also included in this area are a number of pesticides not yet addressed in the monitoring programs, such as significant pesticide metabolites, new pesticides, foreign-used pesticides not approved for use in the United States, and pesticide ingredients categorized as inert. Thus, analytical methods have become one of the limiting factors in enforcing pesticide tolerances in food. The uncertainty over this gray area often is interpreted as a lack of proof of the safety of food and so contributes to public concerns over pesticide residues.

Recent evaluations of Federal pesticide monitoring programs have highlighted the gap between the number of pesticides that could potentially be found in food and the number of pesticides that can be detected by methods routinely used. Although the size and the public health significance of this gap are debatable, a general consensus exists that improved analytical methods could help enhance the effectiveness of monitoring programs.

Toward this end, increasing interest exists, including in the U.S. Congress,[1] in expanding the capability of current analytical methods and developing new methods to detect pesticide residues in food. Emphasis is being placed on making methods more practical, e.g., able to identify increased numbers of pesticides, be less time-consuming, and use equipment commonly found in analytical laboratories. Emphasis also exists on improving methods to address those pesticide residues with the greatest potential health hazards. Furthermore, attention is being given to potential applications of new, emerging analytical technologies, such as new instrumentation, technologies based on biologically produced reagents, more rapid semiquantitative and qualitative techniques, and technologies that could be easily used outside the laboratory.

Although increased interest exists in improving analytical methods, no consensus has yet developed on the importance of doing so. In contrast to the general public's uneasiness over pesticide residues in food, the Federal agencies responsible for regulating foods do not have the same level of concern for the situation as it exists. Based on the low violation rates found in food under current testing programs, the Food and Drug Administration (FDA) of the U.S. Department of Health and Human Services and the Food Safety and Inspection Service (FSIS) of the U.S. Department of Agriculture consider that pesticide residues in foods is not the most important food safety issue.[2] The agencies consider other sources of food contamination such as microbiological and animal drug residues as having higher priority in allocation of their resources.

Because of growing congressional interest in pesticide analytical methods, the Office of Technology Assessment (OTA) was requested by Congress to examine the state of the art of analytical technologies and methods to detect pesticide residues in food and offer options on how Federal agencies, especially FDA, could improve their analytical capability through the adoption or improvement of technologies and analytical methods. This OTA report provides a brief assessment of existing, new, and emerging analytical technologies and methods to detect pesticide residues in food. Second, the report addresses Federal research and programmatic issues relevant to the development and adoption of technologies and methods.[3] Information presented in this report was gathered from 1) telephone interviews with some 50 experts; 2) visits to 7 pesticide analytical laboratories: 3 FDA, 1 State, 2 private, and 1 foreign; 3) OTA staff research; and 4) a 2½-day OTA technical workshop. The workshop participants and observers are listed in appendix A and the 13 peer-reviewed technical papers presented at the workshop are in appendix B.

---

[1]Several bills have been introduced in 1987-1988 of the 100th Congress that include sections on the development and implementation of more "practical" analytical methods for the detection of pesticide residues in food.

[2]FDA believes, and has frequently told the Congress, that the low incidence of illegal pesticide residues in the American food supply and the results of FDA's Total Diet Study indicate that pesticide residues in food do not pose a health hazard (1).

[3]The issue of the actual public health hazard due to pesticide residues in food was outside the scope of this OTA study.

CHAPTER 1 REFERENCES

1. Food and Drug Administration, Office of the Associate Commissioner for Legislative Affairs, official Agency response to OTA June 1988 draft report, June 29, 1988.

2. Food Marketing Institute, *Trends: Consumer Attitudes and the Supermarket* (Washington, DC: Food Marketing Institute, 1988).

Chapter 2
Federal Pesticide Residues in Food Monitoring Programs

CONTENTS

Page

The Legal Basis for Federal Pesticide Monitoring in Foods 7
Federal Monitoring Programs 8
    Environmental Protection Agency 8
    Food and Drug Administration of the
        U.S. Department of Health and Human Services 9
    The Food Safety and Inspection Service of the
        U.S. Department of Agriculture 12
Other Pesticide Residues in Food Monitoring Programs 15
Chapter 2 References 16

Figures

Figure   *Page*
2-1. FDA Pesticide in Food Monitoring Program in 1987 11
2-2. Number of Food Monitoring Samples Analyzed for
      Pesticide Residues in 10 States in 1987 15

Table

Table   *Page*
2-1. Numbers of Compounds Determined or Identified by
      Primary FDA Multiresidue Methods 9

Federal Pesticide Residues in Food Monitoring Programs

THE LEGAL BASIS FOR FEDERAL PESTICIDE MONITORING IN FOODS

Comprehensive Federal food laws are a 20th-century phenomenon, although the States regulated food quality before 1900. The 1906 publication of Upton Sinclair's novel *The Jungle* sparked a consumer reaction against the adulteration and misbranding of food, which resulted in the passage of the Federal Meat Inspection Act (FMIA) of 1906 and the Pure Food and Drugs Act (F&D Act) of 1906 (5). Both statutes have been significantly amended, although they retain their original purposes today. The F&D Act of 1906 was revised into the Federal Food, Drug, and Cosmetic Act (FFDCA) in 1938. The origin of Federal regulation of pesticide use can be traced to this same general period with the Federal Insecticide Act (FIA) of 1910. The FIA was replaced by the Federal Insecticide, Fungicide, and Rodenticide Act (FIFRA) of 1947, which as amended, remains the basis for regulating the use of pesticides today.

Currently, Federal jurisdiction over pesticide residues in food is divided among four bodies—the Environmental Protection Agency (EPA), the Food and Drug Administration (FDA) of the U.S. Department of Health and Human Services, and the Food Safety and Inspection Service (FSIS) and Agricultural Marketing Service (AMS) of the U.S. Department of Agriculture (USDA). Their authority for this work comes primarily from five laws: FIFRA, FFDCA, FMIA, the Poultry Products Inspection Act, and the Egg Products Inspection Act.

EPA, under FIFRA, must register a pesticide before the pesticide can be distributed or sold in the United States (7 U.S.C. Section 136 et seq., 1982 & Supp. IV 1986). The registration includes the specific commodities the pesticide can be used on. In registering a pesticide, EPA balances the risks and benefits associated with the use of that pesticide while ensuring that its use will not cause an unreasonable risk to humans or the environment.[1]

If the pesticide is to be used on food or feed commodities or if its use will lead to residues on these products, EPA, under FFDCA, establishes the legal maximum level of the pesticide residue (including residues of significant metabolites or degradation products) allowed in each specific food or feed (FFDCA; 21 U.S.C. Sections 346A, 1982 & Supp. IV 1986). These levels are known as tolerances. A tolerance, or an exemption from a tolerance, must be granted before such a pesticide is registered. Tolerances cannot be legally exceeded and residues of pesticides are prohibited on foods for which no tolerance has been established or exempted. Commodities that violate these prohibitions are subject to seizure by FDA, USDA, or a State enforcement agency (33).

FDA, under FFDCA, has responsibility for enforcing tolerances established by EPA in food (except meat and poultry) and animal feed moving in interstate commerce and for enforcing prohibition of a pesticide residue in food or feed for which no tolerance has been set or exemption given (21 U.S.C. Sections 331-337, 1982 & Supp. IV 1986).[2]

---

[1]The registration requirements for pesticides are set forth in Section 3 of FIFRA and are defined more fully in EPA regulations (40 C.F.R. Sections 158 and 162 1987).

[2]In some cases, a specific residue may be present on a commodity for which no tolerance exists because of the environmental persistence of the pesticide rather than its direct application on the commodity. If in this type of case FDA considers low levels of such a residue to pose little risk to human health, FDA used to informally set regulatory residue levels called "action levels" at which FDA would take regulatory action and below which the food was not found to be violative (21 CFR Sec-

(continued on next page)

FSIS of USDA is responsible for enforcing tolerances in meat and poultry under authority of the Federal Meat Inspection Act (21 U.S.C. Sections 601-695, 1982 & Supp. IV 1986) and the Poultry Products Inspection Act (21 U.S.C. Sections 451-470, 1982 & Supp. IV 1986). AMS of USDA is responsible for pesticide residue monitoring of raw egg products (dried, frozen, or liquid eggs) and tolerance enforcement at establishments having official USDA egg products inspection service under authority of the Egg Products Inspection Act (21 U.S.C. 1031-1056). Under this act, FDA has jurisdiction over these products outside such establishments.

(continued from previous page)
tions 109 and 509, 1987; FDA Compliance Policy Guides, 1986). The informal process by which these action levels have been set has been vacated by the Federal Appeals Court in the *District of Columbia Consumer Nutrition Institute* v. *Young,* 818 F.2d 943 (D.C. Cir. 1987). EPA and FDA are currently determining how to address these cases.

FEDERAL MONITORING PROGRAMS

Environmental Protection Agency (EPA)

EPA has no direct responsibility for enforcing pesticide tolerances in food; therefore, its monitoring of pesticide residues in food is minimal. EPA's primary responsibilities concerning pesticide residues in food, as noted earlier, are registering the pesticides and establishing pesticide tolerances for food and feed. EPA's pesticide monitoring work is geared primarily toward regulating pesticide levels in the environment (e.g., water, air, and soil) and ensuring that pesticides are being used in accordance with their registration. However, EPA conducts some monitoring for pesticide residues in food as part of its monitoring of pesticides in the environment. Agricultural commodities are occasionally analyzed by EPA as a means of identifying pesticide misuse or pesticide drift from point of application or, if necessary, of obtaining additional residue data for a pesticide under Special Review to determine if a pesticide's registration should be canceled, denied, or reclassified because of adverse effects (32).

The tolerance-setting process is the basis for FDA and USDA regulation of pesticide residues in food. As part of the tolerance-setting process, EPA requires the submission of, among other things, the following: 1) residue chemistry data, e.g., what residues occur and how much of each is present; 2) toxicity data; and 3) an analytical method to detect the pesticide and its toxic metabolites in the foods for which a tolerance is to be set. The first two sets of data are used by EPA to determine the likely level of dietary exposure to the pesticide, level of dietary exposure acceptable for human health, and the tolerance level in each food (33).[3] (For a detailed description of the tolerance-setting process, see ref. 24.)

Limitations of the tolerance-setting process may affect the capabilities of FDA and USDA to monitor for pesticide residues in food. For example, if incomplete metabolism studies were used in setting tolerances, then all the possible metabolites and breakdown products of the pesticide are not known and methods for their analysis may not be available or required (33). A second important limitation (discussed in chapter 7) is the regulatory usefulness of the methods submitted to EPA as part of the tolerance setting process.

[3]The majority of tolerances are established for pesticides on raw agricultural commodities and set to protect the public health while considering the benefits of the pesticide use. A small number of tolerances are set for processed foods. Under FFDCA, if a pesticide concentrates during food processing and therefore occurs in a higher concentration in the processed food than in the raw agricultural commodity, the decision to establish a tolerance must be only risk-based, without the consideration of potential benefits. An additional rule, applying only to processed foods, is that if a pesticide that concentrates during processing also causes cancer in humans or animals, then no tolerance can be granted for the processed food. For pesticides that do not concentrate, the tolerance for the raw agricultural commodity suffices for processed foods. For further details on this distinction see ref. 25.

Food and Drug Administration (FDA) of the U.S. Department of Health and Human Services

FDA enforces pesticide residue tolerances established for a wide variety of raw agricultural food and feed, and for processed products. Commodities sampled do not include meat and poultry, which are the province of USDA. To fulfill its regulatory responsibilities, FDA established a pesticide monitoring program that is designed to identify and quantify pesticide residues in food and animal feed. The two main objectives of this program are: 1) to monitor domestic and imported food and feed commodities for pesticide residues in support of regulatory actions against illegal residues, and 2) to gather information on the incidence and levels of pesticide residues in the food supply (28).

The potential coverage of the FDA's pesticide monitoring program includes approximately 316 pesticides for which tolerances have been established; pesticides whose registrations have been canceled but persist in the environment; pesticides previously exempted from the establishment of tolerance levels but for which safety concerns have subsequently arisen; pesticides with experimental use permits or pending tolerances; pesticides used only in foreign countries; and metabolites, other breakdown products, and impurities of pesticide products (28).

Given that the monitoring of all pesticide/commodity combinations for all of these pesticides would far exceed the resources of the FDA, a selective monitoring approach has been adopted (28). The two primary factors used to determine which pesticide/commodity combinations will be monitored are: 1) analytical method capabilities, that is, largely the capabilities of multiresidue methods; and 2) priorities of monitoring in terms of the likelihood of pesticide application to certain commodities and the potential health risk to the consumer from consumption of a particular pesticide/commodity combination (28). The risk assessment is made primarily on the basis of the FDA Surveillance Index (SI).[4] Table 2-1 shows how much pesticide coverage is provided by the five major multiresidue methods (i.e., methods that can detect more than one pesticide during an analysis of a single sample) routinely used by FDA to monitor pesticide residues in food.

---

[4]At the recommendation of an FDA study group (10), a five-level risk classification was developed on the basis of available toxicological data and potential human dietary exposure. The categories established are as follows: Class I, pesticides posing high health hazards; Class II, pesticides posing a possible high risk; Class III, pesticides posing a moderate hazard; Class IV, pesticides posing a low hazard; and Class V, pesticides posing very little potential hazard (29). A complete description of the process of assigning a pesticide to one of these classes is presented in Reed (29). The Surveillance Index is not yet complete. Two hundred and five pesticides have been ranked thus far.

Table 2-1.—Numbers of Compounds Determined or Identified by Primary FDA Multiresidue Methods[a]

Type of compounds	Total entered in data base	Total[b] for all 5 methods	Number of compounds determined or identified PAM I sec. no.				
			211.1/231.1[c]	212.1/232/.1[d]	232.3[e]	232.4/242/.1[f]	242.2[g]
Pesticides with tolerances	316	163	68	85	55	140	20
Pesticides with temporary or pending tolerances........................	74	10	4	3	4	9	4
Pesticides with no EPA tolerance	56	25	17	21	7	10	0
Metabolites, impurities, alteration products, and other pesticide-associated chemicals[h]	297	92	20	32	31	61	8

[a]As of May 1988.
[b]This number is not cumulative because several methods may detect the same pesticide.
[c]Gas chromatographic method for nonpolar (primarily organochlorine and organophosphorus) pesticides in fatty foods.
[d]Gas chromatographic method for nonpolar (primarily organochlorine and organophosphorus) pesticides in nonfatty foods.
[e]Gas chromatographic method for organophosphorus pesticides and metabolites.
[f]Gas chromatographic method for polar and nonpolar pesticides, using a variety of selective detectors.
[g]Liquid chromatographic method primarily for N-methyl carbamate pesticides.
[h]Only certain of the chemicals in these four pesticide-related groups necessarily occur as residues or are of toxicological concern.

SOURCE: D. Reed, P. Lombardo, J. Wessel, et al., "The FDA Pesticides Monitoring Program," *Journal of the Association of Official Analytical Chemists* 70(3):593, 1987. The 1987 table was updated for OTA by the Center for Food Safety and Applied Nutrition of the Food and Drug Administration in May 1988.

The two major components of the FDA pesticide monitoring program are: 1) general commodity monitoring, and 2) the Total Diet Study.

General Commodity Monitoring

General commodity monitoring is designed to enable the enforcement of tolerances established by EPA and determine the incidence and levels of residues in domestic and imported raw agricultural commodities, processed foods, and animal feed (28). More specifically, the objectives of this program are to: 1) determine on a geographical basis pesticide residue levels of individual food commodities, 2) survey on a nationwide basis pesticide residue levels of selected food commodities, 3) monitor imported food commodities and deny entry to those with illegal pesticide residues, and 4) identify pesticide residues occurring in excessive levels as a basis for compliance followup and enforcement action.

Approximately 15,000 commodity samples were analyzed in 1987 for pesticide residues by 16 FDA laboratories under the general commodity monitoring program. About 47 percent of samples were from domestic sources and 53 percent were imported commodities (22; figure 2-1). Emphasis on imported commodities has increased in the past few years. The majority of samples are collected at random for monitoring purposes and are known as surveillance samples. The remainder, known as compliance samples, are collected after a violation has been found or there is evidence of a likely violation (28). Imports receive more compliance sampling because less information is available on foreign growing areas, pesticide use, and agricultural practices than for domestic commodities (16). FDA's ability to prevent violative food from reaching the consumer is constrained by the amount of time needed for sample transport and analyses. As such, food sometimes is able to reach the market before results of analyses are available (34). FDA can detain imported commodities until compliance analyses are completed but cannot detain domestic commodities (34).

The percentage of samples that violate EPA tolerances is known as the violation rate. FDA believes that violation rates cannot be extrapolated to give the correct level of violations in the general food supply because the biased nature of FDA sampling (both compliance and surveillance sampling) would lead to the calculation of an overly high level of violations (17, 20). First, compliance samples will have a higher violation rate than the general food supply and the surveillance samples because compliance sampling is done only when a violation is suspected. Second, surveillance samples are not conducted in a totally random fashion. Surveillance sampling is biased toward pesticide/ commodity combinations with past residue problems and also contains a greater percentage of fruits and vegetables than exists in the general food supply (17).

For all food samples analyzed by FDA in 1987, the violation rate for surveillance samples was 2.5 percent (1.5 percent for domestic samples and 3.4 percent for imports). The violation rate for compliance samples analyzed that year was 11.7 percent (12.1 percent for domestic samples and 11.6 percent for imports) (17). Additional data on violation rates have been compiled by FDA's Los Angeles laboratory based on 5 years (1982-1986) of its analysis of almost 20,000 samples (93 percent of which were surveillance samples and 67 percent were imports). The majority of these samples were fruits and vegetables. The violation rate for surveillance samples was 2.76 percent (3 percent for domestic samples and 2.6 percent for imports). The violation rate for compliance samples was 17.8 percent (19.7 percent for domestic samples and 17.5 percent for imports) (16). Seventy-five percent of the violations stemmed from pesticide residues on commodities that did not have a tolerance established for the pesticide (20).

The Center for Food Safety and Applied Nutrition (CFSAN) is responsible for much of the direction of the FDA monitoring program, primarily through the development of its annual series of compliance program guidance manuals.

Figure 2-1.—FDA Pesticide in Food Monitoring Program in 1987

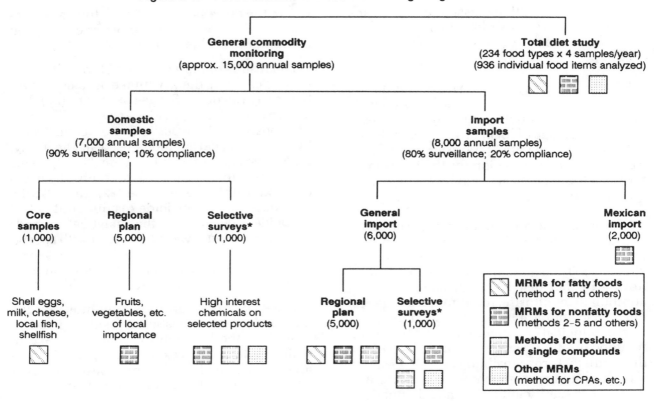

Note that all numbers of samples are approximate. Codes for analytical methods refer to those most often used for analysis of the samples in any category.
Abbreviations: MRM = multiresidue method; CPA = chlorophenoxy acid. Definitions: compliance samples = samples collected from shipments for which there was prior evidence or suspicion of illegal pesticide residues (i.e., subjective samples); surveillance samples = samples collected from shipments for which there was no prior evidence or suspicion of illegal pesticide residues (i.e., objective samples).
*A combination of special emphasis surveys and headquarters-initiated surveys.

SOURCE: B. McMahon and J. Burke, "Expanding and Tracking the Capabilities of Pesticide Multiresidue Methodology Used in the Food and Drug Administration's Pesticide Monitoring Programs," *Journal of the Association of Official Analytical Chemists* 70(6):1073, 1987. The 1987 table was updated for OTA by the Center for Food Safety and Applied Nutrition of the Food and Drug Administration in May 1988.

Four types of sampling plans make up general commodity monitoring: core samples, special emphasis surveys, headquarters-initiated surveys, and regional sampling plans (see figure 2-1, which combines special emphasis surveys and headquarters-initiated surveys into selective surveys).

Core samples, which must be analyzed by each district, are identified by CFSAN. Core samples are of commodities susceptible to environmental contamination and likely to bioaccumulate fat-soluble pesticides (e.g., fish, milk, dairy products, shell eggs, and feed) (28).

Special emphasis surveys permit each district to sample two domestic pesticide/commodity combinations and two imported pesticide/commodity/country-of-origin combinations. CFSAN develops the list of combinations for selection by districts, and districts may propose additional combinations subject to CFSAN approval. These surveys focus on those pesticides neither adequately measured nor regularly analyzed by the five multiresidue methods routinely used. These pesticides may be selected for monitoring because of EPA requests, FDA investigatory reports, a high SI classification for a pesticide, or past violation problems (28).

Headquarters-initiated assignments (or special surveys) are those in which CFSAN instructs a district to analyze a specific commodity.

Finally, regional sampling plans (for domestic and imported food) allow each region to determine what products it plans to sample based on its knowledge of local crops, pesticide use, and coordination with State programs. In 1988, FDA required each region for the first time to write up these plans and submit them to headquarters (19).

Ultimately, the number of samples collected and analyzed for pesticide residues in a district is determined by the available resources provided by FDA headquarters for pesticide monitoring in that district. FDA laboratories, in addition to monitoring foods for pesticide residues, also monitor foods for sanitation and microbiological contamination. Monitoring nonfood products such as medical devices and drugs are their responsibility as well. Pesticide monitoring must compete for resources with these other significant public health functions, and sampling plans are sometimes derailed by emergency situations (e.g., a product tampering incident).

The Total Diet Study

Since the early 1960s, FDA has monitored dietary intake of pesticides in a "market basket" of selected food items (including meat and poultry) that are purchased at the retail level and then prepared ready-to-eat prior to analysis. CFSAN determines the commodities to be sampled, and the analysis is carried out by the FDA Total Diet laboratory in Kansas City, MO. Two hundred thirty-four foods selected to represent the diet of the U.S. population are collected in retail markets four times annually, once from each of four designated geographical areas of the United States (northeast, south, north central, and west) (22, 27, 28). A single collection consists of identical foods from retail stores in three cities within each geographical area (27). Samples are sent to the Total Diet Laboratory,

where the three samples of each food are combined to form a single sample and analyzed using multiresidue methods (27).

The results of the Total Diet Study (TDS) are used to estimate dietary intake of selected pesticides by various U.S. age-sex groups (27). The design of the TDS provides an estimate of public exposure to those pesticide residues detected by the analytical methods used in the study. FDA uses data from the TDS to make judgments about the public health risk presented by pesticide exposure through food (27). In 1987, the TDS detected 53 pesticide residues out of 253 pesticides detectable by the analytical methods used. The residues were compared with acceptable daily intakes calculated by the World Health Organization and none were found to exceed 1 percent of those acceptable levels (18).

The TDS, however, uses only multiresidue methods to detect pesticide residues in food. Therefore, the TDS only provides a partial estimate of total human exposure to pesticide residues in the diet because some pesticides cannot be detected by multiresidue methods.

The Food Safety and Inspection Service (FSIS) of the U.S. Department of Agriculture

The USDA pesticide residue in food monitoring program is part of its National Residue Program (NRP), which addresses residues of pesticides, animal drugs, and environmental contaminants in meat, poultry, and raw egg products. NRP was initiated by the USDA in 1967 and has grown substantially in terms of the numbers of samples analyzed. Overall, approximately 50,000 samples are analyzed annually for about 100 compounds (12, 13, 23). In 1987, the NRP analyzed some 15,260 samples for pesticide residues, and almost 60 percent of these were imported products (15).

The decision of what pesticide to analyze is based on a ranking of the pesticide (based on the pesticide's toxicity and level of human exposure), the capability of testing for the pesticide using a multiresidue method, and past

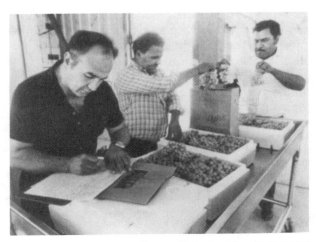

Photo credit: Food and Drug Administration

Samples are collected and shipped to laboratories for analysis. Above, an FDA inspector samples imported fruit entering the United States from Mexico at Nogales, AZ.

residue problems with the pesticide (12). Monitoring decisions are based on a list of approximately 227 ranked pesticides and metabolites that FSIS considers of potential concern (12). Similar to the SI developed by FDA, FSIS established the Compound Evaluation System (CES) in 1985 to improve its ranking of pesticides and bolster support of its monitoring program and analytical methods development work. Pesticide residues are assigned a letter rank for their toxicity (A-D) and a number rank for the degree of human exposure to them (1-4) with A-1 as the highest ranking. Currently, 39 pesticides have been ranked under the CES (30). An advisory board of scientists from EPA, FDA, and USDA was also established in 1985 to help keep pace with new information on compounds of concern (12).

Pesticide residue analysis is accomplished by using multiresidue methods.[5] Normally, a sample is analyzed using one of four multiresidue methods (for chlorinated hydrocarbons, chlo-

rinated organophosphates, organophosphates, and carbamates), which together can detect approximately 40 pesticides (1, 15).[6] FSIS has identified 10 highly ranked pesticides it would like to monitor routinely but cannot using its multiresidue methods (15). In addition, a number of other highly ranked pesticides exist that cannot be detected by multiresidue methods but that FSIS considers less likely to appear in meat (15). FSIS has three laboratories performing pesticide residue analysis and has contracts with 57 non-Federal laboratories that are accredited by FSIS to conduct pesticide analyses as well as analyses of other compounds such as PCBs. These laboratories are accredited only for the pesticide analysis of chlorinated hydrocarbons and they must use an FSIS approved method. FSIS runs a quality assurance program for these laboratories using check samples and onsite reviews (9).

The four components of the National Residue Program are monitoring, surveillance, exploratory projects, and prevention, which are administered by the FSIS (31). Violation rates for the pesticides analyzed in meat products are low. In 1986, no violations were found for the 16 organophosphates tested for in either the monitoring or surveillance programs. For the 13 chlorinated hydrocarbon pesticides tested for in 1986, 9 violations out of 3,498 monitoring samples (a 0.26 percent violation rate) and 18 violations out of 1,071 surveillance samples (a 1.7 percent violation rate) were found (11). Testing for carbamates began in 1987 and results have not yet been compiled. FSIS believes that monitoring data can be used to provide a good indication of violation rates in the general meat supply because monitoring sampling is random (14). However, monitoring data would first have to be adjusted for the difference between the number of samples taken from each animal group and the relative production of each animal to get a proper indication (6). Surveillance data are too biased to be used the same way (14).

---

[5]FSIS requires that its analytical methods be "practical," which it defines as: a) requiring no more than 2 to 4 hours of analytical time per sample (batches of samples may take longer), b) requiring no instrumentation not customarily available in a laboratory devoted to trace drug or environmental analyses, c) having a minimum proficiency level at or below the established tolerance, d) having a quality assurance plan, and e) having undergone an interlaboratory validation study (12).

---

[6]FSIS also analyzes for eight compounds fed directly to animals as larvicides or to kill insects in animal dung. In 1987, 2,914 samples were analyzed for these products (15).

The monitoring program involves random sampling of meat and poultry tissue during routine inspection at slaughter of domestic animals (FSIS personnel are located at processing plants) and of imported products at the port of entry. These samples account for approximately 80 percent (based on 1985 figures) of the total number of samples analyzed (11, 12). The random sampling scheme used in this program is designed statistically to provide 95 percent assurance of detection over the course of a year with a violation rate of 1 percent or more in the national population (12). Monitoring samples are analyzed by the three FSIS laboratories and several of the FSIS accredited laboratories. In most cases, the FSIS monitoring program does not prevent violative products from reaching the consumer because analytical results are not normally available until after the product has reached the marketplace and become difficult to trace (12). Monitoring provides information on the occurrence of residue violation and helps to identify those producers who may be selected for surveillance sampling because of violations.

The surveillance program focuses on the investigation and control of movement of meat and poultry products that are suspected of contamination. Unlike the random sampling conducted under the monitoring program, the sampling conducted under the surveillance program is directed specifically to those meat or poultry carcasses that have been implicated as sources of residues either by the monitoring program, by investigation, or by a prior history of violation by the supplier (31). Carcasses are held until the analysis is complete. Violative meat is condemned and the producer is prohibited from marketing animals until further samples show no illegal residues (26). Analysis of surveillance samples takes precedence over monitoring samples (12). Analysis may be done either by the three FSIS laboratories or else the producer, in order to increase the speed of analysis, may choose to send a meat sample to one of the 57 FSIS accredited laboratories for analysis for chlorinated hydrocarbons. The producer pays for the analysis, and the results go first to the FSIS inspector. Unless there has been a serious contamination event, only a few hundred surveillance samples are analyzed annually for pesticides by the accredited laboratories (2).

Exploratory projects are surveys used to determine if a pesticide not currently detected should be included in the monitoring program. New methods that have not been validated by FSIS may be used in these surveys to detect the pesticides and to evaluate the value of the method (9).

To complement its regulatory work at the slaughterhouse, FSIS has a prevention program based on producer testing and education. Memoranda of Understanding (MOU) are signed with producers who then pay for testing feed, feed additives, litter, and some animals for chlorinated hydrocarbons. About 7 FSIS accredited laboratories perform approximately 2,000 analyses a month and provide FSIS with access to the results (15). Currently, 11 companies (5 beef and 6 poultry producers) take part in this program (3). FSIS has also collaborated with the USDA Cooperative Extension Service to produce educational materials for and provide counseling to producers on how to avoid chemical contamination of animals.

The AMS carries out a small regulatory program for pesticide residues in raw egg products. At its laboratory in Gastonia, NC, approximately 400 to 500 samples are analyzed annually from the approximately 90 domestic, egg-breaking and drying factories and imports using a multiresidue method that can identify 50 pesticides (21). If violations are found in domestic egg products, AMS may analyze raw eggs to find which producer is the source of the violative eggs. Both in 1986 and 1987, AMS found no violations among its monitoring and surveillance samples (21).

OTHER PESTICIDE RESIDUES IN FOOD MONITORING PROGRAMS

Although outside the scope of this report, State and private programs carry out a significant amount of monitoring for pesticide residues in food. Data provided by FDA to the General Accounting Office (GAO) showed that 38 States had such monitoring programs (34). State programs vary widely in the number of samples processed and in the program purpose.[7] For example, Montana's and Florida's programs focus on the most likely cases of overtolerance, e.g., if there has been a major pest outbreak that could lead to overuse of a pesticide; Massachusetts has directed its program to dietary risks (4). Figure 2-2 provides a survey of 10 State pro-

grams and the number of monitoring samples analyzed for pesticide residues. State programs rely primarily on multiresidue methods.

The extent of private sector testing is more difficult to determine. A considerable amount of monitoring by food processors is taking place but remains proprietary information, in part because of fears of the possible negative connotations associated with such testing (7). An example of this work is the National Food Processors Association, which estimates it analyzes approximately 3,000 food samples a year for pesticide residues for its members (8). Federal agencies are interested in using private monitoring data, partly to help set their own monitoring priorities, and EPA has an ongoing project to collect the results of private monitoring.

---

[7]For more information about State programs, see Cusick and Wells, 1988 in appendix B.

Figure 2-2.—Number of Food Monitoring Samples Analyzed for Pesticide Residues in 10 States in 1987

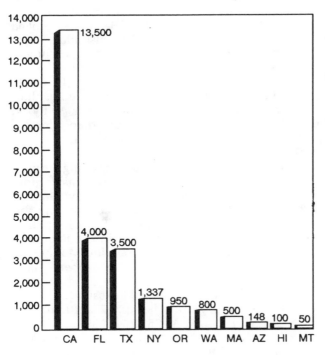

SOURCE: California Department of Food and Agriculture, Pesticide Enforcement Branch. Survey done for OTA, 1988.

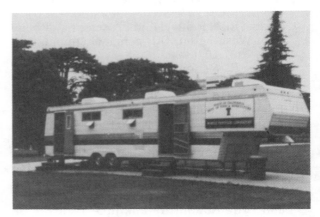

Photo credit: California Department of Food and Agriculture

When a widespread pesticide/commodity problem occurs, the California Department of Food and Agriculture may send one of its three mobile laboratories to assist with monitoring.

CHAPTER 2 REFERENCES

1. Ashworth, R., Chemistry Division, Food Safety and Inspection Service, Washington, DC, personal communication, May 13, 1988.
2. Barth, J., Chemistry Division, Food Safety and Inspection Service, Washington, DC, personal communication, June 29, 1988.
3. Cielo, A., Residue Evaluation and Planning Division, Food Safety and Inspection Service, Washington, DC, personal communication, July 7, 1988.
*4. Cusick, W., and Wells, J., "Pesticide Analytical Methods Development at the State Level," OTA commissioned paper, Spring 1988.
5. Dingel, J.D., "One Goal, Many Agencies: An Assessment of Pesticide Residue Regulation in Animal Feeds and Animal Meat Products," *Food, Drug, Cosmetic Law J.* 41:467-511, 1986.
6. Elder, R., Mathematics and Statistics Division, Food Safety and Inspection Service, Washington, DC, personal communication, July 28, 1988.
7. Elkins, E., National Food Processors Association, Washington, DC, personal communication, Apr. 20, 1988.
8. Elkins, E., National Food Processors Association, Washington, DC, personal communication, Apr. 6, 1988.
9. Ellis, R., Chemistry Division, Food Safety and Inspection Service, Washington, DC, personal communication, July 7, 1988.
10. Food and Drug Administration, Study Group on FDA Residue Programs, "FDA Monitoring Programs for Pesticide and Industrial Chemical Residues in Food" (Rockville, MD: Food and Drug Administration, June 1979).
11. Food Safety and Inspection Service, U.S. Department of Agriculture, *Domestic Residue Data Book, National Residue Program 1986* (Washington, DC: Food Safety and Inspection Service, October 1987).
12. Food Safety and Inspection Service, U.S. Department of Agriculture, *Compound Evaluation and Analytical Capability National Residue Plan, 1987* (Washington, DC: Food Safety and Inspection Service, January 1987).
13. Food Safety and Inspection Service, U.S. Department of Agriculture, "FSIS-18, Facts: The National Residue Program I" (Washington, DC: Food Safety and Inspection Service, revised January 1984).

14. Harr, R., Residue Planning and Evaluation Division, Food Safety and Inspection Division, Washington, DC, personal communication, July 27, 1988.
15. Harr, R., Residue Planning and Evaluation Division, Food Safety and Inspection Service, Washington, DC, personal communication, June 27, 1988.
16. Hundley, H., Luke, M., Cairns, T., et al., "Pesticide Residue Findings by the Luke Method in Domestic and Imported Food and Animal Feeds for Fiscal Years 1982-1986," *J. Assoc. Off. Anal. Chem.*, forthcoming, 1988.
17. Lombardo, P., Pesticide and Industrial Chemicals Branch, Center for Food Safety and Applied Nutrition, Food and Drug Administration, Washington, DC, personal communication, July 27, 1988.
18. Lombardo, P., Pesticide and Industrial Chemicals Branch, Center for Food Safety and Applied Nutrition, Food and Drug Administration, Washington, DC, personal communication, July 13, 1988.
19. Lombardo, P., Pesticide and Industrial Chemicals Branch, Center for Food Safety and Applied Nutrition, Food and Drug Administration, Washington, DC, personal communication, July 8, 1988.
20. Luke, M., Masumoto, H., Cairns, T., et al., "Levels and Incidences of Pesticide Residues in Various Food and Animal Feeds Analyzed by the Luke Multiresidue Methodology for Fiscal Years 1982-1986," *J. Assoc. Off. Anal. Chem.* 71(2):415-433, 1988.
21. Magwire, H., Agricultural Marketing Service, U.S. Department of Agriculture, Washington, DC, personal communication, May 1988.
22. McMahon, B. and Burke, J., "Expanding and Tracking the Capabilities of Pesticide Multiresidue Methodology Used in the Food and Drug Administration's Pesticide Monitoring Programs," *J. Assoc. Off. Anal. Chem.* 70(6): 1072-1081, 1987.
23. Middlekauff, R.D., "Pesticide Residues in Food: Legal and Scientific Issues," *Food Drug and Cosmetic Law J.* 42:251-264, 1987.
24. Moore, J., "Statement Before the Committee on Agriculture, Nutrition, and Forestry, U.S. Senate," *Federal Insecticide, Fungicide, and Rodenticide Act*, hearings before the Committee on Agriculture, Nutrition, and Forestry, Senate, U.S. Congress, May 20, 1987, serial No. S. Hrg. 100-394, Part I (Washington, DC, 1988).

---

*These references are contained in Appendix B.

25. National Research Council, Board on Agriculture, Committee on Scientific and Regulatory Issues Underlying Pesticide Use Patterns and Agricultural Innovation, *Regulating Pesticides in Food: The Delaney Paradox* (Washington, DC: National Academy Press, 1987).

26. National Research Council, Food and Nutrition Board, Committee on the Scientific Basis of the Nation's Meat and Poultry Inspection Program, *Meat and Poultry Inspection: The Scientific Basis of the Nation's Program* (Washington, DC: National Academy Press, 1985).

27. Pennington, J. and Gunderson, E., "History of the Food and Drug Administration's Total Diet Study," *J. Assoc. Off. Anal. Chem.* 70(5):772-782, 1987.

28. Reed, D., Wessel, J., Burke, J., et al., "The FDA Pesticides Monitoring Program," *J. Assoc. Off. Anal. Chem.* 70(3):591-595, 1987.

29. Reed, D., "The FDA Surveillance Index for Pesticides: Establishing Food Monitoring Priorities Based on Potential Health Risk," *J. Assoc. Off. Anal. Chem.* 68(1):122-124, 1985.

30. Rubin, L., Residue Evaluation and Planning Division, Food Safety and Inspection Service, Washington, DC, personal communication, May 16, 1988.

*31. Taylor, S., "Developing Pesticide Analytical Methods for Food: Considerations for Federal Policy Formulation," OTA commissioned paper, Spring 1988.

32. Trichilo, C., Office of Pesticide Programs, U.S. Environmental Protection Agency, Washington, DC, personal communication, June 27, 1987.

*33. Trichilo, C. and Schmitt, R., "Federal Pesticide Monitoring Programs: Analytical Methods Development," OTA commissioned paper, Spring 1988.

34. U.S. Congress, General Accounting Office, "Pesticides: Need to Enhance FDA's Ability to Protect the Public From Illegal Pesticides," GAO/RCED-87-7 (Washington, DC: U.S. Government Printing Office, October 1986).

*These references are contained in Appendix B.

Chapter 3
Contemporary Analytical Techniques for Pesticide Residues in Food

CONTENTS

Page

Sample Preparation. 21
Extraction 22
Cleanup. 23
Determination—Chromatographic Separation. 25
    Gas Chromatography Separations 25
    High Performance Liquid Chromatography Separations 26
    Thin Layer Chromatography Separations 28
    Supercritical Fluid Chromatography Separations 28
Determination—Detection 28
    Gas Chromatography Detectors 28
    High Performance Liquid Chromatography Detectors 30
    Detection Techniques for Thin Layer Chromatography. 31
Conclusion 31
Chapter 3 References 32

Figures

Figure   *Page*
3-1. Simplified Scheme of the Steps in the Analysis of Plant Material for
    Pesticide Residue 22
3-2. Schematic Diagram of a Gas Chromatographic System 26
3-3. Chromatogram of a Gas Chromatograph 27
3-4. Schematic Diagram of a High Performance Liquid Chromatographic
    System 27

Tables

Table   *Page*
3-1. Materials Used for the Preparative Chromatography of Pesticide
    Residues in Food 24
3-2. Comparison of Retention Data for Seven Chlorinated Hydrocarbon
    Pesticides on a Packed Column and on a Wide Bore
    Capillary Column 27
3-3. Gas Chromatography Detectors Used for Pesticide Residue Analysis . . . 29
3-4. Detectors Used in High Performance Liquid Chromatography Analysis
    of Pesticide Residues 31

Contemporary Analytical Techniques for Pesticide Residues in Food

Pesticides may occur in foods in concentrations called trace levels. Trace levels are generally at concentrations of parts per million, that is, one microgram of pesticide per gram of food or less. Measuring such small amounts of pesticides in the presence of enormous amounts of other chemicals that occur naturally in food is a challenge because those chemicals may interfere with measurement. A variety of analytical methods (see ch. 6) are currently used to detect pesticide residues, and all contain certain basic steps in application. The basic steps of an analytical method include the following:

- *sample preparation:* preparation of the sample to be analyzed by chopping, grinding, or separating plant parts;
- *extraction:* removal of a pesticide residue from the sample's other components;
- *cleanup (isolation):* removal of constituents that interfere with the analysis of the pesticide residue of interest, this step includes partitioning and purification;
- *determination—separation:* separation of components, individual pesticides, and sample coextractives according to differential partitioning between a solid or nonvolatile solvent and a liquid or gas carrier that moves through a column (liquid and gas chromatography) or along a coated plate (thin layer chromatography); and
- *determination—detection:* production of a response that measures the amount of the components moving through the column, allowing detection and quantification of each pesticide.

How these steps interact within any particular method is shown in figure 3-1 (1). The cleanup step in figure 3-1 has two parts, partitioning and purification, and the extracting solvent is either acetone or acetonitrile.

This chapter describes existing and new technologies currently used to analyze pesticide residues in food and notes how these technologies can improve the analytical steps described above.

SAMPLE PREPARATION

The first step to analyzing a food sample is to chop, grind, or otherwise separate plant or animal parts. The samples must be handled in such a way as to avoid the loss of volatile pesticide residues and to prevent contamination of the sample with other pesticides or interfering chemicals. If only the edible portion of the sample is to be analyzed, it must be removed from non-edible portions. If several different edible portions of a food are analyzed separately, the portions must be separated from each other in each sample. If, however, several samples are combined to provide a representative composite sample from which one or more subsamples are to be taken for analysis, all samples must be handled in an identical manner to avoid inaccurate results in analyzing the subsamples. Chopping or grinding followed by blending and mixing are manipulations designed to produce a homogeneous composite sample from which subsamples can be taken and to disrupt the gross structural components of the food to facilitate extracting pesticides from the sample. Performing this step can be time-consuming and labor intensive.

Figure 3-1.— Simplified Scheme of the Steps in the Analysis of Plant Material for Pesticide Residue

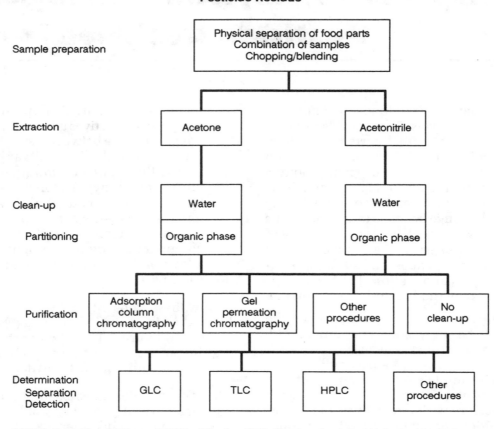

SOURCE: Modified from A. Ambrus and H.P. Thier, "Allocation of Multiresidue Procedures in Pesticide Residue Analysis," *Pure and Applied Chemistry* 58(7): 1035–1062, July 1986.

EXTRACTION

Extraction is performed with a solvent to remove the pesticide residue of interest from other components of the sample. In most analytical laboratories, a solvent such as acetone or acetonitrile is used to extract pesticides from 250 grams or less of the food to be analyzed. The solvent is blended with the food, and smaller amounts can be further homogenized using an ultrasound generator. Salts, such as sodium chloride or sodium sulfate, can be added to absorb water. Or additional water can be added, if desired, so that the resulting aqueous solution can be partitioned with a water-immiscible solvent in a subsequent cleanup step.

Extraction times vary from a few minutes to several hours, depending on the pesticide to be analyzed and the sample type. Problems that occur during the extraction process include incomplete recovery and emulsion formation. Incomplete recovery generally can be remedied by selecting a more efficient solvent. Emulsions, the production of a third phase or solvent layer that confuses the partitioning process, can usually be broken down by adding salt to the sample/solvent combination. Residual amounts of the extracting solvent or partitioning solvent should not be allowed to reach the detector if it is an element-specific detector and the solvent contains that specific element. These problems can be solved by proper solvent selection or by removal of the interfering solvent during the cleanup process.

Supercritical fluids (SFs) may provide a new technique for extracting pesticides. SFs are fluids that are more dense than gases but less dense than liquids. SFs are not yet used in regulatory methods to analyze pesticide residues in food but are gaining favor among analytical chemists and food engineers for the ability to extract a wide variety of chemicals from many sample types. SFs have many advantages over conventional solvents. They yield high recoveries of the extracted chemical in a short time, sometimes as quickly as 10 to 30 minutes at temperatures only slightly above ambient (40 to 50°C). Such temperatures prevent thermal decomposition of the extracted chemical. Since some degree of extraction selectivity can be created by choosing an appropriate pressure, this feature may allow the chemist to separate compounds that may interfere during extraction. Removal of the SF from the dissolved chemical in the gas form is easily accomplished (19). The residual chemical of interest can then be dissolved in a conventional solvent and carried through one of the conventional chromatographic analyses (discussed later). Much remains to be done to explore the usefulness of supercritical fluid extraction (SFE) for rapidly and efficiently extracting pesticides from foods.

CLEANUP

Cleanup or isolation removes the constituents that interfere with the analysis of the pesticide residue of interest. Cleanup is usually achieved by a combination of partitioning[1] and purification, and the latter is usually accomplished by preparative chromatography. The degree of cleanup required is determined by the efficiency with which the partitioning solvent can remove pesticides from the sample extract while leaving behind mutually occurring interferences. Special modification techniques may improve the efficiency of cleanup as well as the efficiency of detection (16).

The preparative chromatography typically used for purification is of the: 1) adsorptive, or 2) gel permeation (or size exclusion) type. Adsorption chromatography is based on the interaction between a chemical dissolved in a solvent and an adsorptive surface. Particles of the chromatographic material are placed in large glass columns (30 cm x 2 cm), the sample is deposited in a solvent on the top of the column and eluted with various types of organic solvents. Separation occurs when the pesticide elutes in fractions different than the sample coextractives. Table 3-1 summarizes the materials that have been used with these two types of preparative chromatographic modes, giving some of their distinguishing features.

Gel permeation (or size exclusion) chromatography is a technique that separates compounds from one another on the basis of differences in molecular size. Preparative-sized columns similar to those used in adsorption chromatography are used, and samples are placed at the top of the column and then eluted with a solvent; larger molecules elute before smaller ones in an ordered fashion. The ordering by size in gel permeation is a result of small holes designed into the particles placed in the column that retard the movement of smaller molecules through the column; such sizing cannot occur on adsorption columns.

The advantages of gel permeation over adsorption chromatography are that no loss of pesticide occurs on the column, either by irreversible adsorption or by chemical reactions. A disadvantage is that a medium-pressure piston-type pump is required to deliver solvent to the column, making a sample injection valve nec-

---

[1]Partitioning is the process of distributing the pesticide between two immiscible solvents so that the pesticide will appear in one phase and potential interferences in another, which then can be discarded.

Table 3-1.—Materials Used for the Preparative Chromatography of Pesticide Residues in Food

Florisil
1. A diatomaceous earth adsorbent; retains some lipids preferentially; particularly suited for cleanup of fatty foods.
2. Good for cleanup of nonpolar pesticides, such as the chlorinated hydrocarbons; produces very clean eluants, removes most interferences when eluted with nonpolar solvents.
3. Difficult to use for fruits and vegetables when moderately polar to polar pesticides are present.
4. Prone to vary from batch to batch.
5. Sometimes oxidizes organophosphates with thio-ether linkages; adsorbs some oxons irreversibly.
6. Most widely used material in the United States.

Alumina
1. Basic alumina can be substituted for Florisil for the cleanup of fatty foods.
2. Does not vary from batch to batch as much as Florisil.
3. Will decompose some organophosphates.
4. Does not effectively separate some plant materials from the pesticide.

Silica gel
1. Particularly useful for isolation of certain polar pesticides without losses.
2. Will not adequately separate some plant coextractives from some pesticides.
3. Will separate some organochlorine pesticides from animal fat well enough to permit thin layer chromatography.

Carbon
1. Unlike other adsorbents, carbon has different elution characteristics due to its lipophilic nature; absorbs preferentially nonpolar and high molecular weight pesticides.
2. Removes chlorophyll well from vegetables but not waxes.
3. Strongly affected by pretreatment; results in literature often not comparable.
4. Difficult to maintain flow rates in columns.

SOURCE: Office of Technology Assessment, 1988.

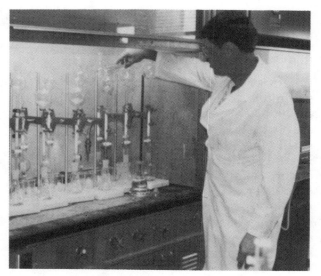

Photo credit: *Food Safety and Inspection Service Laboratory, Athens, GA*

After putting the sample through an alumina packed column, solvent is added to elute the pesticides off of the packing in the column.

essary. The required equipment is more expensive than that used in adsorption chromatography, although such equipment is available in an automated package.

The cleanup step is often a limitation in pesticide residue methods because it generally consumes a large amount of the total analysis time and restricts the number of pesticides that are recovered in some cases, as a result of losses in chromatography, partitioning, and other cleanup steps. New technologies such as solid phase extraction (SPE) (also known as accumulator or concentrator columns) can speed up cleanup as well as extraction. The SPE packing materials or cartridges retain the pesticide when the extract is passed through without retaining potential interferences extracted from

the food. The SPE cartridge is a small plastic, open-ended container filled with adsorptive particles of various types and adsorption characteristics. The pesticide is then eluted and carried forward to an appropriate determinative step. Conversely, SPE may be used to cleanup the extract by retaining coextractives and allowing the pesticide to pass through.

SPE technology is particularly attractive for use in pesticide residue analytical methods, since it often eliminates the need for expensive and environmentally sensitive solvents. These cartridges also have the following advantages: batch sample processing capabilities, small size, adaptability to robotic technology, low cost, and ready availability from many sources. SPEs have the disadvantages of being unproven for many pesticides, unable to handle large sample sizes, and generally are ineffective for extracting water-soluble pesticides and metabolites. As more types of adsorbents become available, however, the last disadvantage may be remedied. Using this type of cleanup sometimes results in losses of pesticides that cannot then be determined chromatographically, but under such circumstances, cleanup steps should be minimized or eliminated. SPE is being used by industry and private laboratories but is not yet routinely used by regulatory agencies to a significant extent. SPE cartridges are being used by several FDA laboratories to clean-up extracts before the detection step to protect the column used in high performance liquid chromatography (HPLC).

DETERMINATION—CHROMATOGRAPHIC SEPARATION

After a pesticide has been extracted and isolated from the sample, it is further separated from other coextractives, usually by either gas chromatography or liquid chromatography or, less frequently, by thin layer chromatography.

Gas Chromatography (GC) Separations

Historically, gas chromatography has been the dominant technique of separation, with at least 40 years of development and refinement. Most multiresidue methods (MRMs) used by the FDA and USDA and most single residue methods (SRMs) are based on GC.

Separations of pesticides and sample coextractives occur in analytical columns within a gas chromatograph; the columns are usually made of glass and are either the type that is packed or the wall-coated, open tubular type known as capillary.

A column filled with particles is called a packed column and has an internal diameter of about 2 millimeters; a column with a thin film on the wall and an internal diameter of about 0.1 millimeter is called a capillary column. Packed columns are typically 2 meters or less in length whereas capillary columns are typically 10 meters and longer, sometimes reaching 50 meters.

A sample of food extract, about 10 microliters or less and either cleaned up or not, is placed at the beginning of the column where the solvent is flash evaporated along with the pesticide. A gas, called the carrier gas, is continually flowing through the column, moving the pesticide along, which partitions between the particles packing the column or the thin film of involatile liquid on the wall of the column if it is a capillary column. The relative affinity of the pesticide for the particles or the thin film determines when it elutes from the column, at which time it goes through the detector where a response is generated and printed out on a recorder. The continuous trace of such responses is called the chromatogram (figure 3-2). Chromatographic peaks appear on the chromatogram; their position on the chromatogram is called the retention time. Quantifications are performed by measuring the area under the peak and comparing its area to that of varying amounts of analytical standards (figure 3-3).

Historically, the packed column has been used by most pesticide residue analytical chemists. As a result, a vast amount of retention data[2] exists for pesticides on packed columns. One way of expressing retention data is the use of "relative retention time" (rrt) for a particular pesticide/column combination. The rrt values are then used to identify an unknown by comparing the rrt to that of a standard. Chlorpyrifos is typically used as the standard for chlorinated hydrocarbon and organophosphate pesticides. The lack of rrt data for capillary columns is a constraint to their use.

Until the mid-1970s, capillary chromatography was used only when packed columns could not fully resolve the many components in the sample undergoing analysis. Today, the availability of a varied and growing selection of capillary columns has increased their popularity. A conventional capillary chromatogram has been more time-consuming to develop (requiring as much as 30 to 45 minutes) than packed column chromatograms (requiring less than 30 minutes) (3). However, the availability of the

---

[2]Retention data are retention time (time required to elute a compound from a chromatographic column) and retention volume (volume of carrier gas required to elute a compound from a GC column).

Figure 3-2.—Schematic Diagram of a Gas Chromatographic System

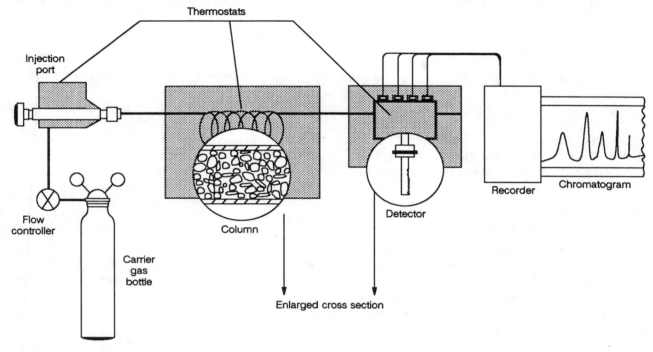

SOURCE: H.M. McNair and E.J. Bonelli, *Basic Gas Chromatography* (Berkeley, CA: Consolidated Printers, 1969).

wide bore capillary column has reduced time. Table 3-2 summarizes retention data for seven pesticides on a packed column and on a wide bore capillary column.

A new generation of hardware gives flexibility in the use of "guard columns," pieces of deactivated but uncoated fused silica tubing used to guard the analytical column from contamination by deposition of involatile food coextractives. Such guard columns could enable capillary column chromatography of relatively unclean food extracts that heretofore could only have been chromatographed on packed columns (2).

High Performance Liquid Chromatography (HPLC) Separations

HPLC for the analysis of pesticide residues is a fairly recent occurrence, but it is becoming the second most frequently used technique after GC. GC depends upon the volatilization of the pesticide, whereas HPLC is dependent on the ability of the chemical to be dissolved in a suitable solvent.

Separations occur on the analytical column packed with uniformly sized and shaped particles with a liquid film of varying polarities or adsorptive sites. A small volume of sample is deposited on the top of the column, and solvent is pumped through at high pressure. As the solvent moves through the column, the pesticide distributes itself between the particles (stationary phase) and the solvent (mobile phase); the pesticides that have a higher affinity for the stationary phase exit the column last (figure 3-4).

Stationary phases are commercially available that can selectively retain any molecular structure—polar, nonpolar, ionic, or neutral; separations can even be made to occur as a function of molecular size (gel permeation). Chemical derivatizations, the synthesis of a chemical derivative of the pesticide, therefore are not required for separations by HPLC. They are used to label molecules that do not respond to con-

Figure 3-3. — Chromatogram of a Gas Chromatograph

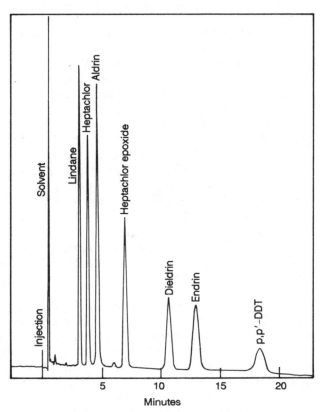

During sample analysis, the results of GC and HPLC chromatographic separation and detection steps appear on the chromatogram as peaks. The time it takes a peak to appear is used to identify the pesticide. The quantity of the pesticide can be determined by measuring the area under the peak.

SOURCE: Alltech Associates, Inc., Applied Science Labs, State College, PA, 1988.

Table 3-2. — Comparison of Retention Data for Seven Chlorinated Hydrocarbon Pesticides on a Packed Column and on a Wide Bore Capillary Column

Pesticide[a]	Retention times (minutes)[b]	
	Packed column[c]	Capillary column[d]
Lindane	2.5	0.7
Heptachlor	3.9	1.1
Aldrin..............	4.8	1.5
Heptachlor epoxide..	6.7	1.9
Dieldrin	9.9	2.8
Endrin	12.0	3.2
p,p' DDT	14.1	4.5
Total analysis time[e]	15.0	4.7

[a]Both columns exhibit comparable resolution between peaks, R=s > 1.0.
[b]Retention time (time required to elute a compound from a chromatographic column) and retention volume (volume of carrier gas required to elute a compound from a GC column).
[c]Glass column, 1.8 M x 0.4 cm; PT 4% SE-30 + 6% OV-210 on Gas Chrom Q, 80/100; 200°C; electron capture detector; nitrogen carrier, flow 90 ml/min; 2 x 10^{-9} grams for each pesticide.
[d]Open tubular column, 10 M x 0.053 cm; RSL/200, 1.2 microns thick; 200°C; electron capture detector; nitrogen carrier, flow 5 ml/min, 15 ml/min makeup; unknown amounts of pesticide.
[e]Represents time at which all pesticides have passed through the column.

GLOSSARY: **Gas Chrom Q**—a white diatomaceous earth that has been screened, acid and base washed, neutralized, and silanized (support for liquid phase); **OV-210**—50% trifluoropropyl, methyl silicone (liquid phase of gas chromatographic column packing material); **PT**—pretested; **R=s 1.0**—Resolution (the true separation of two consecutive peaks) of greater than 1 second; **RSL/200**—polydiphenyldimethylsiloxane (liquid phase); **SE-30**—methyl silicone gum (liquid phase of gas chromatographic column packing material).

SOURCE: Alltech Associates, Inc. "Catalog #150," Avondale, PA, 1988.

ventional analytical detectors. Such labeling usually enhances the detectability of the molecule. Sometimes labeling is done "post column," i.e., after elution from the chromatographic column, as for the N-methylcarbamates and carbamoyl oximes (13). Such labeling permits measurements of these classes of pesticides in the presence of other potential interferences as a result of the specificity of the reaction.

HPLC is not as efficient as capillary gas chromatography for separatory purposes because the chromatographic peaks are broader. However, HPLC columns are more efficient than packed GC columns when columns of equal

Figure 3-4. — Schematic Diagram of a High Performance Liquid Chromatographic System

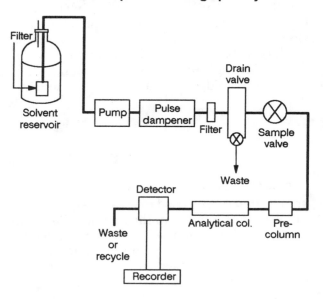

SOURCE: J.M. Miller, *An Introduction to Liquid Chromatography for the Gas Chromatographer* (Bridgewater, NJ: GOW-MAC Instrument Company).

length are considered. HPLC columns usually last longer because they are not subjected to the extremely high temperatures that GC columns are.

Thin Layer Chromatography (TLC) Separations

This technique is based upon partitioning a pesticide between a solvent and a thin layer of adsorbent, which is usually silica or alumina oxide that has been physically bonded to a glass or plastic plate. Samples are applied in a solvent as spots or bands at one edge of the plate and the plate is then placed in a tank containing a solvent. The solvent migrates up the plate by capillary action, taking the pesticide with it and depositing it at a given distance up the plate. The time required for TLC plate development may range from a few minutes to several hours depending on the pesticide, the solvent, and the adsorbent. Following complete development, the plate is then removed from the tank and the spots or bands left by the migration of the solvent are detected using one of several techniques.

As a separatory technique, TLC is much less efficient than either GC or HPLC because the resolution separated by TLC is approximately less than one-tenth of that found using a packed GC column to produce the same separation. Consequently, TLC as a separatory technique has largely been replaced by GC and HPLC. On the other hand, interest exists in using TLCs to develop rapid, semiquantitative methods (see ch. 6).

Supercritical Fluid Chromatography (SFC) Separations

SFs may provide a new technique for chromatographic separation in the regulatory analysis of pesticide residues in food. With SFs as the solvent phase, SFC can chromatograph chemicals that cannot be handled by gas chromatography because of their involatility or thermal instability. Because the chemical undergoing chromatography diffuses more readily in the SF than in the liquid used for HPLC, the solvent can be pumped at a higher velocity, resulting in shorter analysis times. A fringe benefit is that many detectors designed for GC can also be used in SFC. Detectors that have been shown to be effective are the flame ionization, the nitrogen-phosphorus, and the atomic emission spectrometric as well as the UV absorbance detector.

Extraction and chromatographic separation using SFs was recently demonstrated for the analysis of sulfonylurea herbicides (8). This technique, called SFE/SFC, was capable of producing chromatographic responses from extracts of sand, soil, wheat kernels, whole wheat flour, wheat straw, and from a cell culture medium. No recoveries or concentration levels were given.

Such a coupled extraction and analysis using supercritical fluids warrant further examination as a rapid means of analyzing pesticide residues in foods, if automation in general and robotics in particular can be used for sample insertion into the instrumentation.

DETERMINATION—DETECTION

This final step of analysis produces a response that can be used to measure the amount of pesticides moving in the column. There are numerous types of detectors. These detectors operate under various principles and have the ability, in some cases, to detect only certain classes of chemicals.

Gas Chromatography Detectors

Concurrent with improvements in gas chromatographic column technology have been major improvements in detectors. These improvements resulted in a growing number of detector types becoming available, increases in detector sensitivity due to improved design and enhanced electronic stability, and a trend toward detector miniaturization, which makes them more amenable for use in capillary chromatography.

Historically, only five detectors have been used. They are the electron capture detector (ECD), Hall microelectrolytic conductivity detector (HECD), the thermionic detectors (NPD and AFID), and the flame photometric detector. Table 3-3 summarizes their characteristics.

Of these detectors, the ECD was the first to be used for pesticide residue analysis. ECD measures the loss of detector electrical current produced by a sample component containing electron-absorbing molecule(s). Being very sensitive for measuring halogenated pesticides, its value lies in the analysis of chlorinated hydrocarbon pesticides such as aldrin, dieldrin, and DDT. Its sensitivity to such compounds has made ECD attractive for the analysis of polychlorinated biphenyls (PCBs) as well. ECD also responds to portions of organic molecules, other than halogens, which have a large electron affinity, and for that reason the detector sometimes has difficulties analyzing some unclean crop extracts. Recent improvements in related electronics and the incorporation of a high-temperature radioactive source have made the technology less susceptible to fouling from crop coextractives.

The Hall detector can be set to measure chlorine (and other halogens), nitrogen, or sulfur. When set for chlorine, the detector is especially useful for simplifying the detection of halogenated pesticides because nonhalogens are not detected, thus producing a simpler chromatogram to interpret. Similarly, when the detector is set for one mode, it will not detect pesticides that require one of the other settings. This detector is more selective than the ECD, but the ECD is more sensitive. In addition, the Hall detector does not need as clean an extract as the ECD, and therefore its use can lead to faster methods by allowing reductions in cleanup. A drawback is that the Hall detector requires more maintenance than the ECD.

Somewhat less sensitive than the ECD, but essentially nonresponsive to nonhalogenated compounds, the Hall electrolytic conductivity detector also has improved over the last few years. In fact, it has replaced the ECD in some laboratories where extreme sensitivity is not required. The Hall detector can also be set up for nitrogen and sulfur containing compounds.

Both the NPD and AFID measure the presence of nitrogen and phosphorus atoms in the pesticide, with little response resulting from other types of atoms in the molecules. At this time, the NPD has all but replaced the AFID in most residue laboratories due to its more sim-

Table 3-3.—Gas Chromatography Detectors Used for Pesticide Residue Analysis

Type	Selectivity	Approximate limit of detection	Sample destruction	Reliability	Examples of pesticides detected
Alkali Flame (AFID)	Organic P, N	10^{-12} g P 10^{-10} g N	Yes	Fair	Triazine herbicides (atrazine)
Electron Capture Detector (ECD)	Electronegative Containing Groups	10^{-13} g Cl/sec as lindane	Yes	Fair	Organochlorines (methoxychlor)
Flame Photometric	Organic P, S	10^{-12} g P/sec 2×10^{-12} g S/sec	Yes	Excellent	Organophosphate (malathion)
Hall Electrolytic Conductivity Detector	Organic Cl, S, N	$1\text{-}2 \times 10^{-13}$ g CL/sec $5\text{-}10 \times 10^{-13}$ g S/sec $1\text{-}2 \times 10^{-12}$ g N/sec	Yes	Fair	Organochlorines (aldrin)
Nitrogen-phosphorus Detector (NPD)	Organic P, N	$< 0.2 \times 10^{-12}$ g P/sec $< 0.4 \times 10^{-12}$ g N/sec	Yes	Good	Organophosphates (parathion)
Mass Selective Detector (MSD); Ion Trap Detector (ITD)	everything except carrier	10^{-11} g; MID	Yes	Good	All pesticides

SOURCE: Office of Technology Assessment, 1988.

ple operation as well as more reproducible responses from individual detectors.

The flame photometric detector measures sulfur or phosphorus. It is a rugged detector, highly stable, and very selective since it does not detect compounds other than organophosphates and those containing sulfur. The flame photometric detector is less sensitive for phosphorus than the NPD and less sensitive for sulfur than the Hall detector. However, it is useful for the analysis of unclean food extracts.

Conventional mass spectrometers (MS) have been used by some pesticide residue laboratories as gas chromatography detectors and to a lesser extent as high performance liquid chromatography detectors. Their cost ($150,000 and higher) has limited their use. MS is normally used when special techniques are necessary to confirm the identity of a particular pesticide, when conventional detectors cannot detect the pesticide, or for unidentified analytical responses (discussed in ch. 6). Usually an MS is set to the multiple ion detection mode in order to gain sensitivity; the alternative would be to obtain full spectral scans on each chromatographic peak, which is always less sensitive. The use of MS is growing, especially with the development of the more portable and less costly mass selective detector (MSD).

The MSD and ion trap detector (ITD) may become more routinely used for pesticide residue analysis as improvements in their computer software are made and their scan parameters become more suitable for chromatography. Both detectors operate on the principle of mass spectrometry. They differ primarily in the manner in which ions are filtered and in the software that is available for controlling the scan parameters and data acquisition. Both can be set to monitor one or more ions during the development of a chromatogram, and both can take full scans (mass spectra) of chromatographic peaks. Consequently, these detectors can be used to acquire quantitative and structural data on chromatographic peaks; both are compatible with capillary columns.

A large and significant difference exists in the way in which selected ions can be monitored during the chromatography, however. Only the MSD can be programmed to change which ions are being monitored during the chromatogram; this allows the instrument to be set so that as suspected pesticides elute from the column, the ions that give the greatest response and are characteristic of the molecule can be sequentially monitored. The ITD does not have this capability. Both detectors have the disadvantage that if nothing is known about the nature of the sample, they cannot be programmed for selected ion monitoring.

High Performance Liquid Chromatography Detectors

The HPLC detectors used for pesticide residue analysis are the UV absorption, fluorometer, conductivity, and electrochemical. A summary of the characteristics of those HPLC detectors is presented in table 3-4. The fixed wavelength UV absorbance detector is used frequently for trace analysis of pesticides. Many pesticides absorb UV light at the wavelength of mercury discharge (254 nanometers) and can be detected in very small quantities. Unfortunately, many food coextractives do so as well, making this detector nearly useless for trace analysis in foods.

An alternative is the variable wavelength detector, which can be tuned to a wavelength that is absorbed by the pesticide but not by the food coextractives. Several successes have been observed using the variable wavelength detector for "unclean" food extracts, including oxamyl and methomyl on strawberries (15). A newer version of the variable wavelength detector, the photo-diode array detector, is capable of molecular identification for the suspected pesticide because it is capable of taking a complete absorption spectrum on a chromatographic peak during the chromatogram. Recent versions of this detector approach the limits of detection observed for contemporary variable wavelength detectors.

The fluorometer is a highly sensitive HPLC detector for some pesticides. Typically, it is used for pesticides with aromatic molecular structures such as alachlor or paraquat. This detector, however, has limited application to

Table 3-4.—Detectors Used In High Performance Liquid Chromatography Analysis of Pesticide Residues

Type of device	Units	Full-scale sensitivity at + 1 noise	Sensitivity to favorable sample	Temperature sensitivity
UV Absorption	AU[1]	0.001	5x10⁻¹⁰ g/ml	Negligible
Fluorometer			10⁻¹⁰ g/ml	—
Conductivity	μmho[2]	0.05	10⁻⁸ g/ml	2%/°C
Amperometric (Electrochemical	A[3]	5 x10⁻⁹	10⁻¹⁰ g/ml	1%/°C

[1]AU = absorbance units
[2]μmho = unit of conductivity; 1mho=ohm⁻¹
[3]A = amperes

SOURCE: Office of Technology Assessment, 1988.

the detection of most pesticides—those that do not fluoresce appreciably. Two ways exist to avoid this dilemma: labeling the pesticides with fluorescent molecules before chromatography by HPLC or by forming postcolumn fluorescent derivatives (11, 12). Another recent approach is to form fluorescent molecules from pesticides by photolyzing them in a photoreactor (7) and then measuring their fluorescence.

For compounds having photo-ionizable functional groups, the photoconductivity detector is especially advantageous over UV detectors. It has been well studied and used by FDA and other laboratories for residue analysis. The electrochemical detector is also under study for its potential to improve detection of electroactive functional groups.

Detection Techniques for Thin Layer Chromatography

The spots or bands produced after the development of a thin layer plate are detected using one of several techniques such as visualization under UV light. Another technique uses reagents to produce colors resulting from chemical reaction that is specific for the pesticide/reagent combination. Amounts of pesticide can be judged semiquantitatively by comparison with standards that are developed on the same plate as the unknowns. An extensive review of how this technique can be applied to pesticide residues in foods has been published recently (17).

A popular color reaction used to visualize and quantify pesticides separated by TLC is produced by a cholinesterase enzyme-linked chemical reaction (9, 10, 18). Thin layer chromatograms are developed in a tank in the normal way, removed from the tank and sprayed with a solution of the cholinesterase enzyme. The plate is then sprayed with a solution of the color-generating reagent; where inhibition of the enzyme by the pesticide occurs, the reagent is not hydrolyzed, and coloring does not occur in those areas of the plate occupied by the cholinesterase-inhibiting pesticide. Such an enzyme inhibition approach was used in the development of a postcolumn detector for the analysis of carbamate pesticides by HPLC (13). Both techniques are capable of analyzing nanogram amounts of insecticide. More recently, there have been several applications of the enzyme-linked Hill reaction for detecting photosynthesis-inhibiting herbicides, such as the triazines, phenyl ureas, and anilides following TLC separation (4, 5, 6, 14).

CONCLUSION

The techniques currently used in the analysis of pesticide residues in food permit precise and accurate detection and quantification of trace levels of hundreds of these chemicals. The relatively recent development of SFE and SPE promises to increase the efficiency of pesticide removal from food material and reduce analysis time. Technological advances in GC column packing material, composition, wall coatings and size, and detectors have improved not only the sensitivity but also the specificity of the analyses performed. The detection and quantification in foods of an increased number of polar and thermally labile pesticides and metabolites have been made possible by the increased use of HPLC, a technique that has also been improved in recent years. SFC may further enhance the ability to detect this group of pesticides. All of these techniques will continue to be refined not only as discrete and sequential steps in analytical method development, but also as equivalent and parallel steps to increase the number of pesticides that can be determined in a single sample by a single method (e.g., multi-detector systems, e.g., Luke procedure; see ch. 6).

However, as techniques are improved by changes in instrument and hardware design, bringing about more sensitive, selective, and reproducible devices, their costs usually increase, particularly when automated sample handling and data manipulation are included. These additional costs translate into higher costs to implement contemporary pesticide methodologies for food.

CHAPTER 3 REFERENCES

1. Ambrus, A., and Thier, H.P., "Application of Multiresidue Procedures in Pesticide Residues Analysis," *Pure and Applied Chemistry* 58(7): 1035-1062, July 1986.
2. Freeman, R.R., and Hayes, M.A., "Column Considerations When Doing Trace Analysis on Open Tubular Columns," *J. of Chromatographic Science* 26(4):138-141, April 1988.
3. Jennings, W., *Analytical Gas Chromatography* (New York: Academic Press, Inc., 1987).
4. Kovac, J., and Henselova, M., "Detection of Triazine Herbicides In Soil By A Hill-Reaction Inhibition Technique After Thin Layer Chromatography," *J. of Chromatography* 133(2):420-422, March 1977.
5. Kovac, J., and Henselova, M., "A Rapid Method for Detection of Hill Reaction Inhibitors," *Photosynthetica* 10(3):343-344, 1976.
6. Lawrence, J.F., "Simple Sensitive and Selective Thin-Layer Chromatographic Technique For Detecting Some Photosynthesis Inhibiting Herbicides," *J. Assoc. Off. Anal. Chem.* 63(4): 758-761, 1980.
7. Luchtefeld, R.G., "An HPLC Detection System For Phenyl Urea Herbicides Using Post-column Photolysis and Chemical Derivatization," *J. of Chromatographic Science* 23(11):516-520, November 1985.
8. McNally, M.A.P., and Wheeler, J.R., "Supercritical Fluid Extraction Coupled With Supercritical Fluid Chromatography for the Separation of Sulfonylurea Herbicides and Their Metabolites From Complex Matrices," *J. of Chromatography* 435:63-71, 1988.
9. Mendoza, C.E., Wales, P.J., McLeod, H.A., et al., "Enzymatic Detection of Ten Organophosphorus Pesticides and Carbaryl on Thin Layer Chromatograms: An Evaluation of Indoxyl, Substituted Indoxyl and 1-Napthyl Acetates As Substrates Of Esterases," *Analyst* 93 (1102):34-38, January 1968.
10. Mendoza, C.E., Wales, P.J., McLeod, H.A., et al., "Thin-Layer Chromatographic-Enzyme Inhibition Procedure To Screen For Organophosphorus Pesticides In Plant Extracts Without Elaborate Clean Up," *Analyst* 93(1104):173-177, March 1968.
11. Miles, C.J., and Moye, H.A., "Extraction of Glyphosate Herbicide from Soil and Clay Minerals and Determination of Residues in Soil," *J. of Agricultural and Food Chemistry* 36(3): 486-491, May/June 1988.
12. Miles, C.J., Wallace, L.R., and Moye, H.A., "Determination of Glyphosate Herbicide and (Aminomethyl) Phosphonic Acid in Natural Waters by Liquid Chromatography Using Pre-column Fluorogenic Labeling with Fluorenylmethyl chloroformate," *J. of Assoc. Off. Anal. Chem.* 69(3):458-461, May/June 1986.
13. Moye, H.A., and Wade, T.E., "A Fluorometric Enzyme Inhibition Detector For Carbamate Pesticide Analysis By High Speed Liquid Chromatography," *Analytical Letters* 9(10):891-920, 1976.
14. Sackmauerova, M., and Kovac, J., "Thin-Layer Chromatographic Determination of Triazine and Urea Herbicides in Water by Hill-Reaction Inhibition Detection Technique," *Fresenius Zeitschrift fur Analytische Chemie* 292(5):414-415, 1978.

15. Scherer, S.J., Pesticide Research Laboratory, University of Florida, Gainesville, FL, personal communication, Apr. 12, 1988.

*16. Seiber, J., "Conventional Pesticide Analytical Methods: How Can They Be Improved?" OTA commissioned paper, Spring 1988.

17. Sherma, J., "Modern Analytical Techniques," *Analytical Methods for Pesticides and Plant Growth Regulators*, vol. XIV, G. Zweig and J. Sherma (eds.) (New York: Academic Press, 1986).

18. Wales, P.J., McLeod, H.A., and McKinley, W.P., "TLC-enzyme Inhibition Procedure to Detect Some Carbamate Standards and Carbaryl in Food Extracts," *J. Assoc. Off. Anal. Chem.* 51(6):1239-1242, November 1968.

19. Wright, B.W., Wright, C.W., Gale, R.W., et al., "Analytical Supercritical Fluid Extractions of Adsorbent Materials," *Analytical Chemistry* 59:38-44, January 1987.

*This reference paper is contained in appendix B.

Chapter 4
Immunoassay:
An Emerging Technology

CONTENTS

	Page
Introduction	37
The Immunoassay	37
Strengths and Weaknesses	40
Status of Regulatory Use of and Research on Immunoassays	41
The Potential Role of Immunoassays in the Detection of Pesticide Residues in Food	44
Chapter 4 References	45

Box

Box		Page
4-A. Enzyme-Linked Immunosorbent Assay (ELISA)		39

Figure

Figure		Page
4-1. Artist's Conception of Antibody-Antigen Interactions		37

Tables

Table		Page
4-1. Immunoassays for Pesticides Under Development by Regulatory Agencies		42
4-2. Commercially Available ELISA Test Kits for Pesticides		43

Immunoassay: An Emerging Technology

INTRODUCTION

Immunoassays, which use antibodies to detect chemical compounds, are widely used in clinical chemistry but have not been equally applied to the analysis of pesticide residues (4). Yet they seem to have a potentially significant role in analyzing pesticide residues in food. Antibodies can be developed to identify single pesticides or, in some cases, small groups of similar pesticides. Those immunoassays that determine groups of pesticides supply data for the entire group and not the individual pesticides. Immunoassays can also be used to provide quantitative data, similar to that provided by conventional analytical techniques, or they may provide qualitative or semiquantitative

data. The latter type can, in some cases, yield results more quickly than conventional techniques.

U.S. Federal and State agencies do not currently use immunoassays in their pesticide residue regulatory programs on food. However, FSIS has begun implementing the use of an immunoassay to detect a small group of pesticides, and Canada's Department of National Health and Welfare (which regulates pesticide residues in food) will be training laboratory personnel in the fall of 1988 in the use of a specific immunoassay to determine one pesticide (1, 13).

THE IMMUNOASSAY

In higher animals, specialized cells (known as B lymphocytes) recognize substances foreign to the body (known as antigens) and respond by producing antibodies that recognize and bind to the antigens (figure 4-1). The introduction of a pesticide can stimulate an animal's immunological system to develop antibodies that will recognize and bind to that specific pesticide. These antibodies can be obtained from the animal's serum and used for the detection of the pesticide. However, antibodies are so specific that it is important to decide upon the purpose of the antibody before development begins. For example, for pesticides that are metabolized quickly, antibodies may need to be developed for the significant metabolites rather than the original pesticide.

Pesticides are usually made up of molecules too small to induce the production of antibodies. Therefore, pesticides must first be conjugated to a larger carrier molecule, often a pro-

Figure 4-1.—Artist's Conception of Antibody-Antigen Interactions

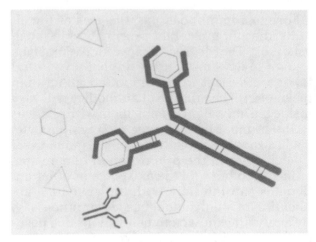

Antibody-antigen interactions result from a precise fit between a surface feature of the antigen and the correspondingly shaped binding sites in the antibody molecules.

SOURCE: Environmental Monitoring Systems Laboratory-Las Vegas, Environmental Protection Agency.

tein. Once attached to the carrier molecule, the pesticide is called a hapten. Where the conjugation occurs will influence the types of antibodies produced. The chemical synthesis of the hapten-carrier conjugate is generally considered to be the most important factor in obtaining useful antibodies for analytical use, and the chemistry involved is a major factor in the cost of immunoassay development (9). The hapten-carrier conjugate is then injected into a vertebrate, e.g., a rodent or rabbit, or for large amounts of antibodies, a sheep or goat. The animal will produce an array of antibodies; some will bind to the carrier molecule, some to the hapten-carrier conjugate, and some to the hapten. Only the last of these is useful for developing an immunoassay to detect the pesticide. These antibodies will be heterogeneous because different B lymphocytes may produce antibodies that bind to slightly different sites on the hapten. These antibodies are known as *polyclonal* because they are produced from a number of different B lymphocyte clones in the animal. They need to be characterized for their affinity for the hapten (the strength of their binding interaction with the hapten) and their specificity (whether they bind only to the hapten or to other related chemicals as well).

For most immunoassays, the greater the affinity, then the greater the sensitivity of the analysis (10). The degree of specificity must be known to determine if the antibody will bind to, or cross-react with, compounds other than the hapten. The mixture of antibodies will vary inside the animal producing them with changes in the number of each type of B lymphocyte; it will also vary between each animal immunized. The changes in the proportion of hapten-specific antibodies and the existence of other antibodies can interfere with the analytical application of a polyclonal-based immunoassay. By analyzing known concentrations of a pesticide along with the unknown concentrations in a sample, these variations can be adjusted for, and successful polyclonal-based immunoassays for pesticides can be developed (10, 11).

The production of *monoclonal* antibodies can offer some benefits over polyclonal antibodies, but some tradeoffs exist. Monoclonal antibodies are produced through a fusion of mouse or rat B lymphocyte spleen cells with myeloma tumor cells to produce hybridoma cells, a small percentage of which will produce the desired antibody. The spleen is normally taken from an animal that has first successfully produced useful polyclonal antibodies. This process takes a minimum of 3 months before large quantities of antibodies can be produced (21). Hybridomas can live almost indefinitely and can produce an unlimited amount of homogeneous monoclonal antibodies without the interfering antibodies that may exist with polyclonal antibodies. And like polyclonal antibodies, hybridomas can be stored in liquid nitrogen and easily distributed between laboratories.

Monoclonal antibodies, however, are not necessarily the better choice for a specific immunoassay. Polyclonal-based immunoassays may be adequate for an immunoassay, and in some cases, they are the more sensitive of the two (3). But for other pesticides, monoclonals may be necessary (3). Production of monoclonal antibodies requires more time, labor, equipment, and training than polyclonal antibodies and can add 25 percent to development costs (7). New techniques now under development may reduce the costs of hybridoma production, however (9).

Polyclonal or monoclonal antibodies are next incorporated into an immunoassay. Immunoassays for pesticides operate by competitive inhibition, or displacement, in which the antibodies are simultaneously exposed to an unknown amount of a pesticide in the sample and to a known quantity of the pesticide separate from the sample. The more pesticide in the sample, the fewer antibodies will bind to the latter pesticide (4).

To allow measurement, some sort of tracer must be attached to either the antibody or the pesticide. Currently, the most widely used tracer is an enzyme that will generate an easily measurable color when an additional substance is added. Other tracers include radioisotopes, fluorescent molecules, and magnetic particles (10). The radioimmunoassay (RIA), while in some ways more effective than the enzyme immunoassay, currently receives less attention for pesticide detection because of the demands and hazards of working with radioactive substances and because enzyme immunoassays have become increasingly practical (13). The fluorescent immunoassay, currently used in clinical applications, potentially may become as, or more, important for pesticide residue analysis in food as the enzyme immunoassay. It can be faster, more sensitive, and more easily automated than the enzyme immunoassay (9).

To determine the amount of pesticide in a sample, a standard curve is prepared. Several different known quantities of the pesticide (called standards) are separately analyzed with the immunoassay. A standard curve is prepared from these results and usually based on the ratio of the amount of pesticide in the standard to the measurement of the tracer (e.g., the intensity of color produced by an enzyme tracer). The measurement of the tracer from an assay of a sample can then be compared against the standard curve to determine the amount of the pesticide in the sample (see box 4-A).

Some extraction and possibly cleanup of the sample may be required before the antibodies can be used. For some aqueous solutions such as juices, immunoassays may be applied directly. Immunoassays for some vegetables and fruits have also been used without a cleanup step (14). However, cleanup is commonly nec-

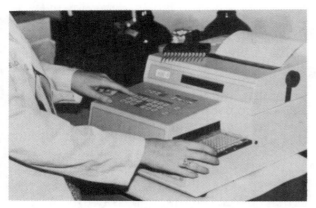

Photo credit: *Environmental Monitoring Support Laboratory-Las Vegas, Environmental Protection Agency*

A microprocessor-controlled photometer automatically reads samples in the 96-well microtiter plate within 2 minutes and provides results in report form.

Box 4-A.—Enzyme-Linked Immunosorbent Assay (ELISA)

ELISA is a common example of an immunoassay using an enzyme tracer. A test tube or well in a 96-well plastic microtiter plate is coated with a known amount of pesticide (conjugated to the carrier molecule) and so the pesticide is immobilized on the surface of the tube or well.

The sample extract containing an unknown amount of the same pesticide is added to the tube or wells. In separate tubes or wells on the plate, known concentrations of the pesticide (the standards) are added instead of the sample extract. The antibody that recognizes and binds to that pesticide is then added. Some of the antibody binds to the immobilized pesticide and some to the pesticide in the sample extract or the standards. How much antibody binds to the immobilized pesticide depends on how much pesticide is in the extract or standard.

The extract is washed away, and the amount of antibody bound to the immobilized pesticide will next be measured using the enzyme tracer. A tracer enzyme may be already attached to the antibody or may be attached by adding a second antibody (that binds to the first) conjugated with the enzyme. If the latter is done, then any unbound second antibody is washed away. A solution of colorless subtrate is added, which will be changed by the enzyme to a colored product (21).

The amount of antibodies bound to the immobilized pesticide is shown by intensity of the color; the greater the intensity, the less pesticide is in the sample. The intensity of the color can be measured through the use of a microspectrophotometer, which may be linked to a computer with data-analyzing software. This measurement is then compared against a standard curve, derived from the standards, to give the amount of pesticide in the sample.

---

essary and time-consuming for food containing oil or fat.[1]

Most immunoassay work has taken place in academic and regulatory laboratories (14). The time to develop an immunoassay can vary.

---

[1]For a more detailed description of the technology see ref. 10.

Polyclonal-based immunoassays generally require 9 months or longer to develop (13), and monoclonal immunoassays may take a year or more (21). However, commercial laboratories having abundant resources and personnel may be significantly faster than smaller laboratories in developing an immunoassay, sometimes as much as 4 to 5 months faster (7).

Another potential application of antibodies is the biosensor, which theoretically can provide real-time, continuous monitoring of pesticides in a matrix. The biosensor uses biological molecules, such as antibodies, to recognize and bind to the desired pesticide and a mechanism whereby the binding generates an electrical signal that can be measured and converted to give the concentration of the antigen (10). Compared to immunoassays, the application of biosensors for the detection of pesticide residues in food is uncertain.

STRENGTHS AND WEAKNESSES

Immunoassays are particularly suited for polar, water-soluble pesticides and their degradation products that are generally difficult to analyze using conventional analytical methods. Because immunoassays can determine biorational pesticides (such as *Bacillus thuringiensis*), they could be important if use of biological pesticides increases (10). They also can be significantly faster than certain conventional methods. Comparisons of quantitative immunoassays with conventional single residue methods using gas or liquid chromatography to analyze specific pesticide/food commodities show that immunoassays can analyze four to five times as many samples in a given time period (15, 16, 17).

The rapid nature of immunoassays is based on a number of factors. The cleanup step can be avoided or abbreviated for aqueous samples (such as juices and milk) and for many fruits and vegetables. The detection step can be faster than in conventional methods. For qualitative and semiquantitative immunoassays, the detection step may take no more than 5 minutes. For quantitative immunoassays, the use of a 96-well microtiter plate and plate reader allows detection and quantification of a large number of samples at one time. Quantitative immunoassays take approximately 4½ to 6 hours to perform on food, from sample preparation to detection. Liquids can take significantly less time. At Health and Welfare Canada, one person can analyze 12 to 16 fruit and vegetable samples in triplicate (along with controls) in one day. This work has been for research, not for regulatory application, and Health and Welfare Canada believes the number of samples could be tripled for regulatory application (14). Therefore, although the quantitative immunoassay procedure may take as long as a conventional method, more samples can be analyzed at one time.

The use of automation and robotics could further increase the number of samples analyzed. The principal steps of an ELISA that can be automated include coating of the wells or tubes with the immobilized pesticide; washing; addition of antibody, standards, and samples; and color reading. Systems are available for automating one or more of these steps. For example, unattended, automated spectrophotometers can read 10 to 25 microtiter plates and record the results in report form. However, because most enzyme immunoassays have long incubation periods, automation of the entire procedure by a single unit is not practical yet (9).

In addition, immunoassays can be simpler to use than conventional techniques, require less skilled personnel, and require minimal instrumentation time and comparatively inexpensive equipment. Technicians can be trained within 2 weeks (8, 13). And given that immunoassays can be more portable and simpler to use, they may be adaptable to field use for food. The actual costs of an immunoassay used on food for pesticide analysis versus a conventional method have not been compared (13). But the costs of analyzing a sample in general and for specific nonfood matrices with an immunoassay are lower than for conventional techniques (9, 22).

Despite these advantages, the use of immunoassays for monitoring pesticide residues in food has been constrained by a number of factors. Immunoassays may not be as sensitive for some compounds as conventional methods, and they can have lower levels of reproducibility. Because immunoassays are compound-specific, they are not suitable for multiresidue analysis. Therefore, while they may analyze more samples in a given time than multiresidue methods, they can detect fewer pesticides.

Characteristics of the food or the pesticide, in some cases, may also preclude the use of immunoassays. For food samples and pesticides requiring considerable cleanup work, immunoassays may be no faster than conventional techniques. In addition, immunoassays may not work well in certain foods. For some pesticides, e.g., those of very small molecules or having nonrigid structures, it may not be possible to develop antibodies. Or if the pesticide has little aqueous solubility, it may not be possible to use an immunoassay.

Not enough is known about possible cross-reactivity of specific antibodies with other chemicals present in food. Problems caused by cross-reactivity are a concern but can be controlled if the antibodies are first well characterized and if blank samples and samples with known concentrations are analyzed at the same time with the sample in question (4). Cross-reactivity can also be a benefit if an immunoassay is needed for a group of similar pesticides.

Another constraint to the use of immunoassays for pesticide residue analysis in food seems to be the reluctance of some analytical chemists to explore the potentials of immunoassays. This is due in part to analytical chemists' general unfamiliarity with the biologically based technology. This constraint may be overcome by validation of the technique and increased training in its use. The speed of doing so will depend on institutional commitment, however.

STATUS OF REGULATORY USE OF AND RESEARCH ON IMMUNOASSAYS

Antibodies have been developed and reported for at least 30 pesticides, though few have been applied to food (for a listing of immunoassays developed for agrichemicals, see ref. 11). Currently, no government agency has used immunoassays for regulation of pesticide residues in food, but many are supporting research and development for immunoassay determination of pesticides, in some cases for matrices other than food (see table 4-1).

Regulatory agencies' acceptance of immunoassays vary. Health and Welfare Canada is the furthest along in the development of immunoassays for pesticide testing in food. Since 1980, Canada has developed seven immunoassays for use in food and is currently developing one for 2,4-D. Canada has focused its work on quantitative polyclonal-based ELISAs for polar compounds in non-fatty foods. Canada's regulatory laboratories are not yet using immunoassays, but a planned fall 1988 training workshop on an ELISA for carbendazim is a first step toward transferring the technology to the field laboratories (13).

FSIS recently has decided that immunoassays can have an important role in its regulatory program. This is in part a response to the National Research Council's recommendations to test more samples and to test for more chemicals using more rapid methods.[2] FSIS is now working on implementing a semiquantitative immunoassay for the rapid detection of a group of five pyrethrin insecticides for regulatory use in 1989 at its Athens, GA, laboratory. Part of

---

[2]In response to a request from FSIS, the Committee on the Scientific Basis of the Nation's Meat and Poultry Inspection Program, Food and Nutrition Board of the National Research Council prepared in 1985 the report *Meat and Poultry Inspection: The Scientific Basis of the Nation's Program* (12), which included technical recommendations for FSIS's inspection program.

Table 4-1.—Immunoassays for Pesticides Under Development by Regulatory Agencies

Agency	Pesticide	Matrix	Type of assay	Type of antibody[a]	Data provided	Contractor (if one)
FSIS	heptachlor & heptachlor expoxide	meat & poultry	ELISA	M	quantitative	Lawrence Livermore Laboratory
	triazines[b]	meat & poultry	ELISA	P	qualitative	
FDA	paraquat	potatoes	ELISA	M	quantitative	Research Triangle Institute (RTI)
	fenamiphos, fenamiphos sulfone and sulfoxide	oranges	ELISA	M	quantitative	RTI
	benomyl, carbendazim, thiophanate methyl	apples	ELISA	M	quantitative	RTI
	glyphosate	soybeans	ELISA	M	quantitative	RTI
EPA.........	paraquat	soil & water	ELISA	P & M	quantitative	
	pentachlorophenol[c]	water	ELISA	M	quantitative	
	atrazine & simazine[d]	soil	ELISA	M	quantitative	
CDFA	molinate	water	ELISA	M	quantitative	University of California—
	thiobencarb	water	ELISA	M	quantitative	Davis & Berkeley
	atrazine & simazine	water & soil	ELISA	M	quantitative	EPA—Las Vegas laboratory[e]
Health & Welfare Canada	2,4-D		ELISA	P	quantitative	

[a]P = polyclonal and M = monoclonal.
[b]FSIS is evaluating a rapid ELISA test for triazines developed by ImmunoSystems Inc.
[c]EPA is evaluating a pentachlorophenol immunoassay developed by Westinghouse Bio-Analytic Systems Company.
[d]EPA is developing the soil extraction technique for the immunoassay under contract with CDFA.
[e]The University of California at Davis is doing the hapten synthesis work and developing polyclonal antibodies. The University of California at Berkeley is developing the monoclonal antibodies. The EPA Las Vegas laboratory is developing an extraction technique for atrazine and simazine in soil samples.
SOURCE: Office of Technology Assessment, 1988.

this work is on completing the extraction and cleanup steps for the immunoassay (1). FSIS has contracted for the development of other ELISAs for heptachlor and a number of animal drugs. In addition to contracting for the development of immunoassays, FSIS also tests commercially developed test kits and is currently evaluating a commercial qualitative immunoassay for triazine herbicides. FSIS's use of immunoassays is made more difficult because it works primarily with fatty commodities—meat and poultry—which normally require significant cleanup.

FDA has no current plans to implement the use of immunoassays for regulatory work. FDA, however, has a 3-year, approximately $500,000 contract begun in September 1987 for the development of six complete, quantitative immunoassay methods based on monoclonal antibodies (2). FDA is taking a somewhat "wait and see" attitude on the results of this research before determining the role of immunoassays in its pesticide regulatory program.

EPA has established a program at its Las Vegas Environmental Monitoring Systems Lab-

oratory on using immunoassays for the detection of hazardous substances, including pesticides, in the environment. The program tests commercially available immunoassays as well as develops immunoassays. EPA does not address food but it has an interagency agreement with FSIS for the development of antibodies of common interest.

The California Department of Food and Agriculture (CDFA) has contracted for the development of three immunoassays for use on environmental matrices: soil, surface water, and groundwater. CDFA has no plans yet to use these immunoassays on food (19).

Agencies have also taken different approaches to the development of immunoassays. FDA, for example, has contracted for the development of entire immunoassays. EPA has cooperative agreements with university laboratories to provide hapten work, antibodies, and in some cases the entire immunoassay. Health and Welfare Canada has developed its immunoassays inhouse. It seems that enough outside expertise exists in antibody development for regulatory agencies to tap using contracts instead of having to develop the capability to do such work in-house. Agencies, however, would need some in-house expertise, at least to identify the types of antibodies needed, to evaluate the results of the antibody development, and to adapt the immunoassay for use on food. This last capability would also allow agencies to take advantage of antibodies developed by others for nonfood matrices.

Because the application of immunoassays to pesticide monitoring in food is new, a great opportunity exists for agency coordination of research. As noted earlier, EPA and FSIS have an interagency agreement, and some of CDFA's work is done at EPA. But neither FDA nor Health & Welfare Canada seem to be well linked with one another nor with the other agencies. Coordination could be stimulated if agencies jointly listed which pesticides need improved methods and then identified those best addressed by immunoassays. In this way, devel-

opment of antibodies useful to all agencies could be done without duplication of effort.

Commercial development of immunoassays for analyzing pesticides is also taking place. A number of rapid immunoassay tests have been developed by small private firms (see table 4-2). Many of these test kits were developed for use on water and require adaptation to food. Currently, FSIS is the only regulatory agency doing adaption work. Quantitative immunoassays for pesticides are also being developed privately, but again they are not aimed for use in regulating pesticide residues in food. Identification by Federal agencies of priority immunoassay needs and communicating these needs to the private sector might stimulate private development of immunoassays for use in food. In some cases, private companies have developed immunoassays for internal use, and Federal agencies could investigate the possibility of obtaining and modifying these immunoas-

Table 4-2.—Commercially Available ELISA Test Kits for Pesticides

Pesticide	Claimed limit of detection[a]	Water & food matrices[b]	Firm
Paraquat	100 ppb	water	Environmental Diagnostics Inc. Burlington, NC
Triazine herbicides (atrazine, simazine propazine)	1 ppb	water, milk, soup, and fruit juices	ImmunoSystems Inc. Biddeford, ME
Chlordane-related pesticides (chlordane, heptachlor dieldrin, aldrin endrin, endosulfan)	1 ppb 200 ppb	water beer	
Benomyl	500 ppb	water, orange and grape juice concentrate	
Carbofuran	1 ppb 25 ppb 100 ppb	water grape juice rice	
2,4-D	1 ppb 100 ppb	water beer	
Triazine herbicides	same as triazines above		Westinghouse Bio-Analytic Systems Co. Rockville, MD
Aldicarb	10 ppb	water and watermelon	
Carbofuran	10 ppb	water	
Parathion	10 ppb	water and fruit juice	
Pentachlorophenol	10 ppb	water	

[a]ppb = parts per billion
[b]These food matrices are ones that the firms have tested their immunoassays on. Some of these immunoassays were developed to analyze nonfood matrices and their modification for use on food may not be a priority of the firm.

SOURCE: Office of Technology Assessment, 1988.

says for agencies' use on food (10). For example, a polyclonal-based quantitative immunoassay for cyanazine (an atrazine herbicide) was developed for soil and water by Shell Oil Company and used to provide data for EPA reregistration of the pesticide. The immunoassay has a detection limit of 0.5 parts per billion and can analyze five times as many samples a day as a conventional method using gas chromatography (18).

As a new technology in the pesticide analysis area, immunoassays require rigorous validation before acceptance by analytical chemists (21). Validation of immunoassays initially could be accomplished through comparisons with established methods, although in time agencies may need new validation and quality control protocols to address the unique properties of immunoassays (3). Standardized methods for using immunoassays and criteria for evaluating data, a general plan for establishing degree of cross-reactivity, and minimum quality specifications for the materials (including antibodies used) would all benefit the validation of immunoassays (9).

As in the case of research, coordinating the validation process for immunoassays among regulatory agencies could be improved, possibly in conjunction with appropriate professional associations such as the Association of Official Analytical Chemists (AOAC). Currently, agencies are conducting validations of immunoassays individually. No official validation studies of immunoassays for pesticide residue detection in food have been submitted to the AOAC. Health and Welfare Canada validated each of its immunoassays by analyzing four to five commodities each with four different concentrations of the pesticide, in duplicate or triplicate, using conventional methods and the immunoassay on each sample (13). EPA used the same process of analyzing each sample by both a conventional method and an immunoassay in its validation of a commercial, quantitative immunoassay for pentachlorophenol. For future evaluations, EPA will prepare individualized evaluation studies based on a statistically significant number of samples analyzed through conventional methods, which will eliminate the need to analyze every sample by conventional methods (20).

THE POTENTIAL ROLE OF IMMUNOASSAYS IN THE DETECTION OF PESTICIDE RESIDUES IN FOOD

Immunoassays have a number of potential regulatory roles. The small number of pesticides each immunoassay can detect means that immunoassays will complement or improve multi-residue methods (MRMs) rather than replace them. For example, development of immunoassays could be focused on those polar, moderate-to-high health hazardous pesticides that MRMs cannot address. Current MRMs might also be improved by analyzing a sample extract with conventional techniques as well as immunoassays, thus increasing the number of pesticides that could be detected by the MRMs. Additional work would be required to overcome possible negative effects of extraction solvents on the immunoassay. For all uses of immunoassays, conventional methods will be necessary

to confirm violations and ensure that the immunoassays are not giving false negative or false positive results.

Advances in immunoassay technology may result in immunoassays being submitted to EPA during the tolerance-setting process to fulfill the requirement for an analytical method. EPA has not formally decided if such a method would be acceptable, and FDA and FSIS would need to provide input because the submitted methods are to be used for regulatory work. Therefore, EPA's, FDA's, and FSIS's capability to use immunoassays could affect the agencies' decision to accept them as submitted methods. In a worst case scenario, EPA might be faced with the submission of analytically acceptable, commercially available methods whose acceptance might be denied because a regulatory agency does not have the expertise or equipment to use them.

Quantitative immunoassays could replace impractical conventional single residue techniques, increase the number of samples analyzed for certain pesticides (even those for which practical conventional techniques exist), and increase the number of special surveys for specific pesticides. Increased automation, including robotics, of the immunoassay would further support these activities. Once accepted, quantitative immunoassays may also be used as a confirmatory single residue technique for analysis by conventional methods.

Semiquantitative or qualitative immunoassays could test large numbers of food samples rapidly for specific pesticides that need to be monitored but that have shown few violations in the past. Thus, more time-consuming and expensive, conventional quantitative methods could be reserved for confirming violative samples. Currently, some private sector food manufacturers, such as certain baby food producers, use rapid ELISA tests to ensure that the products they buy do not have illegal residues of certain pesticides (5, 6). The use of immunoassays in monitoring programs may require some rethinking of objectives because they would enable a greater number of samples to be analyzed but they do not provide the quantitative data some agencies require.

The ability of immunoassays to analyze large numbers of samples would make them useful when a widespread pesticide residue problem is suspected in a specific commodity or commodities. The large number of samples that need to be analyzed in this situation can overwhelm a regulatory laboratory using conventional methods. Such tests could be used to sort out the violative samples and allow the legal samples to reach the market more rapidly.

In time, the portability and simplicity of immunoassays, especially the semiquantitative and qualitative ones, could provide the opportunity to perform testing outside of the laboratory. Issues such as how to address extraction and cleanup needs, training of the field testers, and how such analysis would fit into current regulatory programs would first need to be addressed before field testing was implemented.

CHAPTER 4 REFERENCES

1. Ashworth, R., Chemistry Division, Food Safety and Inspection Service, Washington, DC, personal communication, May 13, 1988.
2. Clower, M., Center for Food Safety and Applied Nutrition, Food and Drug Administration, Washington, DC, personal communication, July 12, 1988.
3. Hammock, B., Gee, S., Cheung, P., et al., "Utility of Immunoassay in Pesticide Trace Analysis," *Pesticide Science and Biotechnology*, R. Greenhalgh and T. Roberts (eds.) (London: Blackwell Scientific Publications, 1987).
4. Hammock, B., and Mumma, R., "Potential of Immunochemical Technology for Pesticide Analysis," *Pesticide Analytical Methodology*, American Chemical Society Symposium Series 136, J. Harvey, Jr. and G. Zweig (eds.) (Washington, DC: The American Chemical Society, 1980).
5. Harvey, R., Beech Nut Nutrition Corporation, Canajoharie, NY, personal communication, May 20, 1988.
6. Hether, N., Gerber Products Company, Fremont, MI, personal communication, May 13, 1988.
7. Hunter, K., Westinghouse Bio-Analytic Systems Company, Rockville, MD, personal communication, July 1, 1988.
8. Hunter, K., Westinghouse Bio-Analytic Systems Company, Rockville, MD, personal communication, Apr. 15, 1988.
9. Karu, A., Hybridoma Facility, College of Natural Resources, University of California-Berkeley, Berkeley, CA, personal communication, June 28, 1988.
*10. Mumma, R., and Hunter, K., "Potential of Immunoassays in Monitoring Pesticide Residues in Foods," OTA commissioned paper, Spring 1988.

*These references are contained in appendix B.

11. Mumma, R., and Brady, J., "Immunological Assays for Agrochemicals," *Pesticide Science and Biotechnology*, R. Greenhalgh and T. Roberts (eds.) (London: Blackwell Scientific Publications, 1987).

12. National Research Council, Food and Nutrition Board, Committee on the Scientific Basis of the Nation's Meat and Poultry Inspection Program, *Meat and Poultry Inspection: The Scientific Basis of the Nation's Program* (Washington, DC: National Academy Press, 1985).

13. Newsome, W.H., Food Research Division, Health and Welfare Canada, Ottawa, Canada, personal communication, May 6, 1988.

*14. Newsome, W.H., and Graham, G., "Pesticide Residue Monitoring in Canada," OTA commissioned paper, Spring 1988.

15. Newsome, W.H., "Determination of Iprodione in Foods by ELISA," *Pesticide Science and Biotechnolology*, R. Greenhalgh and T. Roberts (eds.) (London: Blackwell Scientific Publications, 1987).

16. Newsome, W.H., "An Enzyme-linked Immunosorbent Assay for Metalaxyl in Foods," *Journal of Agricultural and Food Chemistry* 33(3): 528-530, May/June 1985.

17. Newsome, W.H., and Shields, J.B., "A Radioimmunoassay for Benomyl and Methyl 2-Benzimidazolecarbamate on Food Crops," *Journal of Agricultural and Food Chemistry* 29(2):220-222, 1981.

18. Sharp, J., Agricultural Products Department, E.I. DuPont de Nemours & Co., Wilmington, DE, personal communication, Aug. 2, 1988.

19. Stoddard, P., California Department of Food and Agriculture, Sacramento, CA, personal communication, Apr. 18, 1988.

20. Van Emon, J., Environmental Monitoring Systems Laboratory, Environmental Protection Agency, Las Vegas, NV, personal communication, May 3, 1988.

21. Vanderlaan, M., Watkins, B.E., and Stanker, L., "Environmental Monitoring by Immunoassay," *Environ. Sci. Technol.* 22(3):247-254, March 1988.

22. Wie, S., and Hammock, B., "Development of Enzyme-Linked Immunosorbent Assays for Residue Analysis of Diflubenzuron and BAY SIR 8514," *Journal of Agricultural and Food Chemistry* 30:949-957, 1982.

*These references are contained in appendix B.

Chapter 5
Automation in Today's Pesticide Laboratory

CONTENTS

Page

Individual Component Automation 49
  The Role of Automation 49
Multiple Component Automation—Robotics 51
  Robotics in the Pesticide Residue Laboratory 51
  Two Principles for Successful Use of Robotics 54
  Benefits and Limitations of Robotics in the Analytical Laboratory 54
Chapter 5 References 55

Boxes

Box   *Page*
5-A. The Ideal, Fully Automated Analytical Laboratory 49
5-B. Zymate's PyTechnology Robotics System 52

Figure

Figure   *Page*
5-1. Schematic Drawing of Zymate Robotic System...................... 53

Tables

Table   *Page*
5-1. Laboratory Unit Operations (LUOs) of Robotic Systems 51
5-2. Comparison of Robot and Human Generated Data 53

Automation in Today's Pesticide Laboratory

INDIVIDUAL COMPONENT AUTOMATION

Automation has greatly increased analytical productivity of pesticide residue laboratories, and most such laboratories today use some type of automated equipment. Computers, for instance, have made the identification and quantification of pesticides easier. Automated gel permeation chromatography and autoinjection of samples onto chromatographs have allowed unattended work to take place day and night and permitted analysts to do additional work.

The Role of Automation

Despite such advances in automation, the prospect of designing a fully automated analytical laboratory remains an ideal (box 5-A). The procedures for analyzing a food sample are time-consuming, and many steps must still be done manually. A major percentage of the total analysis time is spent in preparation, extraction, and cleanup. Food is generally subsampled, cut into manageable pieces if necessary, and subsequently blended with solvent to extract the pesticide. The sample is then filtered or centrifuged, and the extract is either partitioned with another solvent or concentrated by evaporation. An optional cleanup step to isolate the pesticide may be required. Finally, the sample is injected into a gas or liquid chromatograph for analysis.

Automating the sample preparation and extraction steps would generate the greatest time savings, but these steps are the most difficult to automate because many types of samples require different preparation (10). Consequently, improvements in automation have focused primarily on the cleanup and determination stages of pesticide residues in food analysis.

Several types of automated equipment can be used in the cleanup step. Gel permeation

---

Box 5-A.—The Ideal, Fully Automated Analytical Laboratory

A fully automated laboratory, now existing only on paper, is one that would automatically process a sample from its entrance into the laboratory through the production of a written final report. An automated process of this type would move the sample through a series of operations whereby it could be subsampled, chopped, ground, blended, filtered, centrifuged, and extracted. The extract then could be evaporated, partitioned, redissolved, diluted, dried, chemically treated, subsampled and chromatographed. Data from the chromatograph would go to a computer, which would identify the sample, perform calculations on its abundance, graph the results, collate it with other data, and produce a hardcopy. Leftover sample or sample extracts would automatically be moved back to a refrigerator, freezer or other proper storage area, where it would be available for reanalysis if the computer data did not meet certain quality assurance/quality control standards.

Only very few regulatory laboratories have experience with robotic automation systems. Given the current cost and capability of automation instrumentation and technology, it is not yet possible to automate regulatory laboratories totally.

---

chromatography (GPC) can be automated (16) (for a description of gel permeation chromatography see ch. 3); in fact, FDA and FSIS use automated GPC, primarily for fatty foods. Requirements for quick results may pose a problem, however, because automated GPC processes only one sample at a time.

Further automation of the cleanup step may be possible with the recent development of an evaporation device that can be connected to the automated GPC. This evaporation device replaces the gel permeation solvent with one more suitable for gas chromatography, concentrates the sample through evaporation, and deposits each sample into a sealed vial, which then can be injected into a chromatograph for analysis. Such a device can process various types of pesticides with excellent reproducibility and recoveries (3). At present, FDA has not used automated evaporation equipment, in part because it does not want to use its capital budget to replace still functional manual evaporators and concentrators. FSIS laboratories do, however, use such equipment.

Another automated device for cleaning up food extracts is the DuPont Autoprep System. This device, used by some FSIS labs, uses centrifugal force rather than gas pressure or vacuum, as is done by other devices designed for this purpose. As many as 12 samples can be processed at a time, only small volumes for each wash are required (1 to 5 milliliters), and the pesticide is effectively concentrated for analysis by chromatography or other means.

The detection step has also been automated. Samples to be analyzed using gas or liquid chromatographs can be loaded on sample trays holding as many as 100 miniature vials and capped to seal-in volatile organic solvents and pesticides. These trays can be refrigerated to prevent the decomposition of thermally unstable pesticides. Automated sample injectors, also known as autosamplers, can then inject the sample into an automated chromatograph for unattended analysis. Autosamplers have the added advantage of being more precise in their volumetric sampling than a chemist, resulting in higher quality analytical data. Autosamplers, however, do not appear to be used for the majority of food samples at regulatory laboratories. In some cases, they are considered slower and more expensive than hand injection (9).

Automation of the detection step has been greatly facilitated by computerized data processing. Gas and liquid chromatographs are equipped with computers known as integrators. Integrators determine the retention time of an unknown chemical, necessary for its identification, and the quantity of the chemical. The integrator can then provide this information in report form. An integrator can be programmed to identify any specified retention time, allowing easier analysis of a specific pesticide. Mass spectrometer and infrared detectors are equipped with computers for sample identification that can search a library to match a sample to a known mass spectra. Data processing's importance is seen as increasing with the development of the laboratory information management system (LIMS). The LIMS goes beyond recording data; it produces tables that could be included in reports, it tracks samples, and it provides an electronic "paper trail" for fulfilling the requirements of "good laboratory practices."[1] In addition, a properly designed LIMS can be linked with virtually any type of analytical instrument from any manufacturer and can be used to collect and interpret data from it. Pesticide residue laboratories have not

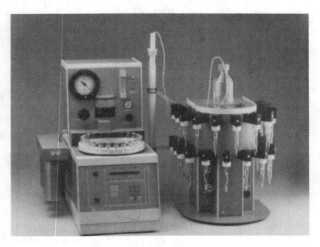

Photo credit: Analytical Bio-Chemistry Laboratories, Inc.

ABC Laboratories' GPC/Autovap® system combines a gel permeation chromatography module with an evaporation module to allow automated sample cleanup and concentration for a maximum of 23 sample extracts.

[1]These are standards describing the quality of instrumental, procedural, analytical, and personnel performance prescribed for laboratories conducting studies that support or are intended to support applications for research or marketing permits for (a) pesticide products regulated by the EPA (40 C.F.R. Section 160) and (b) products regulated by the FDA (21 C.F.R. Section 58).

yet adopted LIMS because of its early stage of application and its high cost (4).

Further improvements in analytical methods are possible through automation, but some constraints exist. Given that much of the automated equipment including robots has high capital costs, Federal regulatory laboratories with low or fluctuating capital budgets may have difficulty purchasing such equipment. Second, manual procedures may be faster than auto-

mated ones on a small scale, although automation may provide other benefits, e.g., reducing analyst exposure to hazardous solvents. Therefore, decisions to increase the use of automated equipment must consider the goals of monitoring programs and the moneys available. For example, if increased sample throughput were the primary goal of a monitoring program, then further advances in automation may be necessary before its adoption.

MULTIPLE COMPONENT AUTOMATION—ROBOTICS

Robotics is a special type of automation that allows mechanical manipulation of an object in a multitask computer-assisted, and reprogrammable manner (6). In the laboratory, the robot uses systems technology to allow multiple devices to perform such simple laboratory operations as weighing, dissolving, diluting, extracting, and so forth. The laboratory robot is a mechanical extension of a computer that allows it to do physical work as well as to process data.

Laboratory robotics is based on the Laboratory Unit Operations (LUOs) concept. LUOs are individual processes that can be linked to each other by hardware and by computer software to achieve a workable, fully automated analyti-

cal procedure. Table 5-1 explains most of the LUOs that robotic systems can now perform. The most popular laboratory robotics system is produced by the Zymark Corporation and is a modular system that combines robotics, programmable computers, and peripheral instruments to carry out laboratory procedures (box 5-B). In this system, the robot itself does little work but simply moves the sample from one workstation to another where the various operations are performed.

Robotics in the Pesticide Residue Laboratory

The presence of automated chromatographs in the laboratory now permits their overnight

Table 5-1.—Laboratory Unit Operations (LUOS) of Robotic Systems

LUO Class	Definition	Example
Weighing	Quantitative measurement of sample mass	Direct measurement using a balance
Homogenization	Reducing sample particle size and creating a uniform sample	Sonication, homogenization, grinding, etc.
Manipulation	Physical handling of laboratory materials	Moving test tube from rack to balance, capping, uncapping
Liquid Handling	All physical handling of liquids—reagents and samples	Dispensing reagents, pipetting sample, large-volume transfer of liquids
Conditioning	Modifying and controlling the sample environment	Timing (start and stop), temperature (heat and control), atmosphere (vacuum or gas blanket), agitation (mix, stir, vortex, shake)
Measurement	Direct measurement of physical properties	pH, conductivity, absorbance, fluorescence, etc.
Separation	Coarse mechanical and precision separations	Filtration, extraction (liquid-liquid, liquid-solid), centrifugation, precipitation, distillation, recrystallization, electrophoresis
Control	Use of calculation and logical decisions in laboratory procedures	Adding calculation volume of solvent based on sample weight
Data Reduction	Conversion of raw analytical data to usable information	Peak integration, spectrum analysis, molecular weight distribution
Documentation	Creating records and files for retrieval	Notebooks, listings, computers

SOURCE: Zymark Corporation, "Laboratory Robotics Handbook," Hopkinton, MA, 1988.

Box 5-B.—Zymate's PyTechnology Robotics System

Zymate's PyTechnology concept of organizing wedge-shaped modules around the central robot is shown in fig. 5-1. In the PyTechnology robotics system, there are 48 positions available, the typical module requiring 2 to 5 positions. Each module is called a PySection and is available for such LUOs as those in table 5-1. Custom modules can also be obtained on special order, designed to meet the user's specifications. Any PySection is simply locked into position with wing nuts, and electrical connection is made at the base of the robot through premounted contacts.

Control of the robot, connected PySections, and other peripheral analytical instrumentation is accomplished through the Zymate controller, consisting of a keyboard, disk drive, and an EasyLab Controller. The EasyLab Controller houses the central processing unit (CPU), a memory board, and module card for each laboratory station connected to the system. A second personal computer can be interfaced with the EasyLab Controller to allow simultaneous acquisition of data and user interaction.

Analytical procedures are programmed into the system via EasyLab Software. Using this software, the chemist programs a series of defined tasks using a "top down" approach. This program has three levels of instructions: the top-level program, the mid-level program, and the robot commands. As the chemist proceeds downward toward the robot commands level, the instructions to the controller become increasingly detailed, so that the last instruction might be something like "open fingers." In addition to having all the software available upon delivery for immediate startup and running "real-world" analytical procedures, the software also can be custom programmed.

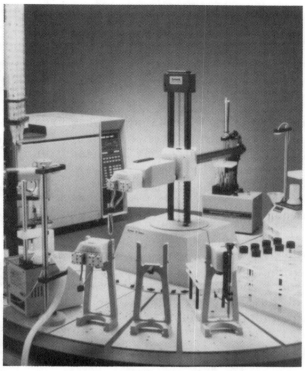

Photo credit: Zymark Corporation

The robot acting as an arm and hand, moves the sample to various modules for different processing steps.

and weekend use; however, many analytical steps are still done manually by highly skilled technicians who perform the tasks of weighing, chopping, blending, filtering, partitioning, and evaporating. If such steps could be done with robotics, these technicians would be free to perform more creative tasks such as data interpretation and method development.

The use of robotics for routine pesticide residue analysis in foods is just beginning. Chemists at the Residues and Environmental Chemistry Section of the Plant Protection Division of Jealotts Hill Research Station in England have successfully devised a robotics system to analyze the pyrethroid insecticide Karate in apples. Portions of apples and pears are carried through weighing, extraction, partitioning, solid phase extraction (SPE) cleanup, concentration, and evaporation steps. Table 5-2 compares recovery data for apples and pears by a robot and by a human. The robot gave more consistent recoveries for all samples studied.

A robotic system for the determination of the herbicide tridiphane in rat chow has been developed as part of a toxicology study on that chemical (7). Recoveries, however, were generally lower using robotics (86.5 percent recov-

Figure 5-1.—Schematic Drawing of Zymate Robotic System

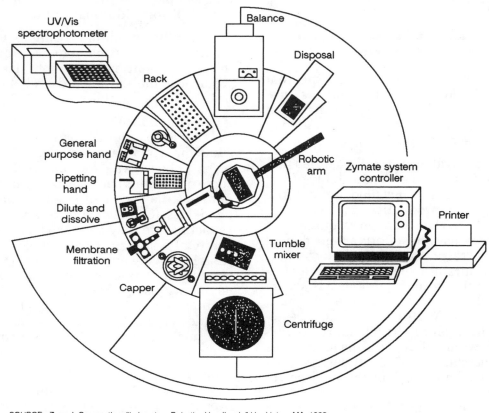

SOURCE: Zymark Corporation, "Laboratory Robotics Handbook," Hopkinton, MA, 1988.

Table 5-2.—Comparison of Robot and Human Generated Data

Sample no.	Robot		Human	
	Internal standard recovery (%)	Residue (mg/kg)	Internal standard recovery (%)	Residue (mg/kg)
1	83	0.10	119	0.10
2	84	0.11	127	0.12
3	83	0.09	111	0.07
4	81	0.08	127	0.07
5	88	0.08	127	0.09

SOURCE: I. Laws and R. Jones, "Generic Sample Preparation System for Automation of Pesticide Analysis," *Advances in Laboratory Automatic Robotics*, vol. 4 (Hopkinton, MA: Zymark Corp., 1984).

ery) than by the manual method (93.0 percent recovery), and 4½ hours were required to process 10 samples by robotics compared with 3½ hours for the manual procedure. On the other hand, the robot can work 24-hour days, whereas the technician normally works only 8. Furthermore, robotic recoveries were more consistent.

A robotic system has been used to isolate a synthetic pyrethroid insecticide from extracts of soil, sediment, fish, and mussel at levels as low as 1 part per billion. Small SPE cartridges packed with Florisil were used to accomplish this, and observed recoveries averaged 85 percent or more for these sample types (1).

Neither FDA nor FSIS uses or is testing the use of robots for analyzing pesticide residues in food, although both agencies are monitoring advances in robotic technology. Health and Welfare Canada is evaluating two robots in its laboratories: one to carry out the liquid-liquid partition step in the Luke method and the other to carry out the extraction and cleanup steps on milk samples undergoing a multiresidue test for organochlorines (12). Early results show the latter robot to be equivalent in accuracy to manual preparation while doubling the weekly output of samples (12).

Two Principles for Successful Use of Robotics

In a recent survey of numerous firms that have installed four or more robotics systems, two principles were mentioned that many felt were necessary for successful incorporation of robotics in a laboratory (8):

- A single motivated and well-qualified person must be given the responsibility of seeing that a system is installed and put into operation in a productive way. That person should be given enough resources and time so that his or her efforts are not diluted with other responsibilities. It may be necessary to hire a chemist with some electronics training or experience, since robotics relies on electronic and computer technologies. Analysts could also be retrained through on-the-job short instruction that would allow persons to improve their understanding of how things are done within the framework of the modern robotics system.
- The selection of an initial application or part of a complex application should have well-understood chemistries so that rapid startup with quickly measurable productivity is realized.

Benefits and Limitations of Robotics in the Analytical Laboratory

The benefits of using robotics in a laboratory include improved test precision, morale, worker safety, and "product" quality (2). Robotics in a regulatory laboratory doing pesticide residue analyses or method development has other advantages as well. It provides exacting timing and uniform sample handling, which ensure precision and accuracy (5). Analytical methods are transportable from laboratory to laboratory, since they are stored on computer diskette and executed by instrumentation that is identical wherever they are implemented (14). Moreover, an electronic "paper trail" is left on the computer for all analytical operations performed on a sample (6, 14). (See Kropscott et al. in appendix B for additional discussion.)

Currently, attention is being focused on designing robots for methods development and the subsequent method optimization. This would lead the way toward a robot specifically designed for pesticide regulatory laboratories.

One common mistake made by those attempting to use robotics in the laboratory is to assume that robots are designed to simulate humans. Robots have a great deal of difficulty with some operations because their parts simply do not have the degree of freedom that a human hand does, for instance. They also do not move as fast nor do they have the load-carrying capacity of a human. For example, robots have trouble moving and processing large fruits or vegetables. They are unable to manipulate some laboratory glassware that is currently in vogue, such as large separatory funnels or evaporative devices. They are better able to manipulate small tubes, pipettes, flasks, and similar containers.

Before robotics can be used in existing MRMs such as the Luke and the Mills-Onley-Gaither procedures, smaller samples, smaller amounts of solvent, and more sophisticated evaporative techniques must be demonstrated to be effective. When necessary, the newer cleanup techniques that reduce sample size requirements, such as SPE cartridges, need to be evaluated. Innumerable successes in the drug and petrochemical industries have demonstrated that great gains can be made in productivity when procedures can be miniaturized.

Robots have significant costs similar to costs of conventional computer systems—estimates range from $60,000 to $120,000 for the purchase of the robot and the renovation of the laboratory (5, 15). In addition to the cost, significant time must be given to adapting the robot to the needs of the laboratory and to familiarizing laboratory personnel with its use. Older model robots had startup times of 3 to 6 months (15), and the Health and Welfare Canada robot now doing milk samples took about a year to set up (11). However, startup times should decrease dramatically with improvements in the robots such as pre-programming and with increased familiarity with their use (13). Lastly, robots are subject to mechanical and electrical breakdowns and require a continuous power supply.

Robotics then should not be viewed as a cure-all for those regulatory agencies now inundated with food samples, but rather as a supplement to conventional manual techniques now being used. It is expensive to acquire, requires a new way of thinking to use it effectively, and suffers from the limitations listed above. On the other hand, it can measurably improve the overall operation of the analytical laboratory.

CHAPTER 5 REFERENCES

1. Akkari, K.H., "Robotic Residue Sample Purification by Solid-Phase Extraction," *Fifth International Symposium on Laboratory Robotics*, Boston, MA, 1987, Abstr. In: *Advances in Laboratory Automation Robotics*, vol. 4 (Hopkinton, MA: Zymark Corp., 1988).
2. Curley, J.E., "Making Robots Fly," *Advances in Laboratory Automation Robotics*, vol. 2 (Hopkinton, MA: Zymark Corp., 1985).
3. Hopper, M.L., and Griffitt, K.R., "Evaluation of An Automated Gel Permeation Cleanup and Evaporation System for Determining Pesticide Residues in Fatty Samples," *J. of Assoc. Off. Anal. Chem.* 70(4):724-726, July/August 1987.
4. Joe, T., Chemistry Laboratory Services, California Department of Food and Agriculture, Sacramento, CA, personal communication, June 3, 1988.
5. Kropscott, B., Dow Chemical Company, Midland, MI, comment at the OTA workshop "Technologies to Detect Pesticide Residues in Food," Mar. 15, 1988.
*6. Kropscott, B.E., Peck, C.N., and Lento, H.G., "The Role of Robotic Automation in the Laboratory," OTA commissioned paper, Spring 1988.
7. Kropscott, B.E., and Dittenhafer, M.L., "Automated Feed Analysis—an Application for Tox-

icology," *Advances in Laboratory Automation Robotics*, vol. 1 (Hopkinton, MA: Zymark Corp., 1984).
8. Laboratory Robotics Handbook (Hopkinton, MA: Zymark Corp., 1988).
9. Luke, M., FDA Pesticide Laboratory, Los Angeles, CA, personal communication, Apr. 26, 1988.
10. McCullough, F., ABC Laboratories, Columbia, MO, personal communication, May 3, 1988.
11. Newsome, W. H., Health Protection Branch, Health and Welfare Canada, personal communication, May 6, 1988.
*12. Newsome, W.H., and Graham, G.F., "Pesticide Residue Monitoring in Canada," OTA commissioned paper, Spring 1988.
13. Paul, A., Zymark Corporation, Hopkinton, MA, comment at the OTA workshop "Technologies to Detect Pesticide Residues in Food," Mar. 15, 1988.
14. Paul, A., Zymark Corporation, Hopkinton, MA, personal communication, May 10, 1988.
15. Peck, C., Dow Chemical Company, Midland, MI, comment at the OTA workshop "Technologies to Detect Pesticide Residues in Food," Mar. 15, 1988.
16. Tindle, R.C., and Stallings, D.L., "Apparatus for Automated Gel Permeation Cleanup for Pesticide Residue Analysis," *Analytical Chemistry* 44(11):1768-1774, September 1972.

*These reference papers are contained in appendix B.

Chapter 6
Pesticide Analytical Methods

CONTENTS

	Page
Introduction	59
Types of Methods	59
Multiresidue Methods	59
Single Residue Methods	61
Semiquantitative and Qualitative Methods	61
Current Needs in Methods Development	64
Cost Considerations of Methods Development Research	69
Needs for Adoption and Use of Methods	69
Chapter 6 References	71

Boxes

Box   *Page*

6-A. The Concepts of Screening and Rapid Testing ... 63

6-B. Ongoing Challenges to Methods Development: Metabolites and
New Pesticides ... 68

Figure

Figure   *Page*

6-1. Decision Tree for Testing Pesticides Through FDA Multiresidue
Methods ... 62

Table

Table   *Page*

6-1. Multiresidue Methods Routinely Used by FDA, USDA, and CDFA ... 60

Pesticide Analytical Methods

INTRODUCTION

The regulatory responsibilities of FDA and FSIS influence the type of methods these agencies use to monitor pesticide residues in food. Methods must provide results that are cost-effective, timely, reliable, and verifiable. The agencies also need methods that can identify as many pesticides as possible in a range of food commodities because they are charged with monitoring all foods for all pesticides. In addition, these methods should use instruments, associated hardware, and reagents that are readily available in the regulatory laboratory or are commercially available and inexpensive.

Regulatory agencies need methods that can give reliable results rapidly—within 24 hours—if violative products are to be kept from reaching the market. Neither FDA nor FSIS has the authority to detain commodities routinely monitored for pesticide residues, but both agencies can detain imports suspected of illegal residues and FSIS can detain suspected domestic meat until the results of analytical testing are received.

Methods must also be able to detect pesticides at, and often below, tolerance levels. They must endure interfering compounds such as other pesticides, drugs, and naturally occurring chemicals and be insensitive to such environmental variations as humidity, temperature, and solvent purity. Chemists with varying levels of training and expertise must be able to use them. There also should be some other means of confirming that a method is accurate.

EPA provides guidance for methods as part of the tolerance-setting process that involves many of these points. According to its Subdivision O Guidelines, submitted methods should 1) take 24 hours, 2) require readily available equipment or reagents, 3) identify the residue in the presence of other residues, and 4) detect the residue at or below the tolerance. EPA's guidelines do not include an emphasis on multiresidue methods (MRMs) or the submission of a confirmatory method.

FSIS also has criteria for methods suitable for its regulatory use: 1) methods must take no more than 2 to 4 hours of analytical time per sample, 2) they must have a minimum proficiency level at or below the tolerance, 3) there must be a quality assurance plan developed for the method, and 4) the method must be successfully validated through an interlaboratory study (6).

FDA does not have a formal listing of guidelines for its methods, but it uses many of the same criteria in evaluating them (13).

TYPES OF METHODS

Multiresidue Methods (MRMs)

MRMs come closest to meeting the method needs of the regulatory agencies. They are designed to identify and quantify a number of pesticides and their toxicologically significant metabolites simultaneously in a range of foods. Their usefulness is based on a combination of three factors:

- determining a broad spectrum of pesticides and their toxicologically significant metabolites in an array of food,

- being sensitive, precise, and accurate enough to be useful for regulatory purposes and acceptable to the scientific community,

- being economical or at least affordable for those laboratories using them.

No single method can optimize each of these three factors; as a result, the MRMs used are a compromise of these elements (see ref. 20 for futher discussion of this point).

MRMs have two other advantages. An MRM may be able to detect, but not measure, a particular pesticide or metabolite in food. The MRM, in such cases, signals the presence of the compound, which can then be analyzed with a single residue method (SRM) (16).

Second, MRMs record the presence of unidentified chemicals, known as an unidentified analytical response (UAR). Once observed, the chemical's identity can be determined by matching its result to a known chemical with a similar chromatographic result or by other techniques such as mass spectrometry. In this way, MRMs can identify the presence of possibly hazardous chemicals that were not expected to be residues in food and might have been overlooked. For example, polychlorinated biphenyls (PCBs) were discovered in meat and animal feed after appearing as UARs on the chromatograms of samples analyzed for the chlorinated hydrocarbon pesticides.

MRMs contain the steps of preparation, extraction, cleanup, chromatographic separation, and detection (as described in chapter 3). All MRMs used today in the United States are based upon either gas chromatography (GC) or high performance liquid chromatography (HPLC) as the determinative step. Of the 10 MRMs routinely used by FDA and USDA, 8 rely on GC as the determinative step (see table 6-1). Thin layer chromatography is still used by several agencies in Europe, but it has lost favor in this country because of its semiquantitative nature (1).

The FDA and USDA have geared much of their pesticide methods research to developing

Table 6-1.—Multiresidue Methods Routinely Used by FDA, USDA, and CDFA

Agency	Method[1]	Food type analyzed	Pesticide groups detected
FDA	GC-multiple detectors (Luke method)	nonfatty	organochlorines organophosphates organonitrogens
	GC-multiple detectors (Mills method)	fatty	organochlorines organophosphates
	GC-multiple detectors (MOG method)	nonfatty	organochlorines organophosphates
	GC-multiple detectors (Storherr method)	nonfatty	organophosphates
	HPLC-fluorescence (Krause method)	nonfatty	N-methyl carbamates
USDA-FSIS	GC-ECD	fat	chlorinated hydrocarbons
	GC-ECD (western method)	liver and fat	chlorinated organophosphates
	GC-NPD (eastern method)	liver	organophosphates
	HPLC-fluorescence	liver	carbamates
USDA-AMS[2]	GC-ECD	fatty (raw egg products)	chlorinated hydrocarbons
CDFA[3]	GC-ECD	nonfatty	organochlorines
	GC-NPD or FPD	nonfatty	organophosphates
	HPLC-fluorescence	nonfatty	carbamates

[1]Methods are identified by the combination of the instruments used for chromatographic separation and detection. Abbreviations for the these instruments are as follows:
 GC: gas chromatography
 HPLC: high performance liquid chromatography
 ECD: electron capture detector
 NPD: nitrogen-phosphorus detector
 FPD: flame photometric detector
 In some cases, a method may also have a name and these are noted in parentheses.
[2]AMS: The Agricultural Marketing Service
[3]CDFA: The California Department of Food and Agriculture

SOURCE: Office of Technology Assessment, 1988.

MRMs over the years. FDA's MRMs appear in Volume I of the Pesticide Analytical Manual (PAM I), and they are considered of high quality and capable of providing data that will withstand challenge during court litigation (for details on the development of FDA's MRMs see ref. 19).

The primary weakness of existing MRMs is that they cannot detect every pesticide. For example, of the 316 pesticides with tolerances, only 163 of them could be analyzed with FDA's five routinely used MRMs. A second weakness is that some MRMs require a great deal of time to perform, thereby reducing the number of samples analyzed and the speed of analysis. For example, certain foods, such as those with high concentrations of fats and oils, are difficult to analyze in a timely manner.

Single Residue Methods (SRMs)

A large number of methods exist that are designed to analyze a single pesticide and, in many instances, its metabolites or degradation products. Although less efficient than MRMs, the use of SRMs is necessary to monitor those pesticides, including a number of high health hazard ones, that cannot be detected by MRMs.

SRMs depend on a number of different techniques and vary widely in terms of reliability, efficiency, throughput (samples per day), degree of validation, and practicality for regulatory use. SRMs are primarily developed by the private sector for submission to EPA as part of the tolerance-setting process. Therefore, a method exists for every pesticide with a tolerance, although methods for some pesticides (primarily the older ones) may not be effective.

Most SRMs, like MRMs, are based on GC using the full array of element-specific detectors. Volume II of the *Pesticide Analytical Manual* (PAM II) consists solely of SRMs, both those that have undergone EPA review and possibly EPA laboratory evaluation, and those that have appeared in a peer-reviewed journal of high quality (these methods are normally similar to ones approved by EPA but adapted for other commodities) (10). In PAM II, those methods

reviewed by EPA are listed with Roman numerals and those not reviewed are lettered.

SRMs are not considered adequate for routine monitoring by the regulatory agencies, although FDA uses them. To monitor one pesticide with an SRM is considered inefficient when an MRM can measure many pesticides using the same resources. In addition, SRMs vary widely even for chemicals of the same class, so a laboratory needs a wide array of glassware, evaporative devices, chromatographs, and detectors to use the SRMs available. There is also dissatisfaction with the performance of some SRMs (24). Some chemists feel they are better served sometimes by 1) going to the scientific literature for methods, 2) borrowing methods from State laboratories, or 3) going directly to the registrant for the newest method. Others feel it is better to develop their own methods or adapt existing methods developed for pesticides of similar structure. SRMs are also not as capable of identifying UARs as MRMs.

In an attempt to reduce the need to use SRMs, EPA now requires that all pesticides requiring a new tolerance be evaluated to see if they can be detected by FDA and USDA MRMs. Only FDA has developed the testing protocols to support such testing. FDA has also devised a "decision tree," showing the order in which the FDA MRMs should be tested using the new pesticide to minimize research time (figure 6-1). The results confirm or deny whether that particular pesticide can be recovered through one of the MRMs. It has not yet been decided whether the EPA will still require development and submission of an SRM if the pesticide can be analyzed by an MRM (23).

Semiquantitative and Qualitative Methods

Semiquantitative and qualitative methods range widely in their ability to quantify the chemical present in a sample. Semiquantitative methods indicate the range of pesticide residue concentration in a sample; qualitative methods show whether or not a particular pesticide exists above some predetermined concentra-

Figure 6-1.—Decision Tree for Testing Pesticides Through FDA Multiresidue Methods

Part A

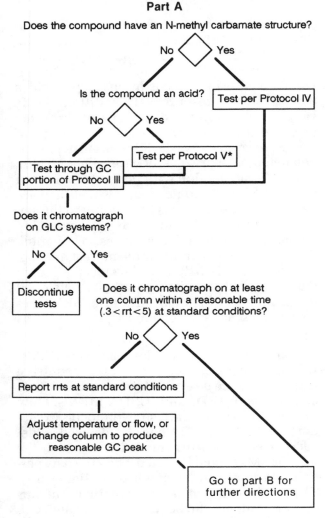

Part B

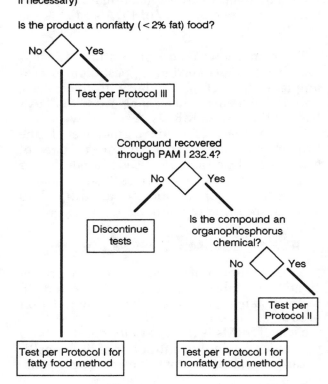

SOURCE: Food and Drug Administration, Division of Contaminants Chemistry, March 1988.

monitoring, although both agencies are conducting ongoing research. Similarly, EPA is conducting research on the use of these methods on nonfood matrices. Given that the majority of these methods have been developed for pesticides in nonfood matrices, significant adaptation research may be necessary for their use on foods.

Semiquantitative and qualitative methods make use of such technologies as thin layer chromatography (TLC), enzyme inhibition, and immunoassay. These three technologies can be moved from the laboratory into the field without losing their ability to detect pesticides. And because sophisticated instrumentation is not required, they are relatively inexpensive compared to quantitative methods.

tion. In this way they differ from the majority of conventional MRMs and SRMs, which fully quantify the amount of pesticide in a sample. (See also box 6-A.)

The benefits of these methods may be their low cost, speed, or ease of use. These benefits can contribute to an increase in the number of samples that could be analyzed, although tradeoffs may exist in the number of pesticides that can be analyzed. Currently, neither FDA nor FSIS is using these methods for pesticide

Box 6-A.—The Concepts of Screening and Rapid Testing

Screening and rapid testing are two terms commonly used when discussing improvements in methods that will determine in a short time whether or not a pesticide or group of pesticides is present in food. The use of these terms often is confusing because they have different meanings to different people, and the confusion can be compounded when the two are used together, i.e., "rapid screen."

The term screening, in general, can be applied to two different types of methods. The distinction between the two methods depends on what is being screened--either a large number of pesticides or a large number of samples.

First, screening can mean a method that can detect a large number of pesticides in a sample, that is, the method screens for pesticides. The multiresidue methods (MRMs) used by FDA and USDA are screening methods under this definition. These "MRM screens" analyze for a large number of pesticides at one time and therefore are the most cost-efficient approach when data on pesticide application are lacking or when a number of pesticides are known to have been used. Also, they can uncover the presence of residues not expected to be in the food. This type of screening method may also be labeled "rapid test" for a number of reasons. These MRMs are faster than single residue methods (SRMs) because they can analyze for more pesticides in a given time period. Some MRMs are considered rapid because they are relatively faster than other MRMs. For example, the Luke MRM used at FDA's Los Angeles laboratory can detect some 200 pesticides and metabolites in 30 samples each day and therefore is considered a rapid screen.

Second, screening is also used to mean a method that can analyze a large number of samples often for one pesticide or a small group of pesticides in a relatively short period of time, that is, the method screens samples. This type of screening method supports efficient identification of violative samples when a known pesticide/commodity problem exists or where a pesticide/commodity combination is known to have a low violation rate. When a method is used in this manner, the speed of analysis in terms of the number of samples that can be analyzed per unit time is emphasized and, in this context, it would then be considered a "rapid screen." Application of such a rapid screen to a large number of food samples thought to contain violative samples would allow nonviolative food to reach the market more quickly and reduce the number of samples that need to be analyzed by more time-consuming and expensive conventional methods. Those samples with positive results would be analyzed by a conventional method.

This type of screening uses technologies that are less expensive and more rapid to use than conventional methods, such as thin layer chromatography, immunoassay, and enzyme inhibition. The lower cost of these techniques stems from their relative speed of analysis and use of less expensive and more simple equipment. These techniques often are called "rapid tests," because of their speed.[1] The tradeoffs of using these techniques are noted in chapters 4 and 6. Neither FDA nor FSIS uses such screening methods for pesticide monitoring in food, although FSIS is actively researching its use.

[1]For more detail on this type of screening, see Ellis 1988 in appendix B.

A drawback of semiquantitative methods is that they do not provide the degree of accuracy necessary for enforcement action, e.g., for use in a court of law. Violations found by a semiquantitative method would have to be verified by a quantitative analytical method—or maybe two. And with the possible exception of thin layer chromatography, none of the semiquantitative techniques provide data that can be used to address UARs.

TLC is used sometimes in Europe for regulatory purposes (see ref. 1 for a bibliography of TLC applications). Thin layer chromatography-based methods have the advantage of an ability to analyze several pesticides simultaneously. As many as 20 pesticides can be tested at once if chromatographic conditions are properly chosen. TLC has been used successfully by FSIS to analyze the drug sulfamethazine in animal tissues; field use by inspectors relatively unskilled in analytical chemistry was also successful. An attempt to use TLC for analysis of chlorinated hydrocarbons in animal tissues has been unsuccessful, however, because of problems in achieving the desired sensitivity and an overly complicated sample extraction procedure for nonlaboratory use (3). Several potentially useful TLC methods are described in chapter 4 of PAM I. They are carryovers from early work at FDA and USDA and require sample cleanup by conventional Florisil or alumina columns. Both FDA and FSIS have ongoing research on TLC applications.

Enzyme inhibition-based color reactions are a means of making the spots and bands of pesticide residues on thin layer chromatographic plates visible in order to measure the pesticide residue either visually or with instruments. Such techniques have been developed for cholinesterase-inhibiting insecticides and photosynthesis-inhibiting herbicides.

In addition to working with TLC, enzyme inhibition may also be used for a "stand alone" test kit. Currently, one such qualitative kit is commercially available for the detection of cholinesterase-inhibiting insecticides (organophosphates and carbamates). The kit is inexpensive and can detect a large number of pesticides in concentrations of parts per million. The kit has been privately used for analyzing food extracts and for analyzing water used to wash skins of fruits and vegetables for pesticide residues (9). This type of kit is not specific unless information about the history of the sample is available. For example, it will give a positive response for a large number of compounds without being able to identify the specific compounds. This type of kit also may suffer from interferences produced by extraction solvents.

Immunoassays have been developed for semiquantitative and qualitative tests, although much immunoassay research has focused on quantitative assays (17). If needed, quantitative immunoassays based on color reactions could be adapted to semiquantitative assays with visual interpretation of the results. Such tests could then be more easily used outside the laboratory. Several qualitative tests are commercially available. Immunoassay-based methods have the advantage of speed since many tests can be performed simultaneously and some analyses take less than a few minutes if extractions are not necessary. They also have the advantage of being extremely sensitive, detecting some pesticides far below their tolerances, and they are usually specific, although sometimes cross-reactions occur that give false positives (17). A drawback is that immunoassays provide analyses for individual or small groups of pesticides.

Current Needs in Methods Development

Improving Existing Analytical Methods

Considerable time and resources have already been invested in developing analytical methods. Rather than devoting resources exclusively to developing new analytical methods, existing methods also can be improved through changes in technologies to reduce analysis time and to increase the number of pesticides that can be analyzed. For instance, improvements could be made in the following ways:

1. simplifying cleanup
2. improving extractions with supercritical fluid extraction (SFE)
3. miniaturization with solid phase extraction (SPE)
4. capillary columns
5. increased use of high performance liquid chromatography (HPLC)
6. use of immunoassay as a detection technique
7. increased automation
8. mass selective detection (MSD)

(1) Simplifying cleanup. Simplifying a method by eliminating sample manipulation in the cleanup step would shorten analysis time, eliminate opportunities for pesticide loss, reduce solvent and consumables usage, and reduce overall analytical costs.

Two FDA MRMs and the three used by the California Department of Food and Agriculture (CDFA) use food extracts that have not undergone any type of sample cleanup. Approximately 80 percent of the food samples analyzed by FDA are examined with the Luke method, and CDFA conducts more analyses with its own three methods than any other State. The trend toward less extensive sample cleanup in these methods has been a result of improving capabilities of element-specific detectors (NPD, FDP, ECD, and Hall).

As sample cleanup is reduced or even eliminated, increased stress is placed on the determinative step. As a result, the chromatographic separation begins to suffer from the presence of large amounts of sample coextractives. Such coextractives may produce a loss of resolution of pesticides in the sample, a loss of pesticide on the chromatographic column, and fouling of the detector. For these reasons, the chemist must weigh the need to shorten analysis time with the instrumentation "down time," that is, time required to clean, repair, and regenerate the instrument to its original operating specifications.

However, because reduction of cleanup steps pays high returns in time saved for a typical analysis by reducing analytical costs and increasing sample throughput, efforts should be made to explore it fully.

(2) Improving extractions with SFE. As more efficient hardware (particularly miniaturized valves, pumps, ovens, and refrigeration devices) becomes available for SFE, the technique may become more practical for extracting pesticides in foods, possibly in the field, e.g., the slaughterhouse. SFE can be coupled to capillary column gas chromatography or supercritical fluid chromatography (see ch. 3) to provide an on-line extraction/determination, although validated methods have yet to be developed using this approach. Since extraction time can be shortened, then selectivity can be gained by leaving potential interferences behind and thermally unstable chemicals can be dealt with. The technique has become attractive for consideration in the future. It may ultimately shorten analysis time while expanding the array of pesticides and metabolites that can be extracted.

Carbon dioxide, a relatively inert gas, has been used as an SF for the extraction of many types of organic compounds. Straight chain hydrocarbons have been selectively extracted from other chemicals present (8). More than 85 percent of such hydrocarbons were extracted in 5 minutes. Extractions can be even more efficient and faster as well as applicable to more polar chemicals by modifying the carbon dioxide with small amounts of polar organics.

(3) Miniaturization with SPE. An opportunity to reduce analysis time, solvent consumption, and overall costs might be through use of miniaturization (20). The philosophy of present miniaturization focuses on the use of small solid phase extractions (SPEs). These cartridges are now commercially available, are inexpensive ($2 to $3 each), and are disposable. Use of SPEs has not been demonstrated yet for MRMs, although they have been successfully used in SRMs (for such pesticides as aldicarb and paraquat). Problems associated with larger adsorption columns, such as the Florisil columns, may still exist with SPEs in MRMs. For example, pesticides may not exit the SPE in distinct groups but may instead be scattered among several fractions. In addition, there still may be a problem of pesticide loss on these extraction columns, depending upon the elution conditions and the pesticide under analysis. Associated with miniaturization are the problems of taking a truly representative sample, so that analytical results will reflect the average concentration of the pesticide in the food (2).

Miniaturization of MRMs might assist in adapting robotics to MRMs (see ch. 5). Present robotic modules handle samples of 1 to 10 grams better than heavier ones of 25 to 100 grams, like those used for conventional MRMs. Similarly, robots dispense and manipulate 5 to 25 milliliters of solvents more easily than the 100 to 250 milliliters typically used in conventional MRMs (12).

Other spinoffs of miniaturization might be that sample preparation could be done in the field (20), as is now commonly done for water samples. Extending this approach to milk, juices, and other fluid foods might be feasible. If some sort of solid sample extraction could be devised in the field, this approach could be extended to other foods.

In addition to miniaturization, the further development of SPE extractions will reduce or eliminate the need to use hazardous solvents. Present use of such solvents creates a health hazard for the chemist and produces a dilemma for their disposal.

Another spinoff of SPEs is that once the pesticide is on them, they can be stored more easily. The requirement for refrigerating potentially explosive solvents is removed, making the storage more safe and economical.

(4) Capillary columns. With the exception of cost, essentially all objections to capillary column chromatography for analysis of pesticides in foods have been removed. Fifteen-meter-long capillary columns of the wide bore variety cost about $250 compared with about $80 for a packed column, a small difference considering the potential savings in analysis time (see table 3-2), the availability of guard columns, and the reusability of columns following a solvent wash (7).

More important, capillary columns usually provide lower limits of detection because the chromatographic peaks are sharper. Lowering the limit of detection also means that smaller food samples (100 grams or less) can be analyzed. Once smaller food samples are used, then analysis becomes more adaptable to robotics.

For capillary columns to become accepted by many regulatory agencies, additional examination and standardization of columns will be needed so that the relative retention time concept of identifying pesticides can be extended to them. Relative retention time will change when compared to packed columns, but selection and detailed specifications of capillary columns and resources to characterize them fully should relieve this problem. However, costs in terms of equipment and time could be great and would have to be considered in light of existing monitoring activities.

(5) Increased use of HPLC. Since pesticide metabolites usually are more polar than their parent molecule and since HPLC is more adept at dealing with polar compounds than GC, it seems that HPLC has potential for analyzing both the parent and metabolites simultaneously. Recent examples include HPLC methods used for benomyl (fungicide), glyphosate (herbicide), and metabolites of fenvalerate (insecticide). All of the sulfonyl urea herbicides are analyzed by HPLC with the photoconductivity detector.

The trend toward more polar pesticides among those under development also makes HPLC worth examining in the development of MRMs and SRMs. Detectors are the constraining factor in applying HPLC to pesticide residue analysis in food. While columns are now available for almost any conceivable type of pesticide, there is a lack of effective detectors when compared to those available for gas chromatography. Particularly lacking are the element-specific detectors for pesticides containing atoms such as phosphorus, sulfur, nitrogen, and the halogens chlorine and bromine, although the photoconductivity detector works for some sulfur- and chlorine-containing pesticides.

(6) Use of immunoassay as a detection technique. Using immunoassays for detecting pesticide residues can have several advantages over conventional methods: They can analyze an increased number of samples in a given period, are simpler to use, require less skilled personnel and comparatively inexpensive equipment, and can analyze samples for less cost than conventional methods. However, widespread use is constrained by several factors, indicating that immunoassays will complement conventional determinative steps for MRMs but are unlikely to replace them. They may also offer a means to improve SRMs. (See ch. 4 for a detailed discussion of immunoassays.)

(7) Increased automation. Continued improvements in analytical methods are possible through automation. Improvements in automation have focused primarily on the cleanup and detection stages of pesticide residue analysis. Although automating the sample preparation and extraction steps would generate the greatest time savings, these steps are also the most difficult to automate because of the many types of food samples requiring different preparation (15).

Automated equipment including robots involves high capital costs, and many Federal regulatory laboratories may have difficulty purchasing such equipment. Manual procedures may still be faster than automated ones, although automation may provide other benefits, e.g., freeing up analysts' time or reducing analyst exposure to hazardous solvents. Therefore, decisions to increase the use of automated equipment must consider the goals of monitoring programs and the moneys available. Robots are not a cure-all for those regulatory agencies now inundated with food samples. However, robots can measurably improve the overall operation of the analytical laboratory. (See ch. 5 for a detailed discussion of automation.)

(8) MSD. The mass selective detector (MSD) may have an increasingly important role as a GC detector in developing MRMs; it is the only GC detector able to detect any pesticide that can be volatilized that has a molecular weight of no more than 650 atomic mass units (20). This may become an important factor in detector selection because it would not be constrained by the need to have a particular atom, such as sulfur, in the molecule. Although still considered a confirmatory tool, MSD has potential as a programmable GC detector that can be set to provide a relatively large degree of selectivity for pesticides at the trace level. The degree of applicability of this detector to samples of unknown pesticide application history—the sample types for which the MRMs are designed—will depend greatly upon improvements in the number of ion programs that can be used during a chromatographic run.

At present, only eight sets of ions can be programmed into the instrument during a chromatographic run, making its usefulness limited for MRM work. As use of this type of detector grows, its purchase cost ($40,000 to $65,000 per unit, depending upon accessories), should drop accordingly. Some laboratories have difficulty justifying such an expensive detection device, particularly when it is dedicated to quantitative work; typical element-specific detectors cost about one-tenth this much. Such an MSD can be used for full mass-spectral scans, however, giving it the capability of being a quan-

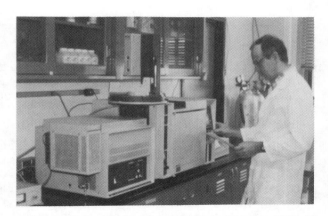

Photo credit: Food Safety and Inspection Service Laboratory, Athens, GA

Bench-top gas chromatograph/mass selective detector combinations are used to confirm a violative residue level in a food sample.

titative and confirmatory tool. MSD devices have been reduced in size compared with mass spectrometers of the 1970s and can be placed on desk or table tops, requiring little more room than the gas chromatograph itself. Space considerations become important when the high costs of supplying a cool, safe, dust-free environment for contemporary analytical instrumentation are taken into account.

Developing New Methods

(1) New MRMs. Research needs to focus on the potential for incorporating more pesticides into existing and emerging MRMs. Significant metabolites of these pesticides—often more difficult to detect than the parent compound—must also be addressed (see box 6-B). As additional data become available, it may become apparent that existing MRMs need to be modified or new methods developed.

It may be more advantageous to develop new MRMs for small numbers of chemically similar pesticides; this has been done for the phenoxy herbicides (PAM I); for the pesticides captan, folpet, and captafol (25); and for the benzimidazole-related fungicides (25). A new MRM is being proposed for collaborative study for analyzing the urea herbicides (11). Restricting new MRMs to such small groups of pesticides would probably not be as efficient for monitoring purposes as adding to existing MRMs or developing new comprehensive ones, but it may provide an interim solution to the ques-

---

Box 6-B.—Ongoing Challenges to Methods Development: Metabolites and New Pesticides

Greatly complicating the issue of developing analytical methods for pesticides in foods is the task of addressing not only the parent compound but also significant metabolites. Since metabolism or degradation of a parent compound generally occurs through cleavage, hydrolysis, conjugation with sugars or other polar compounds, or oxidation, the products so formed are usually more polar than the parent and thus more difficult to detect using conventional multiresidue methods (MRMs).

New pesticides may also pose problems for analysis. Forecasts for emerging pesticide types indicate molecular structures that are similar to those seen today; therefore, current MRMs seem adaptable to many new chemicals. However, analytical difficulties may result from lower applications rates (grams or ounces per acre) of some new pesticides (e.g., the sulfonyl urea herbicides and synthetic pyrethroid insecticides). While the use of this type of pesticide results in low residue levels, its use will require more sensitive analytical methods for detection. In addition, many new pesticides have reduced environmental persistence and therefore rapidly metabolize or breakdown into more polar products. Also, increased use of non-conventional chemical pesticides, such as microbiological and genetic and behavioral biochemicals, will pose difficulties for analysis and require methods development (18).

Analytical chemists are then faced with the current and growing problem of detecting metabolites. In order to provide a method for determining such metabolite residues, a method that is satisfactory for the parent pesticide may have to be altered; such alterations may include chemical derivatization, changes in the nature of the extracting solvent, changes in the chromatographic determinations such as different columns and detectors, and sometimes even going to a different mode for the determinative step. Many metabolites cannot be analyzed by MRMs and will require special procedures (18).

One potential solution to the parent compound metabolite dilemma may be to agree on the use of "indicator compounds"; these may be parent compounds or toxicologically significant metabolites that have been shown by metabolism studies to exist in a predictable manner under certain environmental conditions. Previous studies may also have shown that the relative amounts of the other associated compounds fall within some quantitative boundaries. Knowing the amount of indicator compound present can therefore provide a semiquantitative idea of the amount of other associated compounds present. The use of indicator compounds may, in many instances, obviate the need for using multiple analytical methods to provide information on both parent compound and a list of metabolites (18). Another potential solution would be to develop inexpensive methods to rapidly test whether such residues exist and will need more difficult analysis performed (18).

---

tion of how to handle pesticides of widely different chemical and physical characteristics.

(2) New SRMs. Developing functional SRMs is a balance between the use of innovative approaches and the use of techniques that are practical for regulatory chemists. A successful SRM should be capable of analyzing any of the toxicologically significant metabolites— as defined in Subdivision O of EPA's Guidelines (4)—without separate extractions, cleanup steps, or analytical columns, certainly without incorporating another type of detector. Since most metabolites are more polar than the parent pesticide, this is a challenge for the method developer and will slow the development proc-

ess. Since the method will be used for enforcement only when MRMs are not available, it should use the same glassware, solvents, reagents, and instrumentation as the MRMs. This is currently not a requirement of EPA's Subdivision O Guidelines, but it makes the best use of available resources, obviating the need for having infrequently used equipment sitting around the laboratory.

Frequently, little similarity seems to exist between SRMs presented by tolerance petitioners for individual pesticides with similar structures. This situation might be improved if petitioners made efforts to design "mini-MRMs," that is, methods that would apply to more than one pesticide. This could be accomplished by making only slight modifications to one SRM.

Cost Considerations of Methods Development Research

The costs of sample analysis and research reflect a number of factors. There are the housing and associated upkeep costs for a laboratory that must store toxic and possibly explosive materials and at the same time must maintain an environment suitable for sensitive equipment. A range of glassware and solvents, which must be pure, are required. The sophisticated instruments are a substantial cost, both in the initial purchase and in upkeep. GCs when equipped with detectors and autosamples can cost $32,000 apiece and HPLCs can average $25,000 to $30,000. Together they also require high purity gases or solvents. Service contracts per instrument can cost $2,000 or more a year. The other major cost is analyst time, which accounts for a large part of the cost of each analysis. The cost to analyze individual samples has not been calculated by regulatory laboratories. The closest approximation may be the price charged by a private laboratory, where a single MRM analysis may cost hundreds of dollars.

Over the last 30 years as the sensitivity of instruments has improved, their purchase and upkeep costs have increased; therefore, improvements in analysis are often accompanied by increased costs of analysis (20). New instruments to improve methods also require a high initial capital expenditure although improvements in manufacturing help control cost. Such expenses may slow Federal regulatory agencies from investigating the use of new instruments for improved methods. A further difficulty is if such instruments are used to improve methods, field laboratories will also need to purchase them if these methods are to be used for routine regulatory analyses.

Methods research involves costs beyond those for sample analyses. First are the tradeoff costs of doing research. Equipment and personnel spent on research mean less equipment and analyst time available for sample analyses. Therefore, requirements for more research

need to address requirements for current sampling programs, given that changes in one area can adversely affect the other. Second are the research resources spent unsuccessfully. In the process of improving a method or developing a new one, the analyst attempts to improve the steps involved in the method. Failures in each step or in the entire process use up resources but do not produce results apparent to others. Third are the costs of validating that an improved method is accurate.

Another factor determining the cost of research will be the goals for improving the regulatory programs. Improving MRMs to analyze more pesticides and commodities may be carried out in conjunction with regulatory analysis work. But if the focus is on high health hazard pesticides that cannot be analyzed by existing MRMs, development of new MRMs or practical SRMs may be needed. Longer-term research, high capital costs, and validation costs may be required for introducing new technologies for either improving methods or developing new ones. The same may be true for introducing technologies, such as automation and robotics, that can improve the use of methods. Goals must be set before the level of research resources can be determined.

Needs for Adoption and Use of Methods

Validating Methods

Before any analytical method can be used routinely in the laboratory, it must be validated. Validation is the process whereby one or more individual chemists test the suitability of a particular method for collecting analytical data (21). The suitability of a method will depend in part upon the circumstances of the application. For example, a method that will be widely used will require more validation than one whose use is more confined. The effort expended in validating analytical methods serves to validate the results of sample analyses. Consequently, method validation at several levels (e.g., intralaboratory, interlaboratory, and AOAC collaborative study) is considered inherent to the methods development process.

Intralaboratory validation is the lowest validation level. It requires the developer to demonstrate that the method is reproducible, sensitive, specific, and contains all the qualities needed to meet the method's analytical purposes. The developer then hands the evaluation of the method to someone else within the laboratory for further validation.

Interlaboratory validation is the next level. This level is usually required before a method is used by other laboratories. The laboratory developing the method must find another laboratory to test the method and its written description by analyzing samples with unknown residues and levels. Successful performance of the method by an analyst other than its developer must be provided before the method can be sanctioned for use in monitoring.

A more rigorous validation is undertaken for methods intended for widespread and continuous use. Collaborative study, under the auspices and rules of the Association of Official Analytical Chemists (AOAC), is a major effort involving six to eight laboratories and is usually performed for methods that an organization expects to continue using for many years. Methods are usually not studied collaboratively until they have been in use in several laboratories over an extended period of time and results indicate that they are worth the considerable effort involved. Collaborative studies are far too expensive to be conducted for all methods. If the residue measurements produced in a collaborative study meet the statistical requirements for accuracy and precision, the method is declared official by the AOAC and published in the *Official Methods of Analysis* of the AOAC.

The degree of validation required by FDA and USDA will differ depending upon the application of the method. For the majority of methods, both agencies require an interlaboratory validation involving at least two laboratories. FDA and FSIS encourage the use of AOAC official methods where possible because they are most widely accepted. All five of FDA's routinely used MRMs have received AOAC collaborative study for some commodities and pesticides. In some cases, however, methods validated by an AOAC collaborative study or interlaboratory study may not be available, for example, for pesticides not used in the United States but found in imports or for applying a validated method to a new commodity. A lesser form of validation, such as intralaboratory study, can be used in such cases. As long as the analytical results follow well-accepted principles—sample custody, sample stability, no false positives in control samples, adequate recoveries from fortified samples, and confirmation of results—the method can be used for regulatory enforcement action.

The success of an MRM or group of MRMs is not necessarily guaranteed by the degree of formal validation undertaken. For example, the MRMs used by the California Department of Food and Agriculture (CDFA) have been developed in-house over the past 20 years as a result of information from one of the chemical apparatus supply houses (22). No collaborative studies have ever been done by CDFA (though one is under consideration now) on their in-house MRMs, although they have split samples with FDA laboratories; these split-sample analyses have produced results comparable to those generated in FDA laboratories (22).

Confirmation of Results

When an analysis leads to the finding of a violation, regulatory agencies require that the violation be confirmed by a different technique or method. The most common approach to confirmation is to re-analyze the sample after modifying the original method, for instance, after changing the detector, column, or sometimes both (5, 14). In these cases, confirmation does not require the development of completely new methods.

A second approach to confirmation has been identifying a suspected pesticide residue by its mass spectra. Regulatory agencies are increasingly using mass spectrometers, including the smaller bench-top types, as detectors for GC, and in some cases HPLC, for the confirmation of violations.

When violations are found, confirmatory analyses need to be performed only on certain samples. That is, if numerous tentative positives are uncovered in a group of samples, confirmation is required on only a representative part of these samples.

EPA does not require that pesticides receiving new tolerances have confirmatory methods in addition to the method required for monitoring. Consequently, a second battery of confirmatory methods does not exist. This suggests that some SRMs might not have confirmatory methods and thus can not be used for regulatory purposes.

Overall, however, it appears that confirmatory methods will, for the most part, take care of themselves, assuming that adequate MRMs will be forthcoming for future pesticides and that growth in technologies continues.

CHAPTER 6 REFERENCES

1. Ambrus, A. and Thier, H.P., "Application of Multiresidue Procedures in Pesticide Residues Analysis," *Pure and Applied Chemistry*, 58(7): 1035-1062, July 1986.
*2. Conacher, H.B.S., "Validation of Analytical Methods for Pesticide Residues and Confirmation of Results," OTA commissioned paper, Spring 1988.
*3. Ellis, R., "Techniques for and the Role of Screening Pesticide Residue Analysis," OTA commissioned paper, Spring 1988.
4. Environmental Protection Agency, Office of Pesticide and Toxic Substances, "Pesticide Assessment Guidelines, Subdivision 0, Residue Chemistry," Washington, DC, October 1982.
5. Fong, G., Chemical Residue Laboratory, Florida Department of Agriculture, Tallahassee, FL, personal communication, May 16, 1988.
6. Food Safety and Inspection Service, *Compound Evaluation and Analytical Capability National Residue Program Plan 1987* (Washington, DC: Food Safety and Inspection Service, January 1987).
7. Freeman, R.R., and Hayes, M.A., "Column Considerations When Doing Trace Analysis on Open Tubular Columns," *J. of Chromatographic Science*, 26(4):138-141, April 1988.
8. Hawthorne, S.B., and Miller, D.J., "Extraction and Recovery of Organic Pollutants from Environmental Solids and Tenax-GC Using Supercritical CO_2," *J. of Chromatographic Science* 24(6):258-264, June 1986.
9. Jacobs, W., Enzytech Inc., Lenexa, KS, personal communication, Aug. 10, 1988.
10. Kovacs, M.F. Jr., and Trichilo, C.L., "Regulatory Perspective of Pesticide Analytical Enforcement Methodology in the United States," *J. Assoc. Off. Anal. Chem.*, 70(6):937-940, 1987.
11. Krause, R.T., Center for Food Safety and Applied Nutrition, Food and Drug Administration, Washington, DC, personal communication, May 18, 1988.
*12. Kropscott, B.E., Peck, C.N., and Lento, H.G., "The Role of Robotic Automation in the Laboratory," OTA commissioned paper, Spring 1988.
13. Lombardo, P., Center for Food Safety and Applied Nutrition, Food and Drug Administration, Washington, DC, personal communication, Aug. 1, 1988.
14. Luke, M., Los Angeles Pesticide Laboratory, Food and Drug Administration, Los Angeles, CA, personal communication, May 16, 1988.
15. McCullough, F., ABC Laboratories, Columbia, MO, personal communication, May 3, 1988.
16. McMahon, B.M. and Burke, J.A., "Expanding and Tracking the Capability of Pesticide Multiresidue Methodology Used in the Food and Drug Administration's Pesticide Monitoring Programs," *J. Assoc. Off. Anal. Chem.*, 70(6): 1072-1081, November/December 1987.
*17. Mumma, R. and Hunter, K., "Potential of Immunoassays in Monitoring Pesticide Residues in Foods," OTA commissioned paper, Spring 1988.
*18. Plimmer, J., Hill, K., and Menn, J., "Pesticide Design: Outlook for the Future," OTA commissioned paper, Spring 1988.
*19. Sawyer, L., "The Development of Analytical Methods for Pesticide Residues," OTA commissioned paper, Spring 1988.
*20. Seiber, J., "Conventional Pesticide Analytical Methods: How Can They Be Improved?" OTA commissioned paper, Spring 1988.
21. Taylor, S.E., "Pesticide Monitoring Programs:

---

*These reference papers are contained in appendix B.

Developing New Methods to Detect Pesticide Residues in Food," Report No. 87-413 SPR, U.S. Congress, Congressional Research Service, Apr. 24, 1987.

22. Ting, K.C., Anaheim Laboratory, California Department of Food and Agriculture, Anaheim, CA, personal communication, Apr. 23, 1988.

23. Trichilo, C., Residue Chemistry Branch, Environmental Protection Agency, Washington, DC, personal communication, Apr. 25, 1988.

24. U.S. Congress, Office of Technology Assessment, "Workshop on Technologies to Detect Pesticide Residues in Food," Washington, DC, Mar. 14-16, 1988.

25. Walters, S., Pesticide Industrial Chemicals Research Center, Food and Drug Administration, Detroit, MI, personal communication, May 22, 1988.

*These reference papers are contained in appendix B.

Chapter 7
Federal Methods Development Programs for Detecting Pesticides in Food

CONTENTS

Page

Environmental Protection Agency 75
  Methods Submitted for a Pesticide Tolerance 75
  EPA Research 76
  Supporting Programs 77
Food and Drug Administration 78
United States Department of Agriculture 81
Chapter 7 References 83

Federal Methods Development Programs for Detecting Pesticides in Food

Successful monitoring of pesticide residues depends upon the existence of cost-effective analytical methods for their identification and quantification. A number of Federal agencies are interested in improving methods to test for pesticide residues, but only EPA, FDA, and FSIS programs will be discussed here because their research most directly affects the methods used for analyzing pesticide residues in food. Nevertheless, increased coordination, or at least communication, between all Federal agencies involved in such work would help improve use of research resources.

ENVIRONMENTAL PROTECTION AGENCY

Although EPA currently does not have a significant research program on analytical methods development for pesticide residues in food, EPA supports development of such methods through three activities:

1. Requiring the submission of a pesticide residue method as part of the tolerance-setting process for a pesticide to be used on food or feed and performing a single-laboratory evaluation of many of the submitted methods.
2. Performing a small amount of pesticide methods research that might be applicable to the analysis of food.
3. Administering several programs that support the ability of Federal and State laboratories to conduct pesticide methods research.

Methods Submitted for a Pesticide Tolerance

All pesticides for use in the United States must be first registered with EPA. If a pesticide is to be registered for use on food or feed, or if its use will result in residues on food or feed, a tolerance must be first established for each commodity in which the residue will occur. EPA requires the person or company petitioning for a tolerance to submit an analytical method able to detect and quantify the pesticide residue in every commodity for which a tolerance is to be established. The person or organization petitioning for a tolerance is known as a petitioner or may be called a registrant if the registration and tolerance-setting process occur simultaneously.

EPA's guidelines allow the submission of either a single or a multiresidue method to fulfill this requirement (see EPA, "Pesticide Assessment Guidelines, Subdivision O," October 1982). The petitioner usually submits a single residue method (SRM), which is usually less expensive to develop and more sensitive than a multiresidue method (MRM) (13).

Once a method is submitted, it undergoes a paper review by EPA's Office of Pesticides and Toxic Substances, and then if considered necessary and if resources permit, it is evaluated by an EPA laboratory. The first one or two analytical methods for a specific pesticide in plant commodities and one method for that pesticide in animal commodities normally receive such an evaluation (24). EPA has two laboratories—one in Beltsville, MD and one in Bay St. Louis, MS —that test submitted methods. Methods are initially reviewed on paper at these laboratories.

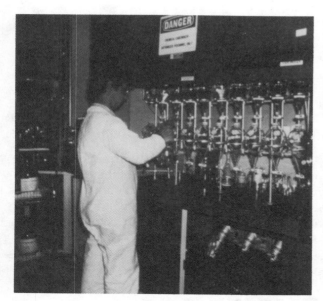

Photo credit: Contractor for the National Aeronautics and Space Administration

EPA has two laboratories that test analytical methods as part of the tolerance-setting process. Here, an analyst at the Environmental Chemistry Laboratory in Bay St. Louis, MS, performs the extraction step of a method.

If deemed unacceptable, the method is returned to the petitioner. If the method is acceptable, an EPA chemist then tests it and makes a recommendation regarding its suitability for enforcing the pesticide tolerance. This process usually takes 3 months. Where necessary, petitioners will make modifications and resubmit the method to the Office of Pesticides and Toxic Substances (16). Once approved, the method is submitted to FDA for inclusion in FDA's *Pesticide Analytical Manual, Volume II: Methods for Individual Residues* (also known as PAM II). Copies of the method can also be obtained from EPA once the tolerance is approved.

The number of methods tested by EPA's laboratories has been increasing over time and outstripping EPA's capabilities, resulting in a backlog of methods to be tested and delays in the registration of some pesticides. For example, in FY 1986, EPA had 25 methods to test but was only able to test 19, carrying the rest over to FY 1987. In FY 1987, EPA was only able to evaluate 24 of 47 methods that needed testing; the rest were carried over to the next year. By

March 1988, EPA had 52 methods to test, had evaluated 17, and expected to receive up to 18 more methods for testing in 1988. In FY 1987, EPA had assigned 7.5 full-time equivalents (FTEs) to testing and expected to assign 10 FTEs in FY 1988, but the backlog still exists (15, 16).

Some SRMs submitted to EPA can be a source of concern for Federal and State pesticide regulatory agencies, because these methods may not be practical for use in Federal and State food monitoring programs for several reasons. First, these SRMs often involve complex and time-consuming analytical manipulations. Regulatory agencies prefer to use the more cost-effective MRMs for routine monitoring and to use SRMs only when intelligence data show that a pesticide residue may be present or when data on the residue level are needed (20). Second, SRMs submitted to EPA need be effective only for the commodities for which tolerances are established and may not be applicable to other commodities (20). Third, some of these SRMs may be analytically flawed, poorly documented, or incapable of analyzing significant metabolites, making them difficult or unusable for regulatory work (5, 17).

EPA has taken several recent steps to improve the quality and usefulness of submitted SRMs (25). It is now mandatory for EPA to test all methods for new pesticides used on foods. User forms have been included in PAM II to alert EPA and others of specific problems with a method. EPA will be requiring an independent evaluation of each method before its submission to EPA beginning August 1, 1989. Also, EPA now requires petitioners to test whether their pesticide can be successfully analyzed through official FDA MRMs, and the test results are sent to FDA. In addition, EPA is considering how to incorporate FDA and USDA input on the regulatory usefulness of submitted methods in the tolerance-setting process.

EPA Research

Methods development at EPA is carried out primarily by EPA's Office of Research and Development (ORD). Although EPA has identified pesticide residues in food as a significant source of human exposure to pesticides, ORD does not have a specific program on methods to detect these residues because regulation of food is outside EPA's mandate.

EPA conducts pesticide analysis and some methods development work at its field laboratories primarily for nonfood matrices. Because of the different matrices involved, the applicability of EPA research on conventional analytical methods for use on food may be limited, especially for extraction and cleanup steps. On the other hand, since EPA uses detection equipment similar to that used in food analysis, EPA advances in the detection step may be applicable to food analysis (3, 18).

EPA's immunoassay work for detecting chemicals may be applicable to food analysis. The Environmental Monitoring Systems Laboratory in Las Vegas, NV, houses a 2-year-old program designed to assess the usefulness of immunoassays for analyzing toxic chemicals, including pesticides. The program's budget for FY 1988 is $450,000 and the program's objectives are to: develop immunoassays, develop criteria for evaluating immunoassays, develop a list of chemicals for which immunoassays can and should be made, and evaluate commercially available immunoassays (28). Although none of this work is aimed at food, immunoassays developed for analyzing soil and water can be adapted for use on food. Further EPA research and the development of an evaluation protocol for immunoassays could be used by FDA and USDA. The Las Vegas laboratory has an interagency agreement with USDA to cooperate on developing antibodies of mutual interest.

Supporting Programs

EPA has several programs that support development of pesticide residue methods at Federal, State, and other laboratories. These programs include the Pesticide and Industrial Chemicals Repository and a training program for State laboratories under contract with EPA.

The Pesticide and Industrial Chemicals Repository provides samples of approximately 1,600 pesticides (foreign and domestic) free of charge to Federal, State, private, and foreign laboratories. Having a chemical of known concentration and purity, known as a standard, is necessary to develop new methods and to check that existing methods used in regulatory work are correctly identifying pesticides. Standards are provided by chemical manufacturers, stored at the repository, and distributed one sample per chemical per year to a requesting laboratory, although greater quantities will be supplied to Federal laboratories upon request (12).

The repository is funded by three EPA programs: Superfund, Solid Wastes, and Pesticides. For FY 1988, the repository had a budget of about $3 million and 22 full-time employees. The pesticide part of the repository costs about $630,000 a year to operate. Because the EPA pesticide program wants to reduce its contribution to the repository's budget, the repository has recently restricted its distribution of pesticide standards. As of July 15, 1988, pesticide standards will no longer be provided to university, private, and foreign laboratories (3, 11).

To further defray costs, EPA is interested in having recipients such as FDA and USDA, who are the largest users of pesticide standards, provide additional support for this activity. FDA is interested in expanding the repository to include an additional 150 foreign pesticides not registered in the United States but that might exist on imported foods (12).

In addition to supplying analytical standards, EPA provides a quality assurance and training program for State laboratories to improve analysis of pesticides in the environment. Currently, EPA has contracts with 52 State laboratories and Puerto Rico, some of which also analyze for residues in foods as part of their own program. EPA helps maintain the quality of analysis of these laboratories through two means. First, EPA performs laboratory quality assurance tests by sending out samples containing known quantities of pesticide residues for the laboratories to analyze. Second, EPA's Denver Regional Office provides weeklong hands-on training workshops for State personnel on the use of specific methods. On average, three workshops are held a year with a limit of 12 participants for each. Demand for the workshop often exceeds available space (10). States have expressed the need for more such training courses (2), including training in the area of analyzing for residues in foods, but this is outside EPA's training goals.

FOOD AND DRUG ADMINISTRATION

Because of FDA's mandate to monitor and enforce pesticide tolerances in food, it is the lead Federal agency for the development of pesticide analytical methods specifically for food. FDA's research concentrates on MRMs as a result of FDA's need to determine the presence or absence of many pesticides in food commodities for which little information exists on pesticides application.

In general, FDA's methods development research can be divided into two broad types: 1) that which deals with immediate program needs, and 2) that which is directed to future goals of greater scope to solve particular problems or to improve overall effectiveness or efficiency. Most of FDA's effort is the first type (7).

Pesticide methods research is primarily conducted in-house at three levels within the agency: in the 16 field laboratories, in two special research centers, and at the Center for Food Safety and Applied Nutrition (CFSAN) in Washington, DC. The CFSAN and two research centers conduct the bulk of methods research because field laboratories normally spend at least 90 percent of their time on regulatory work. FDA does little outside contracting of methods research, although in late 1987 it awarded a contract for immunoassay development because of a lack of in-house expertise.

FDA's pesticide methods research agendas are planned on a year by year basis. These agendas are open to interruption as emergencies arise, e.g., the recent EDB problem.[1] Formal planning sessions with headquarters and field participation are held each year, research projects are printed in the annual technical plan, and their progress reported quarterly.

Research priorities are influenced by factors such as the Surveillance Index, Pestrak,[2] domestic and foreign pesticide use data, new toxicological information, gaps in monitoring coverage, and pesticide registration cancellations. Mechanisms for setting research priorities are currently informal, and detailed listings of long-range priorities have not been prepared (14). No formal list of priority pesticides requiring research action exists. However, an informal list of pesticides requiring methods research in 1988 was developed at the annual planning meeting for the research centers in 1987. Responsibility for the work was divided among the research centers and the Los Angeles field laboratory. The list was a combination of pesticides identified by CFSAN and ongoing work at the research centers (1). Currently, CFSAN is developing a long-term research plan to be completed in 1988. The level of field and outside input into the draft plan is not clear.

CFSAN has the largest concentration of pesticide analytical expertise in one place in the FDA system, with six FTEs carrying out pesticide methods research for food in its laboratory. CFSAN develops a separate annual technical plan containing its own research projects. Current research ranges from expanding MRMs to cover additional pesticides, their metabolites, and additional food commodities to evaluating new technologies and attempting to fit them into existing methods. CFSAN also develops new MRMs on pesticides that cannot be tested with existing MRMs. As the focal point, CFSAN also provides research direction and advice to the research centers and field laboratories. Representatives from CFSAN sit on the committees that approve field laboratory research projects.

---

[1] Improved analytical techniques, in 1984, led to the identification of a large number of illegal EDB residues in grain products.

[2] Pestrak is a computerized data base used to track whether pesticides can be analyzed using one of FDA's five routinely used MRMs.

CFSAN has been a leader in the development of MRMs. Its work has led to the development of four of the five MRMs routinely used by FDA. Based on OTA's observations, however, field laboratories may not consider the bulk of CFSAN's current work to be addressing their analytical methods needs. In addition, CFSAN's research activities do not seem to be meeting the regulatory needs of field laboratories in a timely fashion, and because of the lack of a long-term research plan, CFSAN may not be effectively addressing future monitoring needs.

FDA has two research centers developing methods for analyzing pesticides and other industrial contaminants in foods. Headquarters and research center staff meet annually to set the centers' research agendas, and the centers request research suggestions from the field laboratories. These two centers—the Total Diet Research Center (TDRC) in Kansas City, MO and the Pesticide and Industrial Chemicals Research Center (PICRC) in Detroit, MI—were established in 1980 to meet the analytical needs of field regulatory laboratories. Combined they have six FTEs doing research and one FTE for management.

The TDRC's work primarily supports the Total Diet Study (TDS) carried out by the Total Diet laboratory in Kansas City, MO. The Total Diet Study is not under the same time constraints as many of the field laboratories and requires more sensitive methods than those used by the field laboratories. Thus, some of TDRC's methods development work done for the Total Diet laboratory may not be appropriate for field laboratories' needs.

In several cases, TDRC's work has benefitted specific field laboratories; for example, the use of gel permeation chromatography and wide-bore capillary chromatography, and the development and expansion of two newer MRMs that detect a small number of chlorophenoxy acids or phenylurea herbicides (19). TDRC has also conducted research assigned by CFSAN that addresses field laboratories' specific regulatory needs. For example, TDRC tested a method for ETU (a breakdown product of EBDC fungicides) and found it applicable to only a few commodities (19). TDRC also has a project that uses mass spectrometry to identify or characterize pesticide residues that cannot be analyzed by conventional chromatographic approaches. This project, however, does not seem to be well linked with similar efforts at FDA's Los Angeles and New York laboratories.

PICRC is the center with primary responsibility for supporting FDA field laboratories' analytical methods needs for pesticide residue detection. Much of its work has focused on developing methods for detecting important non-pesticide chemical contaminants in foods, such as dioxin and PCBs. In the area of pesticides, PICRC focuses on classes of pesticides not determinable by existing MRMs.

PICRC has developed methods for the detection of captan, folpet, and captafol using wide-bore capillary gas chromatography and for the benzimidazole-related fungicides (benomyl, carbendazin, thiophanate-methyl, and thiabendazole) using high performance liquid chromatography. The latter work was in support of an assigned field laboratory monitoring program in 1987 and a compliance program in 1988. In response to a contamination problem in dairy products caused by heptachlor expoxide-contaminated feed, PICRC developed a method that allowed the Minneapolis District in 1986 to analyze fatty samples more rapidly than by using the existing official method (27). PICRC has also worked on applying capillary column technology to the analysis of pesticide residues in food and has been instrumental in the Detroit field laboratory's adoption of capillary columns (21). Ongoing research addresses methods for the detection of the "quats" (paraquat, diquat, and difenzoquat) and triphenyltin and its metabolites.

As noted, PICRC's work has supported specific method needs of individual field laboratories. However, OTA observed that several field laboratories do not find the majority of PICRC's work as relevant to their regulatory needs. In part, PICRC was viewed as not having strong enough ties to the field laboratories, especially when compared with its ties to CFSAN. To some extent, the field laboratories

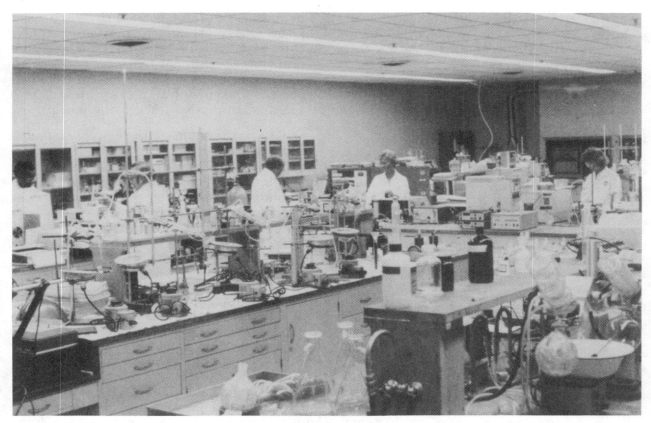

FDA's Pesticide and Industrial Chemicals Research Center is responsible for addressing pesticide analytical methods needs of the field laboratories.

contribute to this problem by not working more closely with PICRC on the type of research PICRC could conduct. For example, only four of sixteen field laboratories responded to PICRC's request for research proposals for FY 1988 (27).

A total of about seven FTEs carry out pesticide methods research at the field laboratories through short-, medium-, and long-term work (6). In the past, medium- and long-term research were approved by separate committees, but starting in FY 1989, a single committee composed of laboratory directors, science advisers, and personnel from CFSAN and the Office of Regulatory Affairs (ORA) will approve this work. This committee also will oversee the work of the two research centers. Much of the field laboratory research work focuses on evaluating whether additional pesticides can be analyzed through existing MRMs. But field laboratory research can make more significant contributions. The most widely used MRM, the Luke method—which was used in 80 percent of FDA's 1987 pesticide residue analyses—was developed at FDA's Los Angeles laboratory (20).

For short-term research, FDA provides 50 hours of "discretionary research" per operating laboratory analyst. The laboratory director normally determines how the time will be divided among analysts and priority topics. "Discretionary research" is used as the need arises for short-term projects and is often, in the area of pesticides, aimed at extending an existing MRM to a new commodity.

With regard to medium-term research at the field laboratories, a pool of research time made up of 150 hours per operating analyst is set aside for research projects. Projects usually require 300 hours and might address expanding a known method to several commodities or developing a new method for a class of pesticides. Project proposals from field laboratories, the two research centers, and CFSAN are ranked by a research committee, reviewed by the director and deputy-director of the ORA (which has line authority over the field laboratories), and final approval rests with the Associate Commissioner for Regulatory Affairs.

Long-term research at the field laboratories takes place through the Science Adviser Research Associate Program (SARAP). Field laboratories may contract with one to two persons from the academic community who then work with laboratory personnel. Field analysts in conjunction with the science adviser may propose long-term research projects (6 to 12 months), often to be done outside the laboratory at the adviser's academic institution sometimes with additional training for the analyst. Approval must be received from the laboratory, the district, the research committee, the ORA, and the Associate Commissioner for Regulatory Affairs. Normally five SARAPs exist at one time, and they may be for any of the methods areas in which FDA works (e.g., microbiology), not only for pesticide residues in food.

A significant amount of resources are used for pesticide methods research being conducted by different groups at FDA. However, based on OTA observations, much of the work conducted by CFSAN and the two research centers is not adequately supporting the needs of regulatory laboratories for fast, practical methods for analyzing pesticide residues in food.

This situation could be addressed by existing groups taking the research responsibilities for which they seem best suited. Normally free from regulatory "fire-fighting" work and away from the "front lines," CFSAN could use its nucleus of expertise to focus primarily on long-term, future-oriented research. To increase the regulatory relevancy of the research centers' work, their research could be more responsive to field needs as identified by the field laboratories rather than by CFSAN. In support of this, field laboratories could expend increased effort in communicating their needs to the research centers, especially to PICRC. Although field laboratories are usually too busy analyzing samples to conduct research, whatever research does take place is perhaps the most immediately relevant for regulatory action. Perhaps more time should be allocated to field laboratory analysts to conduct research, but this would require additional resources to allow laboratories to keep up with their regulatory workload.

UNITED STATES DEPARTMENT OF AGRICULTURE

Development of residue analytical methods by USDA comes under the purview of the FSIS, and pesticide residue research is currently conducted by the Chemistry Division and Field Service Laboratories Division in the Science Program. FSIS's pesticide methods development program currently emphasizes the expansion of existing MRMs complemented by the development of faster methods, many of which are based on immunoassay techniques. These faster methods will allow the weeding out of a large percentage of samples that do not have violative residues without having to analyze them with the more expensive conventional method. This emphasis is, in part, a response to recommendations by a 1985 National Academy of Sciences report and a 1987 General Accounting Office study (9, 23).

FSIS monitors food solely with MRMs and does not depend on SRMs because generally it considers SRMs as too time-consuming and expensive to be practical in a large-scale monitoring program. Therefore, FSIS works primarily to incorporate additional pesticides under its MRMs rather than to improve SRMs. All methods used by USDA in its monitoring programs are subjected to in-house validation, which includes at least three analysts at two laboratories with a minimum of 12 to 18 analyses per analyst for each pesticide-meat tissue combination (4).

In 1985, FSIS closed down its central laboratory at Beltsville, MD (a counterpart of FDA's CFSAN laboratory), which conducted research on analytical methods for detecting pesticide residues in food. Methods research has since been conducted by FSIS field laboratories, through contracts with private organizations, through the Agricultural Research Service (ARS) of USDA, and through interagency agreements. In addition, the Chemistry Division in Washington, DC, is also seeking commercially available rapid test kits.

FSIS has three field laboratories, two of which are currently working on pesticide residue methods (located at Athens, GA, and Alameda, CA). Each laboratory has a methods division unit, and regulatory personnel may also conduct methods work. In-house work on pesticides totals approximately $200,000 per year and 5.5 FTEs (8), with the majority of the work conducted at the Athens, GA, laboratory. Examples of current work include the following:

- Setting up a new, conventional analytical method for four triazines for regulatory

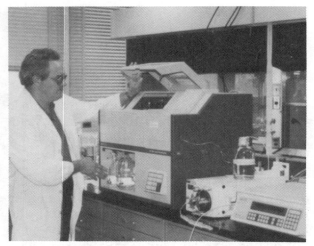

Photo credit: Food Safety and Inspection Service Laboratory, Athens, GA

Much of FSIS' pesticide methods research takes place at the field laboratories. Here, a new methodology using high performance liquid chromatography is being evaluated.

work and testing a commercial rapid immunoassay kit to detect triazines in order to weed out the large percentage of samples that are not violative.
- Expanding an existing MRM for organophosphates, and evaluating a commercial, rapid cholinesterase enzyme kit that tests for organophosphates.
- Setting up a quick semiquantitative immunoassay method for five synthetic pyrethrin insecticides that makes use of solid phase extraction for cleanup.
- Expanding the number of pesticides that gel permeation chromatography can be used for cleanup of meat products.

FSIS also contracts out research with private organizations and other Federal agencies. Current contracts for pesticide residue methods total approximately $285,000 and include the following:

- The Department of Energy's Lawrence Livermore Laboratory's work on an immunoassay for heptachlor-related chlorinated pesticides. This laboratory also developed the pyrethrin immunoassay now being implemented at the Athens laboratory.
- The Colorado School of Mines is investigating supercritical fluid chromatography for aniline-based pesticides.
- The University of Washington is working on the use of thin layer chromatography as part of a quantitative assay.

In addition to outside contracts, ARS also does work for FSIS on pesticide residue methodologies. Currently, ARS in Peoria, IL, is working on the use of supercritical fluid extraction and chromatography in low-fat meat products, and ARS in Beltsville, MD, is researching a quantitative method using gas chromatography for the detection of synthetic pyrethroids (26).

The Cooperative State Research Service of USDA provides funds to four land-grant university laboratories that support the registration of pesticides for use on minor crops. These laboratories may develop SRMs as part of their application for tolerances for the pesticide residue on minor crops (22).

CHAPTER 7 REFERENCES

1. Carson, L., Division of Field Science, Food and Drug Administration, Rockville, MD, personal communication, July 14, 1988.

*2. Cusick, W., and Wells, J., "Pesticide Analytical Methods Development at the State Level," OTA commissioned paper, Spring 1988.

3. Delarco, M., Office of Research and Development, U.S. Environmental Protection Agency, Washington, DC, personal communication, May 5, 1988.

4. Ellis, R., Chemistry Division, Food Safety and Inspection Service, Washington, DC, personal communication, Apr. 6, 1988.

5. Environmental Protection Agency, Office of Pesticides and Toxic Substances, "Notice to Manufacturers, Formulators, Producers, and Registrants of Pesticide Products," PR Notice 88-5, 1988.

6. Food and Drug Administration, U.S. Department of Health and Human Services response to OTA questions, May 1988.

7. Food and Drug Administration, Pesticide and Industrial Contaminants Branch, "Development of Analytical Methods for Pesticide Residues," internal document provided to OTA by FDA, April 1987.

8. Food Safety and Inspection Service (Office of Science), U.S. Department of Agriculture, response to OTA questions, Apr. 29, 1988.

9. Food Safety and Inspection Service, U.S. Department of Agriculture, "FSIS Future Agenda: Response to the NAS Recommendations," Washington, DC, June 1986.

10. Gillis, J., NEIC Center, U.S. Environmental Protection Agency, Denver, CO, personal communication, May 1988.

11. Kantor, E., Environmental Monitoring Systems Laboratory, U.S. Environmental Protection Agency, Las Vegas, NV, personal communication, July 21, 1988.

12. Kantor, E., Environmental Monitoring Systems Laboratory, U.S. Environmental Protection Agency, Las Vegas, NV, personal communication, Apr. 29, 1988.

13. Kimm, V., Office of Pesticides and Toxic Substances, U.S. Environmental Protection Agency, personal communication, July 18, 1988.

14. Lombardo, P., Center for Food Safety and Applied Nutrition, Food and Drug Administration, Washington, DC, personal communication, June 29, 1988.

15. Marlow, D., Chemicals Operations Branch, U.S. Environmental Protection Agency, personal communication, Washington, DC, June 16, 1988.

16. Marlow, D., Chemicals Operations Branch, U.S. Environmental Protection Agency, personal communication, Washington, DC, Apr. 14, 1988.

17. McCasland, W., Texas Department of Agriculture, Brenhan, TX, comment at OTA Workshop "Technologies to Detect Pesticide Residues in Food," Mar. 16, 1988.

18. Mitchum, R., Environmental Monitoring Systems Laboratory, U.S. Environmental Protection Agency, Las Vegas, NV, personal communication, May 16, 1988.

19. Salmon, G., Total Diet Laboratory, Food and Drug Administration, Kansas City, MO, personal communication, June 29, 1988.

*20. Sawyer, L., "The Development of Analytical Methods for Pesticide Residues," OTA commissioned paper, Spring 1988.

21. Schneider, L., Detroit Laboratory, Food and Drug Administration, Detroit, MI, personal communication, Apr. 22, 1988.

22. Seiber, J., Department of Environmental Toxicology, University of California, Davis, CA, personal communication, June 16, 1988.

*23. Taylor, S., "Developing Pesticide Analytical Methods for Food: Considerations for Federal Policy Formulation," OTA commissioned paper, Spring 1988.

24. Trichilo, C., Residue Chemistry Branch, U.S. Environmental Protection Agency, Washington, DC, personal communication, June 27, 1988.

*25. Trichilo, C., and Schmitt, R., "Federal Pesticide Monitoring Programs: Analytical Methods Development," OTA commissioned paper, Spring 1988.

26. U.S. Department of Agriculture, Agricultural Research Service, "Annual Report of Research Programs on FSIS Needs," Washington, DC, March 1988.

27. Walters, S., Pesticide and Industrial Chemicals Research Center, Food and Drug Administration, Detroit, MI, personal communication, June 29, 1988.

28. Van Emon, J., Environmental Monitoring Systems Laboratory, U.S. Environmental Protection Agency, Las Vegas, NV, personal communication, Apr. 14, 1988.

*These reference papers are contained in appendix B.

Chapter 8
Summary and Options

CONTENTS

	Page
Reasons for Needing Additional Methods Work	87
Examples of What Can Be Done	89
Multiresidue Methods	89
Single Residue Methods	90
Semiquantitative and Qualitative Tests	91
Validation: Important for Technology/Methods Adoption	92
Findings and Options	92
Finding 1: Federal Agencies' Pesticide Methods Research, Development, and Adoption Could Be Improved	93
Finding 2: Research Coordination and Cooperation Could Be Increased	98
Finding 3: Pesticide Methods Submitted for Tolerance Setting Could Be Improved for Regulatory Use	101
Finding 4: The Quantity and Quality of the Analyst Workforce Need To Be Maintained	103
Chapter 8 References	105

Box

Box	Page
8-A. Related Issues	94

Table

Table	Page
8-1. Summary of Options to Improve Federal Detection of Pesticide Residues in Food	93

Regulatory laboratories analyze pesticide residues in food by one of two ways:

- multiresidue methods (MRMs) or
- single residue methods (SRMs)

Both the Food and Drug Administration (FDA) and Food Safety and Inspection Service (FSIS) rely on MRMs for the bulk of their testing.

These methods provide quantitative data on a large number of pesticides. FDA supplements its MRM testing with SRMs that also provide quantitative data. A potential third way to analyze residues in food is by using rapid semi-quantitative and qualitative methods. Currently, the majority of such tests developed for pesticides are for nonfood matrices, e.g., water, and are not yet applicable to food.

REASONS FOR NEEDING ADDITIONAL METHODS WORK

If analytical testing is to remain the basis of Federal pesticide residue regulatory programs, then new and improved analytical methods will be needed to carry out the mandate of preventing illegal residues in food from reaching the consumer. The need for improved methods arises from constraints on existing methods used today by regulatory agencies in the following areas:

- *Coverage*: the ability to test for all significant pesticides.
- *Resources*: the availability of sufficient resources (e.g., personnel, instrumentation, and laboratory facilities) necessary to test for all significant pesticides.
- *Confirmation*: the ability to verify that a violation exists.
- *Regulatory action*: the ability to analyze samples in a timely manner so that violative commodities can be stopped before they reach the marketplace.
- *Metabolites, new pesticides, and inert ingredients*: the ability to test for pesticide metabolites and breakdown products, for new pesticides having different characteristics than those analyzed using existing methods, and for significant inert ingredients (if determined necessary).

Analytical methods exist today to analyze for each pesticide residue on the food for which a tolerance has been established. These methods, almost all SRMs, are contained in the *Pes-ticide Analytical Manual Volume II* (PAM II). SRMs are not suitable for everyday monitoring of the food supply for several reasons: a large number of pesticides are commercially available, more than one pesticide is commonly applied to a particular commodity, a pesticide residue may occur on a commodity for which the commodity has no tolerance, and regulatory laboratories work with samples whose pesticide history is unknown (14).

To maximize coverage with given resources, FDA and FSIS rely on MRMs for the majority of their analyses. These MRMs can detect only certain pesticides that may occur in food, including some pesticides of primary concern to Federal agencies (31). FDA's and FSIS's MRMs can test for no more than half of the currently known pesticides. In addition, development of MRMs has not kept pace with the number of new pesticides approved for use on food and feed (14). The five MRMs[1] used by FDA can detect 163 out of 316 pesticides with EPA tolerances and a number of pesticides with temporary or pending tolerances, pesticides with no tolerances, and metabolites that could be found in food (8, 22, see table 3-1 in ch. 3). FSIS's four MRMs can detect approximately 40 pesticides and metabolites of the 227 FSIS lists for consideration (1, 10).

---

[1]In addition to FDA's five primary MRMs, several additional MRMs exist that can analyze a small number of similar pesticides (e.g., chlorophenoxy acetic acids or phenylurea herbicides).

Some pesticides do not require routine monitoring because they pose low risk to human health. But not all higher health hazard pesticides can be analyzed through MRMs. Pesticides that can be analyzed by MRMs are linked through similarities in chemical structure and behavior, not through the degree of health hazard they pose. The General Accounting Office found that FDA's MRMs could not detect 33 pesticides with moderate to high health risks (31). FSIS has identified 10 highly ranked pesticides it would like to monitor routinely but cannot with its MRMs (11). A number of other highly ranked pesticides exist that cannot be analyzed using the MRMs but FSIS considers them less likely to appear in meat (11).

Many pesticides not detected by FDA's and FSIS's MRMs require the use of specific SRMs for analyses. SRMs can be as time-consuming and costly to conduct as MRMs, making them comparatively expensive and inefficient for routine monitoring. Thus, they are used sparingly, usually to test for a pesticide known or suspected to be a problem, to confirm the results of an MRM, or to conduct special surveys that monitor one-time levels of a specific pesticide residue in food. For some pesticides, practical SRMs do not yet exist.

When a violation is found, it must be analytically confirmed before enforcement action is taken. Confirmation is done by analyzing the sample with a different method or with the same method originally used but technically modified. A confirmatory method generally exists for an MRM because modifications can be made by using a different column and/or detector. Confirmation methods do not exist for some SRMs and so may constrain their use.

Existing analytical methods, when combined with sampling and reporting requirements, generally do not provide results fast enough to prevent perishable commodities from reaching the market even after violations are found. Frequently, it takes considerably more than 2 days from the time a sample is collected to the time analytical results are available (31). In many cases, the food is sold during this interval.

Some pesticides may break down to metabolites or degradation products hazardous to human health. Analyzing for the parent compound and its metabolites (or only its significant metabolites) may be outside the capability of existing methods or the available resources of regulatory agencies. For some older pesticides, the metabolism data is flawed and significant metabolites have not been identified (30). In addition, existing MRMs are not designed to detect many polar (water soluble), nonvolatile, and nonpersistent compounds. Many new pesticides are designed to be less persistent in the environment than older ones; therefore, they metabolize or degrade more quickly, producing breakdown products that are more polar and thus more difficult to detect using existing methods. New classes of compounds, such as synthetic pyrethroid insecticides and sulfonylurea herbicides, also are not easily analyzed by existing methods, although they should not be too difficult to detect using available technology (20). This trend suggests that current MRMs will need to be modified or that new MRMs be developed to analyze new pesticides coming on the market.

In addition, pesticides contain a number of chemicals used for purposes other than pest control, e.g., colorants and drift control agents. Currently, these chemicals are categorized under Federal regulation (CFR 180.1001) as "inert ingredients" and are exempted from the tolerance process and Federal monitoring. In some cases, inerts are potential or known toxic substances, and increasing attention is being paid to them as possible health hazards. If Federal monitoring for inerts—or for only those considered a health risk—is determined necessary, existing MRMs will have to be modified to address the larger number of chemicals requiring monitoring.

EXAMPLES OF WHAT CAN BE DONE

Multiresidue Methods

MRMs will remain the foundation of regulatory analysis. They are superior in terms of cost, coverage, and quantified data they provide. Several ways exist to improve the use of MRMs:

- Expand the number of pesticides and commodities that existing MRMs can analyze.
- Develop new MRMs for pesticides not detected by existing MRMs.
- Use new technologies to reduce the resources necessary to perform an MRM.

Existing MRMs can be expanded to analyze additional pesticides as well as additional commodities. The research has not yet been done to determine whether an existing MRM can be used to detect a large number of pesticides without modification. Both FDA and USDA are currently conducting research in this area. For example, FDA's Los Angeles laboratory is determining if the Luke method can be used to analyze an additional 80 older, domestic pesticides and 50 foreign ones (15). And FSIS is trying to adapt its MRMs to analyze an additional seven pesticides (1). The expansion of an MRM to analyze other pesticides and foods may also require some methodology modification. In some cases, subtle modifications such as substituting one solvent for another can increase the number of pesticides an MRM can determine.

Adding new technologies into an existing MRM can also expand the number of pesticides that can be analyzed. For example, new detectors, such as photoconductivity for high performance liquid chromatography (HPLC), can detect additional pesticides, and capillary columns for gas chromatography (GC) can separate individual pesticides that normally might be seen as one peak on a chromatogram from a packed column. Theoretically, immunoassays could be used on an extract prepared for an MRM to identify pesticides the MRM cannot detect. Thus, immunoassays would function as an additional detector for the MRM.

Current MRMs might also be expanded by using different combinations of existing technologies. For example, the ability of the Luke method to detect a large number of pesticides is based in part on the use of two to six combinations of packed columns and detectors (15). Smaller laboratories, however, may not have the equipment for such combinations. Further work on other combinations of technologies could lead to increased coverage of pesticide-matrix combinations.

Another way to expand an MRM might be to develop ways to analyze those parts of the sample now discarded, e.g., the water and cellulose fractions. Theoretically, some highly polar compounds might end up in the water and thus would not be analyzed. FDA's Los Angeles laboratory found daminozide in the water released during extraction of fruits and vegetables (15). Herbicides can be bound to plant material, not extracted with existing methods, and lost when cellulose is discarded. The importance of these bound pesticides to human health has not been established, although initial work shows that the majority are of little concern (34). The relative merits of spending resources for this type of research have not been determined, but developing techniques for the extraction of bound herbicides is seen as an expensive research project (34).

Developing new MRMs can help address the problem of pesticides that cannot be analyzed by existing MRMs. New MRMs are applicable to fewer residues than existing MRMs because such residues will be from pesticides with widely varying chemical structures. In short, new MRMs will analyze smaller groups of chemically related pesticides (25). For example, FDA's Pesticide and Industrial Chemicals Research Center (PICRC) is researching how to expand the use of high performance liquid chromatography (HPLC) to develop new methods that can identify small groups of pesticides not easily detected through GC (32).

New methods may also result from emerging technologies. For example, supercritical fluid extraction (SFE) may simplify sample extraction and cleanup, and supercritical fluid chromatography (SFC) may improve chromatographic separation. The coupling of SFE/SFC could lead to new MRMs capable of detecting small groups of pesticides that are thermally labile or polar (13). Although not now in regulatory use, SFE/SFC is being researched under FSIS contracts for use on pesticides and drugs in meat products.

New technologies may also reduce the time necessary to perform an MRM, thereby freeing up time for analysis of additional samples, a broader analysis of each sample, or additional research. Automated gel permeation chromatography (GPC), autoinjectors, and data processors are already routinely used to free analysts from time-consuming and tedious laboratory activities. Solid phase extraction (SPE), automated evaporators, and other technologies are being developed and used for their ability to save time during sample cleanup.

Robotics is an emerging automation technology that might free large segments of analysts' time now spent on repetitive laboratory procedures; robots are expensive, require substantial design modification, and work best for large numbers of similar samples undergoing the same analysis. Health and Welfare Canada is evaluating the use of a robot in a milk survey for 32 pesticides, metabolites, and PCBs to carry out the extraction and cleanup steps. Early results show that the robot can contribute to a doubled weekly sample output, in part due to its ability to work at night (17). Some U.S. private companies are also using robots for pesticide residue analysis.

In addition to new technologies, new approaches may also reduce analysis time. For example, ongoing FDA research on reducing the size of the sample prepared for analysis could cut extraction and cleanup times.

Single Residue Methods

SRMs will be required to test for pesticides that cannot be analyzed by MRMs, especially those pesticides with significant health hazards. SRMs can be made more practical for regulatory analysis through improvements in their accuracy, cost, and timeliness.

A first step could be to determine if existing SRMs (listed in PAM II) are practical and effective. Those SRMs found wanting would be candidates for improvement or replacement through Federal research or potentially by the petitioner who submitted the method. To ensure that new PAM II methods did not suffer from the same problems, EPA could tighten its requirements for acceptable methods and increase the testing of such methods (for more details, see Finding 3).

Many of the same technologies available for improving MRMs or developing new MRMs could also be used to improve or develop new SRMs. Technical advances have taken place since many SRMs were developed. In some cases, technologies may be more applicable to SRMs than MRMs. For example, SPEs reduce cleanup time but may also cause the loss of pesticides; newer SPEs suffer less from this problem than older ones. Reducing the loss of pesticides can improve the usefulness of a technology for an MRM but not for an SRM, since SRMs only detect one pesticide at a time. Automation and robotics can also be used in SRMs, especially if an SRM is used to analyze large numbers of similar samples for a particular pesticide, as in the case of a special survey. Because of insufficient research resources, the need for improving an individual SRM could be evaluated on the basis of the pesticide's health hazard and the possibility that an MRM could be adapted to test for the pesticide.

The quantitative immunoassay is an emerging technique that could lead to important new SRMs, particularly for those pesticides that do not need extensive cleanup and that cannot be detected easily by existing analytical techniques or when large numbers of samples need analysis. Quantitative immunoassays' potential to analyze more samples in the same period of time than conventional methods, to lower training and equipment costs, and to potentially lower analysis costs combine to make their development attractive for analyzing those health hazardous pesticides that cannot be analyzed by MRMs. Currently, Health and Welfare Canada is taking steps to implement the regulatory use of an immunoassay SRM on food that will give quantifiable results in its field laboratories.

Semiquantitative and Qualitative Tests

Development of semiquantitative and qualitative tests promises to complement existing approaches while also changing them. Qualitative rapid tests identify a residue if it occurs at concentrations above a pre-established level, while semiquantitative methods identify residues over a pre-established concentration and determine the range of their concentrations. Both may test for a single pesticide residue or a group of related ones. In the latter case, the test can identify only the pesticide group, not the specific pesticides. The advantages of such methods are that they can provide fast results at lower cost than conventional methods and may be portable. Their disadvantages are that they usually analyze only a small number of pesticides, and they do not provide quantitative data.

The lack of quantitative data is a major institutional drawback. Regulatory agencies like FDA use methods that can detect and quantify pesticide residues at below-tolerance levels to collect data on the incidence and levels present in food. Such quantitative data are used by EPA in special reviews of pesticides, in pesticide tolerance revocations, and in re-registration of pesticides and are of interest to other groups. FDA is concerned that the use of such tests would adversely affect its data-gathering responsibilities, especially to EPA. To overcome the quantitative data obstacle, FDA could meet

with EPA to determine EPA's actual data needs, how such tests could take place without affecting those needs, and what other data needs might be filled by such tests (e.g., identifying that a pesticide residue commonly exists in a specific food that was thought to be pesticide free).

A number of possible uses exist for these tests, which make use of such technologies as thin layer chromatography, enzyme inhibition, and immunoassay. In cases of a widespread residue problem in a commodity, these tests might identify violative samples more quickly and less expensively.

Secondly, such tests could be used to analyze large numbers of samples for a particular pesticide or small group of pesticides that are expected to have low violation rates. The small number of samples identified as violative could then be analyzed by quantitative methods to confirm and measure the violation. In this way, significantly hazardous pesticides could be routinely monitored while minimizing the use of more expensive SRMs. Along these lines, FSIS is evaluating a commercial immunoassay kit for qualitatively analyzing triazines; this kit could complement a new conventional method for analyzing triazines that provides quantitative results (1). Where applicable, these tests might also be applied to sample extracts prepared for an MRM to analyze additional pesticides. FSIS is developing and evaluating several such tests to analyze triazines, synthetic pyrethroids, and organophosphates in meat products, and FDA is developing a method using thin layer chromatography for organotins (1, 32).

Semiquantitative and qualitative tests may prove applicable for non-laboratory testing if scientific obstacles can be overcome. The benefits of such an approach would include reducing the costs associated with laboratory analysis (including transporting the sample to the laboratory) and speeding up identification of violative samples. Drawbacks would include the training and equipment needs for the inspectors who would do the testing and the additional time they would need to carry out tests. FDA has evaluated one commercial kit for on-site use, but the kit produced an unacceptable number of false negative results (33).

For all these uses of such tests, conventional methods would have to be used to confirm any violation detected and to provide assurance that the tests were not providing unacceptable levels of false negatives or false positives. Nevertheless, given the pressure for broader monitoring with fixed resources, the appropriate role of semiquantitative and qualitative rapid tests in Federal monitoring programs needs to be determined.

Validation: Important for Technology/Methods Adoption

Validation is an important consideration for the adoption of any new technology or method (see ch. 6). Validation is the verification that a technology or method provides useful analytical data and operates within acceptable performance parameters (for a description of these parameters see ref. 4). There are several levels of validation including the following: intralaboratory, interlaboratory, and a collaborative study. FSIS requires a minimum of three analysts and two collaborating laboratories for validation. FDA requires at least two collaborating laboratories to test the method or technique but in some cases may be forced to use an intralaboratory validated method if no other is available. Validation requires time and trained personnel—two scarce components of regulatory work.

Collaborative study involves six to eight laboratories under the auspices of the Association of Official Analytical Chemists (AOAC) and is the most rigorous form of validation. (Methods that have been validated in this way are termed "official" by the AOAC.) The length of time involved to carry out this type of validation (1 to 3 years) (26) and the difficulty in finding enough laboratories to volunteer their resources restrict the number of methods validated in this way. Even the most widely used FDA MRMs are official for only some of the commodities. FDA, in particular, emphasizes the use of official methods where possible. The emphasis on official methods and the limits on performing collaborative studies may make it difficult to adopt a new technology or method if an official one already exists.

To avoid delays in adopting new technologies and ensure the availability of resources for validations, Federal agencies and non-Federal organizations, such as the AOAC, could jointly determine how the speed of official validation could be increased and how to expand participation of additional laboratories. For example, private or academic laboratories could take a greater part in interlaboratory studies.

Immunoassays (discussed in ch. 4) pose a specific validation need. They will require rigorous validation as a new technology for analyzing pesticide residues, and as they are unfamiliar to most analytical chemists. At the same time, pesticide chemists' unfamiliarity with the technology may make it difficult to find the necessary number of analysts needed to perform collaborative studies. In addition, collaborative studies designed for conventional methods may not be applicable to certain immunoassay applications. Therefore, Federal agencies and organizations such as AOAC could determine the protocol for immunoassay validation for pesticide analysis and promote means to overcome obstacles to their validation.

FINDINGS AND OPTIONS

OTA has identified specific options for improving the capability of Federal programs to analyze pesticide residues in foods. The options are summarized in table 8-1 and organized under four categories:

- improving Federal agencies' pesticide methods research, development, and adoption;
- increasing research coordination and cooperation;
- improving the regulatory usefulness of ana-

**Table 8-1.—Summary of Options to Improve Federal Detection of
Pesticide Residues in Food**

Improve Federal agencies' pesticide methods research, development, and adoption	• FDA[a] and FSIS[b] could establish long-term research plans including priority lists of pesticides requiring improved methods. • FDA could improve the organization of its research. • GAO could conduct an evaluation of Federal analytical methods research programs for analyzing pesticides in food.
Increase research coordination and cooperation	• Federal agencies could create a methods research and development advisory committee for pesticide residues in food. The committee could include appropriate non-Federal representatives. • FDA, FSIS, and EPA could establish a methods workgroup for pesticide residues in food. • Federal laboratories could increase coordination with State pesticide residue laboratories. • Federal agencies could improve their use of private sector expertise. • Federal agencies could increase coordination with appropriate agencies of foreign governments.
Improve the regulatory usefulness of analytical methods submitted to EPA as part of the tolerance-setting process	• EPA[c] could require an independent test of pesticide analytical methods before their submission to EPA. • FDA and FSIS could validate submitted methods. • EPA could require the testing, development, or adaption of a multiresidue method for any pesticide requiring a tolerance. • EPA could revise its regulations and guidelines for submitted methods. • FDA and FSIS could review and revise existing methods catalogued in PAM II.[d]
Maintain the quality and quantity of the analyst workforce	• Federal agencies could revise their hiring practices and find ways to give laboratories increased flexibility in hiring new recruits. • FDA and FSIS could increase continuing education and training programs for Federal analysts. • FDA and FSIS could sponsor analytical methods training workshops for State analysts.

[a]FDA: Food and Drug Administration of the U.S. Department of Health and Human Services
[b]FSIS: Food Safety and Inspection Service of the U.S. Department of Agriculture
[c]EPA: U.S. Environmental Protection Agency
[d]PAM II: *Pesticide Analytical Manual*, Volume II, (Washington, DC: Food and Drug Administration).

lytical methods submitted to EPA as part of the tolerance-setting process; and

• maintaining the quantity and quality of the analyst workforce.

Although the options could require congressional action, most of the options can be implemented by the relevant Federal agencies without new or amended legislation. However, a number of these options would require budget increases or realignments in agencies' priorities. In addition to improving analytical methods, the effectiveness of monitoring pesticide residues in food could be enhanced by addressing related issues (box 8-A).

In general, the barrier to expanding the detection of pesticide residues in food seems to stem less from the scientific arena than from the policy one. Individual agencies have given lower priority to such research because of pressing demands to address other matters. In addition, lack of adequate incentives and resources slows progress in this area, including the detection of moderate to high health hazard pesticides not now detectable by existing MRMs.

FINDING 1: Federal Agencies' Pesticide Methods Research, Development, and Adoption Could Be Improved.

Option 1.1: FDA and FSIS could establish long-term research plans including priority lists of pesticides requiring improved methods.

Box 8-A.—Related Issues

In the process of assessing technologies for the detection of pesticide residues in food, certain other issues arose that influence the effectiveness of Federal agencies' monitoring of pesticide residues in food. Although these issues were outside the scope of this OTA study, they warrant brief discussion because they affect the technical capability and research direction of the Federal pesticide regulatory programs. They are the following:

- Intelligence data on pesticide use
- Sampling
- Perception of food safety

Intelligence Data. Analytical chemists can focus their analysis better and improve their ability to detect pesticide residues if they know what pesticides have been used on the crop. For instance, FDA's most widely used MRM, the Luke method, comprises six different column/detector combinations to detect a range of pesticides. Without intelligence data, each of the six combinations would have to be used to check the food sample. With intelligence data, the number of combinations used can be reduced to focus on those pesticides thought or known to have been applied to the crop. Having such intelligence data thereby can free equipment for analyses of additional samples.

The lack of intelligence data today is greater for imports than for domestic foods. FDA laboratories obtain information on domestic pesticide use, for example, from State agencies, land grant universities, USDA's extension service, domestic growers, and pesticide applicators. Information on foreign pesticide use is more scarce. FDA uses the Battelle World Pesticides Program database, which provides country-level data on fungicide, herbicide, and insecticide use in 22 countries. Information may also be obtained from such sources as foreign agencies making pesticide application recommendations and weather reports. Improvements in intelligence data, especially for imports, would increase the analytical effectiveness of regulatory analyses while improving the use of fixed laboratory resources. Improved intelligence data would require additional funds and raise the question of who—regulatory agencies or the private sector—should bear the increased costs.

Sampling. Decisions on how much sampling should take place and what type of commodities should be sampled affect analytical methods development. For example, a decision to increase sampling could lead to an emphasis on making current methods faster, introducing new and more rapid methods, and using semiquantitative or qualitative methods to screen out nonviolative samples quickly. A decision to increase sampling might also lead to requirements for private testing to reduce the burden on Federal regulatory laboratories. Such a step could require Federal quality control and assurance programs for private laboratories performing the analyses. The resulting increase in private testing could lead to increased private development of analytical technologies and methods suitable for regulatory testing.

Correspondingly, a decision to maintain the current level of sampling but increase the number of pesticides analyzed could promote research on expanding the scope of existing MRMs and on developing new MRMs and more practical SRMs. A decision to sample a wider variety of commodities might require increased work on adapting existing methods to new commodities.

Perception. A difference of opinion exists with regard to the actual importance of pesticide residues in food in relation to human health. A significant level of consumer concern and congressional interest exist on the issue. However, the regulatory agencies, FDA and FSIS, do not consider pesticide residues as a high priority issue for food safety. Most regulatory chemists and laboratory directors OTA spoke with believe the food supply is safe with regard to the level of pesticides residues present, and other areas of food regulation should have priority for any new funding. The regulatory agencies' stand on this point has led to their allocation of fewer resources and incentives for the development of improved methods for the detection of pesticide residues in food.

Federal methods research for pesticide residues in food suffers from a lack of long-term planning. For example, neither FDA nor FSIS has a long-term pesticide methods research plan. Instead, each relies on annual research plans that include multiyear projects directed toward short-term program needs. A percentage of research is necessary to address short-term emergency-oriented research. But regulatory work could benefit from long-term planning designed to provide research direction to overall needs and monitoring goals. More specifically, a long-term plan would identify potential future problem areas (e.g., emerging pesticides), develop strategies to address the problem areas, and forecast resources (i.e., skills, time, and funds) necessary to carry out the strategies. Currently, FDA's Center for Food Safety and Applied Nutrition (CFSAN) is developing a long-term research plan to be completed in 1988.

An important element of such a research plan would be the development of a list of top-priority pesticides requiring improved analytical methods. To generate such a list would require developing a formal means to rank pesticides for regulatory action, ranking the pesticides, and then identifying those pesticides that cannot be easily detected by existing methods and those pesticide-matrix combinations for which existing methods are unsatisfactory. By gathering this information, Federal agencies could then develop long-term methods research plans to help identify and measure the most important pesticides of health concern. This list would also assist State and private researchers in setting research priorities. The priority list would be subject to continual revision as new pesticides and new uses were introduced, older pesticides and their uses were ended, and new pesticide data (e.g., metabolism and toxicological) were developed. FDA and USDA may need separate lists because of the different food matrices with which they work. A comparison of those lists with an EPA list of pesticides in environmental matrices would reveal areas of mutual concern and offer an opportunity for coordination of research.

Much of the work needed for development of such a list has already been done by the three agencies. FDA and FSIS have taken steps toward developing such a list, but a list of top-priority pesticides requiring methods development is not available to other agencies nor to the private sector.

FDA began ranking pesticides on its Surveillance Index (SI) in 1981 based on such factors as pesticide toxicity, production and usage, human exposure, and environmental fate (23). Under the SI, pesticides are placed in one of five categories of health hazard. The SI was developed primarily to help set monitoring priorities but has also been used to highlight methods research needs. Currently, 205 pesticides of approximately 316 pesticides with tolerances have been ranked, with the remainder still to be considered (9). An additional 120 pesticides that could be in food will not be ranked because they have low toxicological effects, do not produce residues in food, are no longer manufactured, or are used only in foreign countries on foods not intended for export to the United States (23). Ranking the remaining pesticides with tolerances (and those pesticides that do not have tolerances but have high potential to occur as residues in food) is of some concern because only 10 pesticides per year were ranked in 1986 and 1987 vs. the proposed 30 to 50 (9, 23). FDA also has set up a database, Pestrak, to identify those pesticides that cannot be analyzed through its MRMs.

FSIS has listed 227 pesticides and metabolites of concern and has given each a letter ranking that represents the potential for harmful residues to occur in animals at slaughter. In 1985, FSIS instituted a new ranking system for pesticides, the Compound Evaluation System (CES), using a letter-number ranking code to represent potential toxicity and human exposure. Of the 227 pesticides, 39 have been ranked under the CES, though none have been ranked so far in 1988 (24). Ranked pesticides are then checked for suitable analytical and confirmatory methods. If highly ranked pesticides are found not to have suitable methods for their identification and quantification, research priorities can be adjusted to address the problem. Although the CES is being used to help set research priorities, it is currently too small to provide an overall priority list.

EPA's need for a list of priority pesticides in foods is less because its regulatory responsibilities concern the environment, not food (although it has responsibility for some game animals). A similar listing for the pesticide matrices EPA regulates, however, could be useful to support internal EPA coordination of methods work as well as coordination with other agencies.

Option 1.2: FDA could improve the organization of its research.

Recent studies of deficiencies in pesticide monitoring programs point to the need for an aggressive methods research and development program (28, 31). FDA conducts the majority of Federal research on pesticide residue methods for food. OTA has observed that problems in the organization of FDA's methods research adversely affect the agency's research program.

The basis for OTA's observations was interviews with persons inside and outside the FDA. Within the timeframe and mandate of this work, OTA was unable to evaluate FDA's pesticide methods research program in depth. Because OTA's observations raise significant concerns about the FDA research program, *a more detailed evaluation of the program as well as those of FSIS and EPA conducted by the General Accounting Office would be useful* to gauge the importance of OTA's observations and, if necessary, to identify remedial actions. While OTA did not make similar observations of FSIS's or EPA's programs, an analysis of FSIS's decentralized research approach, EPA's methods evaluation process, and the level of coordination with FDA would be important to obtain an overall picture of Federal methods research on pesticide residues in food.

Pesticide methods research is conducted by four organizational bodies within FDA:[2]

---

[2]Pesticide methods research is conducted in conjunction with industrial chemicals methods research, e.g., PCBs and dioxin. Therefore, the total research FTEs given overstate the number of persons working solely on pesticide methods.

- CFSAN laboratory, which has six FTEs for pesticide methods research.
- Two research centers, the Pesticide and Industrial Chemicals Research Center (PICRC) and the Total Diet Research Center (TDRC), which together have six FTEs for pesticide methods research.
- The 16 field laboratories, which together have approximately seven FTEs for pesticide methods research.

CFSAN has the greatest concentration of research personnel in one place. Research at CFSAN has led to development of four of the five MRMs used by FDA. OTA observed that FDA field laboratories considered CFSAN's current research not geared to regulatory needs, including the timeliness needs, of field laboratories. Little field involvement seems to exist in setting CFSAN's research agenda, which primarily addresses current problems rather than upcoming issues. CFSAN is the proper body to prioritize overall pesticide methods needs, and it does so annually but not in a fashion easily accessible by other Federal agencies, State programs, or the private sector.

FDA's research centers—PICRC and TDRC—were established in 1980 to address the research needs of field laboratories in analyzing pesticides and industrial contaminants. TDRC's primary function is to support the Total Diet Program, and PICRC's is to support other regulatory field laboratories. These centers have developed a number of methods in support of the field laboratories' needs, and a number of specific cases exist of individual field laboratories benefiting from this work.

OTA observed that field laboratories consider a large part of the research centers' work as not being applicable to their regulatory needs. Again, it seems that field laboratories have little involvement in setting the centers' research agendas especially compared to CFSAN. This lack of field laboratory appreciation for the centers' work may in part stem from a failure of the field laboratories to devote the resources needed to work with the centers on appropriate research agendas.

Pesticide methods research at field laboratories is done primarily through short- and medium-term projects. The strength of field research is its immediate relevance to problems at hand. Field research may also significantly improve FDA's analytical work. For example, the Luke MRM was developed at the Los Angeles laboratory, and in 1987 was used in approximately 80 percent of all FDA pesticide analyses. One weakness of field research is that the first priority of field laboratories is regulatory work, and if the need arises, research time will be sacrificed to deal with emergencies. As noted earlier, field laboratories may not be making the effort to help set relevant research agendas for the research centers. Field research also may not be well coordinated between laboratories, leading to duplication of effort or lack of productive interchange.

Although the current structure of FDA research (CFSAN, research centers, and field research) seems to be workable, OTA believes that modifications in the responsibilities of each research body might lead to increased productivity results. As mentioned earlier, a long-term research plan for pesticide methods research would help FDA address the most important needs of its regulatory program, develop improved coordination inside and outside the agency, and address the research responsibilities of FDA's research organizations. Any plan should be based on significant input from FDA field laboratories and from outside experts and should be subject to modification as new needs arise.

CFSAN's research capabilities may be required to address the immediate needs of the regulatory laboratories. If so, then modifications could help make that work more appropriate for meeting field needs. Possible approaches would be to increase field pesticide staff involvement in setting CFSAN's research agenda or to have CFSAN research staff periodically spend time at the field laboratories to improve their understanding of field needs.

On the other hand, CFSAN, as a central laboratory with no line authority over the field laboratories and removed from daily regulatory work, could focus on addressing some longer-term and broader-scope research issues. CFSAN has the time and resources to identify and evaluate new and existing technologies for their application to pesticide residue analysis. Where in-house expertise is lacking, such work might be done through contracts. Contracting allows access to specific expertise but it needs to be done in ways that ensure the work is geared to regulatory needs and is transferable into the FDA system.

CFSAN also has a key role to play in the area of methods development for new pesticides. Changes in the types of new pesticides are seen as making regulatory work more difficult. By tracking the development of new pesticides and addressing the analytical needs for them, CFSAN could help FDA keep up with its regulatory responsibilities and avoid possible future crises.

If CFSAN were to be less involved in research for immediate regulatory needs, then the research centers or the field laboratories might need additional research resources. Ranking pesticides that require methods development research and then coordinating that research are functions that a central laboratory may be best able to accomplish. CFSAN's location enables it to tap EPA's and USDA's pesticide data and research agendas easily, a factor necessary to carry out coordination of priority setting.

The research centers' primary purpose is to support the field laboratories, to be involved in the day-to-day regulatory needs. One way of helping to ensure that research centers are doing so would be to involve field laboratory staff more formally, especially the pesticide specialists, in setting the research centers' agendas. In addition, research center personnel could interact more with field laboratory staff through personnel exchanges, workshops, and increased visits to field laboratories. The centers could assume increased responsibility in technology adoption by adapting and disseminating to the field new methods development work done at CFSAN, at the centers, and at individual field laboratories.

Field laboratories seem best suited to conduct research that meets their individual regulatory responsibilities, such as extending existing methods to analyze additional pesticides and commodities. They are also able to refine new technologies or methods for their own particular situation and validate new methods or techniques. In one case, field laboratories have demonstrated the capability of developing new MRMs. The modifications detailed above would demand increased field participation in setting research agendas for the research centers and possibly for CFSAN and could require additional research to be carried out by field laboratories. Such a redirection of resources would require a corresponding increase in pesticide laboratory personnel to maintain the current level of regulatory work. Therefore, the expansion of field research would require an overall increase in FDA's pesticide methods research expenditures or an internal redistribution of research resources.

FINDING 2: Research Coordination and Cooperation Could Be Increased.

The amount of resources available for methods research for pesticide residues in food increases the importance of coordination between research organizations. Failure to share research plans and results makes it difficult for agencies to be familiar with each others' ongoing work and to benefit from that work. Knowledge of what other agencies are doing can help minimize gaps in pesticide monitoring coverage, facilitate information transfer, provide early warnings of upcoming concerns, and reduce duplication of efforts. For example, FDA let a contract to develop monoclonal antibodies for immunoassays without consulting experts at EPA and Health and Welfare Canada. Antibodies, albeit polyclonal, had already been developed for two of the pesticides included in the contract by Health and Welfare Canada and the University of California at Davis.

Coordination could be increased at all levels: among Federal agencies; among Federal, State, and the private sectors; and between the United States and other countries, in particular, Canada. Resources would have to be redirected in support of measures to increase coordination. Means of increasing coordination include the following:

Option 2.1: Establish a methods research and development advisory committee for pesticide residues in food.

This committee could include representatives of Federal and State regulatory programs as well as representatives of private companies, agricultural producers, consumers, environmental organizations, academic institutions, and pesticide registrants. This committee could include two subgroups: one to deal with policy issues, which would include the chemistry program administrators, and one to deal with scientific issues, which would include the principal chemists. This committee could be mandated to advise the Federal government on current problem areas, support the exchange of results of ongoing government-sponsored projects, and recommend areas of methods research. Another approach that could stand alone or complement the advisory committee would be to follow the Canadian approach of holding workshops with participants from the relevant groups to address specific methods needs when a problem emerges (3).

Option 2.2: FDA, FSIS, and EPA could formally establish a methods workgroup on pesticide residues in food.

Currently, research coordination takes place on a formal and informal bases between EPA, FDA, and FSIS. For example, FDA and USDA use information provided by EPA to help make decisions on what pesticides should be monitored.

Currently, a pesticide analytical methods advisory group with a representative from each of the three agencies meets on an irregular basis. Past meetings led to improvements in the methods program, for example, the inclusion of a user review form in the PAM II to encourage chemists to report problems they had with specific methods. Overall, the advisory group does not have authority, resources, nor commitment to coordinate the pesticide residue methods research of the agencies.

Therefore, a more formal workgroup meeting on a regular basis could improve coordination of the methods research of the three agencies. Effective coordination already exists between FSIS and FDA in another area of regulatory research—animal drugs. FDA's Center for Veterinary Medicine and FSIS have a formalized system for coordinating their work on veterinary drugs through a 2½-year-old working group that puts research needs in priority, and coordinates methods research and validation of new methods (6). In addition, FDA has established project advisory groups with FSIS participation to address veterinary drugs for which residue methods are not available, to contract methods research, and to review the resulting methods (2). Similar coordination on developing research priorities and carrying out methods research and validation could be established between FSIS and FDA in the area of pesticide residue methods.

As part of the workgroup, EPA could continue to supply data for priority setting and increase its use of FDA and FSIS input to ensure that methods submitted during tolerance setting are practical for regulatory work. EPA's role in coordinating research with the other two agencies may be smaller but still important. This is because EPA's methods research does not address food and thus may be of less value to the other agencies. EPA's extraction and cleanup processes may not be applicable to food, especially fatty foods. But since all three agencies use similar detection equipment, advances in such instruments could be used by all three agencies (16). Also, immunoassay research on pesticides can be used by the three agencies because once a pesticide-specific antibody is developed, each agency can then conduct application research to adapt the antibody to matrices of particular concern. Currently, FSIS has an interagency agreement with EPA's Las Vegas laboratory to promote coordination on antibodies of mutual interest.

Option 2.3: Coordination between Federal and State pesticide residue laboratories could be increased.

State regulatory personnel, like Federal analysts, have firsthand knowledge of the needs of field laboratories and could provide guidance for appropriate methods research. Currently, some Federal-State coordination exists. For example, in some FDA districts, FDA and State laboratories divide monitoring responsibilities for certain foods. FDA laboratories also use State pesticide-use data to decide which pesticides and commodities to test. EPA provides pesticide standards to State laboratories and conducts methods training workshops on nonfood matrices for 52 State laboratories. Currently, the California Department of Food and Agriculture (CDFA) and FDA's Pacific Coast Region are developing a Memorandum of Understanding that may include coordination of methods development and quality assurance procedures. Further coordination could include FDA use of State-generated residue data and training of State personnel in pesticide residue methods for food by FDA, similar to the program now run by EPA.

Since most State programs are too small to conduct methods research, opportunities for Federal-State coordination of research on residue methods may be small. But those States with small programs are still knowledgeable of regulatory needs, and their analysts could be consulted. Several States have large-scale pesticide residue monitoring programs and at least one, California, has a significant methods research program. The CDFA recently established a three-person research group to evaluate emerging technologies. It also gave out contracts for developing three immunoassays for pesticide residues in the environment. Increased Federal coordination with State programs like CDFA would expand the scope of overall methods research efforts. It also would help ensure that California establish an effective and efficient program that would complement rather than duplicate the Federal programs.

Option 2.4: Federal agencies could improve their use of private sector expertise.

A tremendous amount of research and development on technologies for detecting pesticides in food is conducted by the private sector. The private sector's contribution to improve analytical methods for regulatory use could be increased in the following ways:

- Creating incentives to stimulate private research and development of methods.
- Tapping the technical expertise of private industry and academia through training and technology transfer.

In addition to the private sector's provision of analytical methods, primarily SRMs, as part of the tolerance-setting process, the private sector also develops new and innovative pesticide residue techniques in response to the market. Analytical instrument makers innovate partly in response to Federal analysts' needs. The development of biologically based technology for the analysis of chemicals has led to private development and marketing of testing kits.

Federal agencies could promote private sector involvement by making clear their own needs. Commercial firms would more likely venture into analytical methods development for pesticides in food if they perceive that a market exists for their products. By making available a list of what methods are needed (e.g., pesticide-matrix combinations) and the type of method needed (qualitative, semiquantitative, or quantitative) for regulatory work, Federal agencies would provide the private sector with needed research direction and some assurance that commercial products indeed have a market among regulatory agencies. For example, FSIS is trying to tap and stimulate the private development of rapid test kits, although these efforts may not be focused enough to convince the private sector that an assured market exists (18). In addition, a common validation procedure would help assure the private sector that acceptance of the technology would require one validation study, not several, for new technologies that are to be used by several Federal agencies.

Along with stimulating market development of methods, the agencies can provide the private sector with seed money in the form of contracts to encourage increased methods research and development. With initial seed money for methods research, the private sector may then be willing to expend its own money for further development. Contracts also will allow agencies to take advantage of expertise not found in-house. FSIS has much of its research done through contracting, while FDA relies primarily on in-house expertise. With the development of new technologies, however, agencies like FDA will need either to increase their contracts to address new developments or bring the expertise in-house, which may be an expensive process. The downside of contracting is that agency personnel must often spend significant amounts of administrative time developing and monitoring the contract. It is sometimes difficult to transfer the results directly because of the nature of regulatory work and lack of in-house expertise.

A large amount of methods development research occurs at U.S. universities, but much of it is devoted to the analyses of environmental matrices, e.g., water, soil, and air, in part because funding is available for such types of work. These methods are of potential use for food analysis. Redirection of university research to food might take additional Federal funding. FDA might improve their use of the four university laboratories funded by USDA to develop methods for pesticides requiring tolerances for use on minor crops (27).

In addition to providing seed money for methods development in the private sector and markets for products, Federal agencies can also tap the expertise that exists in the private sector. Private sector laboratories of pesticide manufacturers and food processors are ahead of Federal regulatory agencies in the use of certain technologies, e.g., robotics and capillary columns. They also may have made improvements in existing methods or developed new techniques of which the Federal agencies are unaware. In some cases, these advances may not be applicable to regulatory usage. On the other hand, Federal and State laboratories have turned to the pesticide manufacturer for advice on methods after encountering difficulty in pesticide analysis.

Federal agencies could obtain additional methods expertise from the private sector through joint public/private sponsorship of technical "hands-on" laboratory workshops. A model may be the annual pesticide residue workshops sponsored by the State of Florida or the EPA method workshops held for State analysts and often taught by private sector personnel using privately supplied equipment. FDA does tap the academic community through contracting science advisers from universities at the field laboratories. The majority of science advisers, however, are not experts on pesticide analytical methods.

Option 2.5: Federal agencies could increase coordination with foreign agencies.

FSIS and FDA have programs whereby foreign scientists work at Federal laboratories to gain experience in analytical methods and to pass on their expertise to Federal analysts. Foreign government pesticide regulatory agencies may have certain methods, research expertise, and knowledge that might be relevant to the United States and vice versa. For example, Health and Welfare Canada has a small pesticide methods research program that seems to be advanced in several areas such as immunoassays and robotics. Yet little interaction exists between that agency and U.S. agencies in the area of immunoassays. Canada has developed seven immunoassays for use on fruits and vegetables. U.S. agencies could take advantage of this expertise and avoid duplicating Canada's work. One easy way to facilitate information transfer between the two countries would be for U.S. agency personnel to attend the Fall 1988 workshop on immunoassays held for personnel from Canada's regional laboratories.

FINDING 3: Pesticide Methods Submitted for Tolerance Setting Could Be Improved for Regulatory Use.

All pesticides used in the United States must be registered by EPA. If a proposed use of a pesticide may result in residues in food or feed, a tolerance (or exemption from tolerance) is required. As part of the tolerance-setting process, EPA requires that the person or organization (known as a petitioner) requesting a tolerance provide an analytical method that can be used to enforce the tolerance set for each pesticide/food combination. To meet this requirement, SRMs, commonly developed to gen-

erate data required for pesticide registration and tolerance setting rather than to meet regulatory needs, are submitted. In some cases, these methods have not been laboratory tested by EPA. Thus, some submitted methods have proved complex, time-consuming, costly, and sometimes cannot be replicated by another laboratory, thus rendering them impractical for regulatory work.

Several courses of action exist that could be taken to ensure that methods submitted for the tolerance-setting process are more useful for enforcement purposes. The majority of these actions, noted below, include stricter EPA requirements on submitted methods to make them more practical for regulatory work. In conjunction with any of these actions could be improved communication between EPA and the pesticide manufacturer as to what kind of methods or information would be most useful for the government. Improved communication could save the company time by focusing its chemists' time, and it could provide agencies with methods more appropriate for regulatory work.

Option 3.1: EPA could require an independent check of pesticide analytical methods before their submission to EPA.

This requirement would increase the likelihood that a submitted method really works. The petitioner could contract with an independent laboratory or have an in-house laboratory carry out the evaluation (if the in-house laboratory were not involved in the development of the particular method). The results from the independent test would be used by EPA in its own evaluation of the method. This action places the cost of additional testing on the person petitioning for a tolerance.

EPA has just implemented this requirement for the first tolerance petition for a pesticide and for any tolerance petition using a new method or a significantly changed method. Beginning August 1, 1989, such petitions are required to include the results of an independent evaluation of the submitted method on six samples (two control samples, two samples fortified with the pesticide at the proposed tolerance, and two samples fortified at 2 to 5 times the proposed tolerance). If more than one commodity is being proposed for a tolerance, the independent evaluation of the method must be on the commodity most difficult to analyze (7).

Option 3.2: FDA and FSIS could validate methods submitted for tolerance setting.

Increased Federal validation would increase the likelihood that a submitted method would be practical for regulatory use. FDA or FSIS could, in addition to EPA, provide a desk review or laboratory evaluation of all or a selected number of submitted methods. Criteria for selecting certain pesticides could be based on such factors as the health hazard of the pesticide, degree of difficulty of the method, or the use of a new technology or procedure. FDA or FSIS could evaluate petitioners' methods as to their applicability to regulatory work, provide EPA with results of the evaluation, and if necessary, EPA could require the appropriate modification of the method before a tolerance was granted.

This action would place an additional resource burden on FDA and FSIS. FDA probably would disagree with the redirection of resources (staff time and funds) for such work, in part because it depends primarily on MRMs not SRMs, and thus probably would not consider validation of petitioner methods a high priority.

Option 3.3: EPA could require the testing, development, or adaptation of a multiresidue method for any pesticide requiring a tolerance.

FDA and FSIS do not have the needed resources to use SRMs routinely and so depend upon MRMs for the bulk of their testing. Therefore, it may be reasonable to have petitioners address the development or adaptation of an MRM to analyze their pesticide. In 1984, EPA added the requirement to its tolerance-setting regulations that petitioners must determine whether their pesticide can be analyzed by FDA's and USDA's MRMs (40 CFR: part 158.125). In 1986, FDA made method protocols available for four of its MRMs, which were needed before such testing could be done and the new regulation became practical (Federal Register,

51(186): 34249, Sept 26, 1986). None of the four MRMs have to work for the pesticide but the results must be provided to EPA, which gives them to FDA. As of May 1988, 12 pesticides had gone through this procedure. As part of re-registration, EPA requires registrants to supply similar testing data on older pesticides if they are not already available. USDA has not published method protocols for its MRMs, and therefore methods submitted for tolerances for meat products have not been tested through FSIS's MRMs.

This requirement could be taken one step further by requiring that for all tolerances, or some subset such as tolerances for new pesticides, an MRM be developed or adapted for the analysis of the pesticide. While this requirement would increase the capability of Federal monitoring of pesticide residues in food, it could also lead to new problems with the regulation of pesticides and could increase costs for pesticide development.

First, if this requirement applied to all pesticides requiring tolerances, a decision would have to be made on pesticides now having tolerances that cannot be analyzed through existing MRMs. In some cases, new pesticides that might have lower health hazards and fewer adverse environmental effects than existing pesticides might not be able to be analyzed through existing MRMs. The requirement could thereby slow down or prevent the introduction of safer pesticides.

Second, the additional research to develop or adapt an MRM would increase the cost of pesticide development and might increase the time before registration is approved. Changes could be made, however, to prevent the delay in the pesticide's entry into the marketplace. A "conditional registration" could be granted based on submission of an SRM with the proviso that the registrant submit an MRM within a given time period. Because it can take several years for a new pesticide to achieve widespread distribution, the MRM would be developed in time for the routine analysis for that pesticide. Another time-saving alternative is for EPA to expedite its review process. Currently, it takes

EPA about 12 to 18 months to respond to a submission. Expeditious review, whether through additional staffing or improvements in efficiency of the review process, could compensate for the additional time required to develop an MRM.

Option 3.4: EPA could revise its regulations and guidelines for submitted methods to ensure that these methods are practical for regulatory work.

EPA has both regulations and guidelines concerning the submission of methods during the tolerance-setting process. EPA could review these regulations and guidelines and make appropriate changes to increase the regulatory usefulness of submitted methods.

EPA's regulations require the following: a method be submitted whenever a tolerance is required (or for most exemptions to a tolerance), the method must not be confidential, and the pesticide be tested through FDA and USDA MRMs (40 CFR: part 158.125). EPA's guidelines (EPA, "Pesticide Assessment Guidelines, Subdivision O," Oct 1982) include certain technical requirements for submitted methods but do not carry the same legal weight as the regulations.

The regulations and guidelines could be tightened in a number of ways to make submitted methods more practical and more appropriate for enforcement work rather than research. For example, the regulations could address the need for practical regulatory methods and either define what is meant by practical or refer to the guidelines for that explanation. The guidelines could be rewritten to set stricter limits on the cost of using a method and the time required for analysis (possibly to the point of setting maximum times for extraction, cleanup, and detection), and the need to analyze for significant metabolites. They could also require improved and more detailed writeups of the methods, require the use of U.S. measurements, and require the use of technology easily available to U.S. regulatory agencies. Currently, revision of regulations and guidelines is not a priority at EPA and so resources are not available to carry it out.

Option 3.5: FDA and FSIS could review and revise existing PAM II methods.

PAM II contains the methods submitted during the tolerance-setting process and approved by EPA. Regulatory analysts have found that PAM II methods can be impractical to use. The usefulness of PAM II is further compromised by a recent EPA decision to discontinue funding (as of FY 1988) for the provision of submitted methods by EPA to FDA for publication in PAM II.

Several steps could be taken to increase the utility of PAM II. First is the continuation of funding at EPA and FDA for PAM II work. Second would be the updating of PAM II by FDA (which maintains PAM II) and FSIS to winnow out impractical methods, possibly through desk reviews and user comments. A further step would be the replacement of existing methods with up-to-date methods that are sometimes available from the pesticide manufacturer. This work would require FDA and FSIS to redirect resources. Updating could concentrate on methods for those pesticides that cannot be analyzed by MRMs and possibly those pesticides of moderate to high health hazard in order to be more cost-effective for regulatory needs.

FINDING 4: The Quantity and Quality of the Analyst Workforce Need To Be Maintained.

Of importance to analytical methods research efforts is the availability of a high quality workforce. The pool of analytical chemists, however, is decreasing as fewer students are entering the field and many experienced chemists (especially at regulatory agencies) are approaching retirement (26). The concern about the potential shortage of chemists is growing and is shared by government agencies and the private sector alike (18).

Option 4.1: Federal agencies could revise their hiring practices and find ways to give laboratories increased flexibility in hiring new recruits.

Regulatory agencies are especially hard-pressed to attract high quality people because of low starting salaries compared with salaries offered in the private sector. Some smaller State programs are severely affected by this problem. In addition, Federal hiring guidelines, encumbered by hiring freezes, short windows of hiring opportunity, and long hiring procedures, seem to make it more difficult to hire people when they are available (29). The Agricultural Research Service has partly avoided this problem by having a quick recruitment process for post-doctoral candidates (19).

To build up this workforce would probably require active promotion and incentives to enter the field of analytical chemistry. This problem is acute in the analytical chemistry specialty of pesticide residue analysis. Many academic institutions that once trained students in this specialty have left the field due to declines in the availability of research funds (much of which went to graduate student stipends) or because other areas, such as environmental toxicology or chemistry seemed to offer more opportunities for their students (27).

Some States (e.g., California and Florida) have already taken steps to attract future chemists by implementing programs for college students to work at or visit their regulatory laboratories. Private industry carries out similar programs. For example, Proctor & Gamble provides short courses to undergraduates on careers in analytical chemistry (5). Federal regulatory agencies have similar programs. For example, under an FDA program, undergraduate students split their year between attending university and working in a FDA laboratory (12). Federal agencies could benefit from taking a more active approach to recruit entry-level chemists.

Another way to attract students to the field would be the establishment of scholarships and fellowships for undergraduate and graduate education. To implement this last option would require additional funding.

Option 4.2: FDA and FSIS could increase continuing education and training programs for Federal analysts.

Concerns also exist about maintaining the quality of the regulatory workforce. Many analysts have been out of school for a number of years, may not be up-to-date on new developments, and may require some retraining (6). FSIS now holds an annual workshop on technology development, has a continuing education program and a competitive training program at the University of Georgia, and has training provided by contractors doing research (6). FDA has fewer external training connections (one exception is the Science Advisory Research Associate Program) and provides most of its training internally. A significant FDA forum is the annual pesticide workshop, which brings together pesticide analysts from the regulatory laboratories, research centers, and CFSAN. Overall, there seem to be additional opportunities for Federal agencies to make increased use of private sector and university expertise in staff training. For example, personnel exchanges with industry and universities could be supported.

Option 4.3: FDA and FSIS could sponsor analytical methods training workshops for State analysts.

Availability of training is even more important for State laboratory personnel, especially for individuals in small State laboratories (21). Analysts in many States do not have the opportunity to learn about the newest advances in pesticide use and analysis because of lack of time and funds to attend meetings.

One effective training program for State personnel, administered by EPA, provides training in analytical methods, though not specifically applicable to pesticides in food. It seems to be popular and highly regarded by the States, and there is a waiting list for attendance. A similar program on pesticide residue methods could be modeled after EPA's program and implemented by FDA and FSIS. Currently, only State personnel near FDA laboratories have the opportunity to receive FDA training.

Some States also have set up their own training programs. For example, for the last 24 years, Florida has held a pesticide residue workshop at which State personnel learn of advances in the use of methods to detect pesticides in foods and the environment. Federal and foreign personnel also attend. California is considering establishing a similar workshop for the western States in conjunction with the University of California.

Support for State analysts training would cost FDA and FSIS additional resources, but it would improve the overall regulation of pesticide residues in food while supporting closer Federal-State cooperation.

CHAPTER 8 REFERENCES

1. Ashworth, R., Chemistry Division, Food Safety and Inspection Service, U.S. Department of Agriculture, Washington, DC, personal communication, May 13, 1988.
2. Barnes, C., Center for Veterinary Medicine, Food and Drug Administration, Beltsville, MD, personal communication, May 16, 1988.
3. Conacher, H., Health Protection Branch, Health and Welfare Canada, Ottawa, Canada, comment at OTA workshop "Technologies to Detect Pesticide Residues in Food," Mar. 16, 1988.
*4. Conacher, H., "Validation of Analytical Methods for Pesticide Residues and Confirmation of Results," OTA commissioned paper, Spring 1988.
5. DePalma, D., Proctor & Gamble Company, Cincinnati, OH, comment at the OTA workshop "Technologies to Detect Pesticide Residues in Food," Mar. 16, 1988.
6. Ellis, R., Chemistry Division, Food Safety and Inspection Service, Washington, DC, comment at OTA workshop "Technologies to Detect Pesticide Residues in Foods," Mar. 16, 1988.
7. Environmental Protection Agency, Office of Pesticides and Toxic Substances, "Notice to Manufacturers, Formulators, Producers, and Registrants of Pesticide Products," PR Notice 88-5, Washington, DC, 1988.
8. Food and Drug Administration, Center for Food Safety and Applied Nutrition, Washington, DC, May 1988 update of Table 1 from Reed, et al., "The FDA Pesticides Monitoring Program," *J. Assoc. Off. Anal. Chem.* 70(3):591-595, 1987.
9. Food and Drug Administration, response to OTA questions, April 1988.
10. Food Safety and Inspection Service, U.S. Department of Agriculture, *Compound Evaluation and Analytical Capability National Residue Program Plan 1987* (Washington, DC: Food Safety and Inspection Service, January 1987).
11. Harr, J., Residue Evaluation and Surveillance Division, Food Safety and Inspection Service, U.S. Department of Agriculture, Washington, DC, personal communication, June 27, 1988.
12. Hundley, H., Los Angeles Laboratory, Food and Drug Administration, Los Angeles, CA, personal communication, July 20, 1988.
13. Lee, M., Chemistry Laboratory Services, California Department of Food and Agriculture, Sacramento, CA, personal communication, June 7, 1988.
14. Lombardo, P., Center for Food Safety and Applied Nutrition, Food and Drug Administration, Washington, DC, personal communication, June 29, 1988.
15. Luke, M., Los Angeles Pesticide Laboratory, Food and Drug Administration, Los Angeles, CA, personal communication, April 26, 1988.
16. Mitchum, R., Environmental Monitoring System Laboratory, Environmental Protection Agency, Las Vegas, NV, personal communication, May 16, 1988.
*17. Newsome, W.H. and Graham, G.F., "Pesticide Residue Monitoring in Canada," OTA commissioned paper, Spring 1988.
18. Office of Technology Assessment, "Technologies to Detect Pesticide Residues in Food," workshop held in Washington, DC, Mar. 14-16, 1988.
19. Plimmer, J., Agricultural Research Service, U.S. Department of Agriculture, Washington, DC, comment at OTA workshop "Technologies to Detect Pesticide Residues in Food," Mar. 16, 1988.
*20. Plimmer, J., Hill, K., and Menn, J., "Pesticide Design: Outlook for the Future," OTA commissioned paper, Spring 1988.
21. Polli, R., Vermont Department of Agriculture, personal communication, Montpelier, VT, Mar. 7, 1988.
22. Reed, D., Wessel, J., Burke, J., et al., "The FDA Pesticides Monitoring Program," *J. Assoc. Off. Anal. Chem.* 70(3):591-595, 1987.
23. Reed, D., "The FDA Surveillance Index for Pesticides: Establishing Food Monitoring Priori-

*These reference papers are contained in appendix B.

ties Based on Potential Health Risk," *J. Assoc. Off. Anal. Chem.* 68(1):122-124, 1985.

24. Rubin, L., Residue Evaluation and Surveillance Division, Food Safety and Inspection Service, Washington, DC, personal communication, May 16, 1988.

*25. Sawyer, L., "The Development of Analytical Methods for Pesticide Residues," OTA commissioned paper, Spring 1988.

26. Sawyer, L., Center for Food Safety and Applied Nutrition, Food and Drug Administration, Washington, DC, comment at OTA workshop "Technologies to Detect Pesticide Residues in Food," Mar. 16, 1988.

27. Seiber, J., Department of Environmental Toxicology, University of California, Davis, CA, personal communication, June 20, 1988.

*28. Taylor, S., "Developing Pesticide Analytical Methods for Food: Considerations for Federal Policy Formulation," OTA commissioned paper, Spring 1988.

29. Trichilo, C., Residue Chemistry Branch, Environmental Protection Agency, Washington, DC, comment at OTA workshop "Technol-ogies to Detect Pesticide Residues in Food," Mar. 16, 1988.

*30. Trichilo, C. and Schmitt, R., "Federal Pesticide Monitoring Programs: Analytical Methods Development," OTA commissioned paper, Spring 1988.

31. U.S. Congress, General Accounting Office, "Pesticides: Need to Enhance FDA's Ability to Protect the Public From Illegal Pesticides," GAO/RCED-87-7, October 1986.

32. Walters, S., Pesticide and Industrial Contaminants Research Center, Food and Drug Administration, Detroit, MI, personal communication, Apr. 22, 1988.

33. Wilkes, P., "Evaluation of Enzytec (TM) Pesticide Detection System for Regulatory Use," *Laboratory Information Bulletin*, Number 8, August 1987.

34. Worobey, B., Health Protection Branch, Health and Welfare Canada, Ottawa, Canada, personal communication, May 5, 1988.

---

*These reference papers are contained in appendix B.

Appendixes

Contents

Page

Appendix A. OTA Workshop Participants and Observers 109
  OTA Workshop Participants: Technologies to Detect
    Pesticide Residues in Food, Mar. 14-16, 1988 109
  List of Observers for the Pesticide Residue Workshop 110
Appendix B. OTA Workshop Papers 112
  The Development of Analytical Methods for Pesticide Residues . .112
  Pesticide Design: Outlook for the Future 123
  Validation of Analytical Methods for Pesticide Residues
    and Confirmation of Results 136
  Conventional Pesticide Analytical Methods: Can They Be
    Improved? 142
  Techniques for and the Role of Screening Pesticide
    Residue Analysis 153
  The Role of Robotic Automation in the Laboratory 163
  Potential of Immunoassays in Monitoring Pesticide
    Residues in Foods 171
  Federal Pesticide Monitoring Programs: Analytical
    Methods Development 182
  Pesticide Analytical Methods Development at the State Level 192
  Pesticide Analytical Methods Development in the Private Sector . .202
  Pesticide Residue Monitoring in Canada 211
  Pesticide Residue Monitoring in Mexico 217
  Developing Pesticide Analytical Methods for Food:
    Considerations for Federal Policy Formulation 219
Appendix C. Glossary of Terms 230

OTA Workshop Participants: Technologies to Detect Pesticide Residues in Food, Mar. 14-16, 1988

Henry Conacher
Chief, Food Research Division
Health and Welfare Canada
Ottawa, Canada

John Cowell
Senior Research Group Leader
Environmental Sciences Department
Monsanto Co.
St. Louis, MO

William Cusick
Branch Chief
Chemistry Laboratory Services
Department of Food and Agriculture
Sacremento, CA

Richard Ellis
Director, Chemistry Division
Food Safety and Inspection Service
U.S. Department of Agriculture
Washington, DC

Silvia Canseco Gonzalez
Plant and Animal Health Office
Agriculture Department
Cozoacan, Mexico City, Mexico

Kenneth Hill
Research Chemist
Environmental Chemistry Laboratory
Agricultural Research Service
U.S. Department of Agriculture
Beltsville, MD

Kenneth Hunter
President
Westinghouse Bio-Analytic Systems Corp.
Rockville, MD

Lyle Johnson
Vice President
Laboratory Operations
Analytical Bio-Chemistry Laboratories, Inc.
Columbia, MO

Bruce Kropscott
Research Chemist
Analytical and Environmental Chemistry
Dow Chemical Co./USA
Midland, MI

Harry Lento
Director, Corporate Analytical Chemistry
Campbell Soup Co.
Camden, NJ

Julius Menn
Associate Deputy Area Director
Plant Science Institute
Agricultural Research Service
U.S. Department of Agriculture
Beltsville, MD

Ralph Mumma
Professor of Chemical Pesticides
Pesticide Research Laboratory
Pennsylvania State University
University Park, PA

W. Harvey Newsome
Head, Pesticide Section
Food Research Division
Health and Welfare Canada
Ottawa, Canada

Cynthia Peck
Senior Research Chemist
Analytical and Environmental Chemistry
Dow Chemical Co./USA
Midland, MI

Jack Plimmer
Research Leader
Environmental Chemistry Laboratory
Agricultural Research Service
U.S. Department of Agriculture
Beltsville, MD

Leon D. Sawyer
Chemist
Center for Food Safety and Applied Nutrition
Food and Drug Administration
U.S. Department of Health and Human Services
Washington, DC

Jim Seiber
Professor and Associate Dean
Department of Environmental Toxicology
University of California
Davis, CA

Sarah Taylor
Analyst of Life Sciences
Congressional Research Service
The Library of Congress
Washington, DC

Charles Trichilo
Chief, Residue Chemistry Branch
Office of Pesticides and Toxic Substances
Environmental Protection Agency
Washington, DC

OTA Staff
Walter Parham
Susan Shen
H. Anson Moye
Allen Ruby

List of Observers for the Pesticide Residue Workshop

Raymond Bowers
General Mills

Jerry Burke
Center for Food Safety and Applied Nutrition
Food and Drug Administration

William Cahill
Sandoz Crop Protection

Lou Carson
Division of Field Science
Food and Drug Administration

Jeff Carter
Iowa Specialty Grains

Bernie Chong
Residue Metabolism
Rohn Haas Co.

Marion Clower
Center for Food Safety and Applied Nutrition
Food and Drug Administration

Paul Corneilussen
Center for Food Safety and Applied Nutrition
Food and Drug Administration

Jack Czarnecki
Hoechst Roussel Agri-Vet

Richard A. DePalma
Procter and Gamble

Jim Devine
American Cyanamid Co.

Ed Elkins
National Food Processors Association

Bob Epstein
Food Safety and Inspection Service
U.S. Department of Agriculture

Bruce Ferguson
ImmunoSystems, Inc.

George Fong
Florida Department of Agriculture

Bob Foster
Adolf Coors

Willa Garner
Environmental Protection Agency

John Gillis
EPA/NEIC Center
Denver Federal Center
Environmental Protection Agency

Robert Graves
Environmental Monitoring Systems Laboratory
   (Cincinnati)
Environmental Protection Agency

Anthony Gross
Nabisco Brands, Inc.

Janet Hathaway
National Resources Defense Council

Donald Hughes
Hazelton Laboratories

William Jacobs
Enzytech

Ian Kelly
Northern Chemical Co.

Milton Luke
Los Angeles District Laboratory
Food and Drug Administration

Pasquale Lombardo
Center for Food Safety and Applied Nutrition
Food and Drug Administration

William McCasland
Texas Department of Agriculture

Albertha Paul
Zymark Corp.

Pete Price
Assembly Office of Research
California State Legislator

Richard Schmitt
Residue Chemistry Branch
Environmental Protection Agency

Susan Shellabarger
Ensys Inc.

Terry Spittler
Department of Food Science and Technology
Cornell University

John Scott Warner
Battelle

Richard Wiles
Board on Agriculture
National Academy of Sciences

Robert K. Williams
CIBA-GEIGY Corp.

Crystal Willis
Grocery Manufacturers of America, Inc.

Albert Yamada
Mike Masaoka Association, Inc.

Congressional Staff
Michael Hoffman
Senator Proxmire's Office

Debra Jacobson
House Committee on Energy and Commerce
   Subcommittee on Oversight and Investigations

Mary Dunbar
Senate Committee on Agriculture, Nutrition,
   and Forestry

Jerilyn Hoy
Cynthia Rasmuseen
General Accounting Office

OTA Workshop Papers

The Development of Analytical Methods for Pesticide Residues

Leon D. Sawyer, Pesticides and Industrial Chemicals Branch, Division of Contaminants Chemistry, Center for Food Safety and Applied Nutrition, U.S. Food and Drug Administration, Washington, DC

Contents

	Page
Abstract	112
Multiresidue Method Development: Background	114
Mills and Mills, Onley and Gaither Methods	115
Storherr Method	116
Luke Method	116
Krause Method	117
Multiresidue Method Development: Summary	118
Multiresidue Method Development: The Future	119
Impacts of Laws and Regulations	120
References	121

Abstract

The U.S. Food and Drug Administration's (FDA) objectives of enforcing tolerances for pesticide residues in foods and feeds and of determining incidence and levels of pesticide residues in the food supply are driving forces in FDA development of residue analytical methods. In turn, such method development is influenced by development of analytical instrumentation, by changing chemical characteristics of new pesticides, and by the constant need to analyze additional food samples for more and varied potential residues.

FDA's chronology of methods development is therefore presented as an example of how the availability of appropriate technology can either advance or hinder development of a needed method. Evolutionary development of five multiresidue methods is discussed, starting with recognition of an analytical need through effects of available instrumentation or determinative systems, development of extraction and cleanup procedures, verification of overall method performance, and extension of such established methods to additional residues and commodities beyond those in the original method study. Reference to interlaboratory validation of each method is also included.

Laws and regulations have affected the limits of determination at which analytical methods must be valid and have dictated coverage for metabolites as well as parent compounds. Future methods development will continue to be driven substantially by such forces and will include new demands for efficiency in application. The search for improved efficiency will dictate exploration of such new approaches as immunoassays, rapid cleanup techniques, improved instrumentation, and automation. Incorporation of these techniques will depend on the degree to which they prove beneficial in a given laboratory situation.

The Food and Drug Administration (FDA) samples and analyzes a wide variety of raw agricultural food and feed products (hereafter referred to as food) to enforce maximum limits, or tolerances, established for pesticide residues. Commodities sampled do not include meat and poultry, which are the province of the U.S. Department of Agriculture (USDA). Residue levels detected, even though they may be below tolerance levels, are quantified and recorded in a central data base. Results of analysis may provide the basis for regulatory actions or may serve the Environmental Protection Agency (EPA), World Health Organization and other groups that have an interest in the historical incidence and levels of pesticide residues in food.

Over the past 25 years, the number of samples analyzed annually by FDA has varied between about 7,000 and 30,000. In fiscal year 1987, about 15,000 samples were analyzed. Also during this year, FDA responded to 26 separate requests from EPA and USDA regarding levels and incidence of residues for 95 chemicals (1). Additionally, FDA's Center for Food Safety and Applied Nutrition responded to 28 Freedom of Information Act (FOI) requests for pesticide monitoring data (1). FDA field offices also routinely respond to a number of similar FOI requests each year.

Since the early 1960s, the FDA has also monitored dietary intake of pesticides in a "market basket" of selected food items (including meat and poultry) that are purchased at the retail level and then prepared ready-to-eat prior to analysis. Results from this Total Diet Program provide the only information available in the United States on types and amounts of pesticides that remain in or on food as it is consumed. These results are compared with Acceptable Daily Intakes and serve as a measure from which food safety judgments can be made. The data also provide a means to identify trends and detect isolated contamination sources. In addition to pesticide residue data, the program also provides dietary intake information for radionuclides, toxic elements, essential minerals, and several types of industrial chemical contaminants. Emphasis, however, has been on pesticide residue data. Pennington and Gunderson (2) and Lombardo (3) provide in-depth discussions of the history and significance of this program. Reed et al. (4) discuss the design and purpose of all FDA pesticide monitoring activities. These references should be consulted for more details on FDA program goals.

This paper addresses FDA's analytical methods development history and does not attempt, in the brief space allotted, to review the entire field of pesticide residue methods. Analytical methods used in its regulatory activities include those with the capability to detect and measure several residues in a single analysis as well as those that detect a single residue or a limited number of related residues.

In most cases, single residue methods are supplied to EPA by the registrant of a pesticide during the process of approval for food use. Applicability of such methods need only be demonstrated on food items for which a residue tolerance is set. These methods are published in Volume II of FDA's Pesticide Analytical Manual (PAM) (5). They often involve complex and time-consuming analytical manipulations. Therefore, resources dictate that single residue methods are generally used only when it is known that a pesticide chemical, not recoverable by a multiresidue method, has been used or when information on its potential residue level is needed. In these situations, PAM II methods if applicable are used in selected surveys. A recent example is the use of a PAM II method for daminozide in apples.

On occasion, residue information and regulation are needed for a pesticide for which no adequate method exists, e.g., ethylene dibromide (EDB). Resources are then diverted to developing and validating a single residue method. Overall, single residue methods are employed, out of necessity, to analyze for selected residues by the FDA and other organizations seeking to test for suspected residues in a given food or category of foods. Judicious use of such methods is an important part of the FDA pesticide monitoring program.

Since spray history or environmental background of most samples is unknown, FDA method development efforts have concentrated on multiresidue methods. This work has continued for approximately 30 years and has sought to take advantage of advancements in analytical technologies as they have become available. Consultation of the scientific literature and contact with other researchers has allowed FDA to stay abreast of new approaches to analysis. Continuing interaction among analysts in FDA's 16 field laboratories and in headquarters has led to refinements that have improved reliability and efficiency.

Analytical method studies usually fall into one of the following categories: development of a new method or technique; expansion of an existing method's applicability to additional analytes and sample types; integration of new technology into an existing method; and validation of a method, technique, or modification. This paper provides an overview of the historical development of five multiresidue methods and illustrates how FDA's research in these categories has been applied to evolution of the methodology.

FDA investigators developing residue methods publish their findings in the scientific literature. Multiresidue methods most commonly used by FDA, along with associated supporting information, are compiled in Volume I of the PAM (5). Once analytical methods are developed, published, and proven reliable by a number of laboratories, a more formal process of validation usually occurs. Collaborative study under the auspices of the Association of Official Analytical Chemists (AOAC) is undertaken for selected methods and analyte/food combinations. Successful collaboration results in the method's adoption as "official" and publication in the AOAC's *Official Methods of Analysis* (OMA) (6).

Hill and Corneliussen (7) have published a comprehensive discussion on the needs and considerations related to official pesticide residue method validation. They emphasize that validation of methods and changes in methods are a long standing regulatory policy. Aside from being a usual laboratory practice, validation is mandated to ensure that analytical results will withstand scrutiny resulting from public overview and possible legal actions that may occur. By regulation (8, 9), both the OMA and PAM contain official validated methods for regulatory use. However, the degree of validation for inclusion in the OMA is more stringent than that required by the PAM.

Space in this paper does not permit extensive discussion of the application of methods. Two recent publications should be consulted, however, for discussions of why FDA develops analytical methods. Reed et al. (4) describe the goals and strategies of FDA pesticide programs, and McMahan and Burke (10) describe the application of analytical methodology in those programs. Topics critical to the valid application of the methods are covered in the latter; this includes discussions on limits of quantitation and quality assurance in the FDA laboratories.

Multiresidue Method Development: Background

Analytical methods for pesticide residues generally require a procedure for extracting residue(s), "cleanup" procedures to isolate residues of interest from other components, and techniques to measure residue level and confirm its identity. In a review article by Dewey (1), reference is made to use of pesticide bioassay as early as 1933 (12) for measuring residues of rotenone and its breakdown products. Though this may not be the genesis of pesticide residue analysis, it provided precedence for extensive research and application of bioassay techniques that continued until about 1960. This means of determination was both highly sensitive and multiresidue in scope. It also demonstrated good accuracy and sensitivity if a single pesticide residue were present and its identity known. However, for samples of unknown spray history, it could only be used to indicate whether a toxicant(s) was present. This type of information is of little use for regulatory purposes or for gathering exposure data. Con-

sequently, research activities were initiated to adapt sample extracts to other sensitive determinative techniques that would simultaneously offer qualitative and quantitative information. This need was fulfilled by chromatographic separation followed by a detection step.

Applied research in chromatographic separation and detection of multiple pesticide residues provided the greatest impact in evolution of current methodology. Initial work with paper and thin layer chromatographic (TLC) systems provided semiqualitative and semiquantitative information. Relatively poor chemical separations were achievable with a single chromatographic development and quantitation relied on visual estimations. These procedures were rapidly replaced with gas chromatographic (GC) systems that provided improved qualitative separations and quantitation capabilities with sensitive (and selective) electronic detectors. TLC continued to be used but primarily to confirm the identity of residues first detected by GC.

Ever since GC applications became commonplace, a continual growth has occurred in detector and column technologies. Many advances have been incorporated into FDA multiresidue applications only to be replaced by still newer refinements. It is expected that many of the current GC applications will again by replaced by capillary column technologies that currently provide greatly increased separation capabilities, once the latter are validated or defined to the extent needed for FDA regulatory purposes.

Multiresidue methods generally include single or multiple steps to extract, purify (clean up and concentrate) and detect several potential residues simultaneously. During the early developmental stage, each individual step is tested to illustrate and document its applicability and limitations. This testing is done with all, or at least several, representative chemicals and sample types for which the method is intended. Continual refinement then follows during routine applications as additional sample types and chemicals are tested. During this time, changes, additions, or minor modifications in the originally proposed steps can occur to expand the method's applicability.

The continual changes that have occurred in multiresidue methodologies are reflected by numerous revisions issued for PAM I. This manual was issued in 1963 and was updated with yearly changes until 1967. In 1968, it was completely revised, and the second edition was published. Twenty-five major and minor revisions have been issued since that time.

In the following discussions, specific examples of the evolution of the five principal multiresidue methods will be presented. Each method is published in PAM I and the OMA. The OMA version reflects applicability of the method as it was collaborated. The PAM version offers guidance to additional applications and options. Methods to be discussed are commonly referred to by the name(s) of the researcher(s) that is (are) recognized as the developer(s) of the originally proposed extraction and purification steps. The discussions will follow this convention.

Mills and Mills, Onley and Gaither Methods

These two methods are discussed together because several similarities exist in both their analytical principles and historic development. Collectively, they have been studied more than all other FDA multiresidue methods combined, and knowledge gained benefited development of later methods.

The Mills fatty food (13) was originally developed for determining residues of organochlorine (OC) pesticides in both fatty and nonfatty food products. Published in 1959, the method used paper chromatography in the determinative step. The nonfatty extraction steps were refined and resulted, in part, in the Mills, Onley and Gaither (MOG) nonfatty food method (14) in 1963. The extraction and cleanup steps described for fats, oils, cheese, milk, and animal tissue in the 1959 Mills paper are basically the same as those currently used for these products. Both the fatty food and MOG methods use a similar solvent partitioning step and an adsorption (Florisil) chromatographic purification step to clean up the extract. The original MOG method provided two determinative techniques, paper chromatography or GC.

The extensive expansion of these two basic procedures has been reviewed by Burke (15). In his article, Burke chronologically details, with supporting precedent data, the development and evolution of FDA's multiresidue methodology from its inception in 1959 to 1970. Most of the paper's 103 references are related to these two methods and include 21 different studies on variables in the method (e.g., Florisil quality, effect of moisture content of sample), 19 method extension reports, and nine AOAC collaborative studies that eventually led to recognition and expansion in the OMA. There were 24 reports describing GC applications, 11 describing related identity confirmation tests, and 19 for other reference purposes.

During this period, the number of chemicals that were known to be recovered by the original Mills fatty food method had expanded from 11 to 59 OC pesticides. Additionally, recoveries of nine organophosphorus (OP) pesticides were documented. The MOG procedure was initially published with a demonstrated ability to recover 5 representative OC pesticides from 11 products. By 1970, the recoverability of 84 pesticide (and related) chemicals was documented; 15 of these were OP pesticides. The combined methods were known to be applicable to about 450 different food products.

By 1970, the determinative step for both procedures had evolved from semiquantitative paper chromatography to quantitative GC determinations with an ever-expanding selection of element-specific or element-selective detectors. During 1959-1970, the following detectors were developed and applied to pesticide analysis: microcoulometric, electron capture (EC), alkali flame ionization (KC1TD) and its simultaneous operation with EC, flame photometric (FPD), and electrolytic conductivity. Mass spectrometry was also applied for confirmation of residue identity. Also during this period, GC behavioral characteristics of many pesticide chemicals (at specified conditions) were determined and tabulated to aid in identifying GC responses. This was accomplished primarily with two general purpose GC columns, but other specialty columns began to be developed for difficult separations and difficult-to-chromatograph polar chemicals.

Since 1970, expansion of the methods' proven capabilities has continued with five AOAC collaborative studies (16-20) and recovery information for additional pesticides and commodities. New chromatographic technologies continue to be introduced and older ones replaced. The methods have also been expanded for use in determining residues of industrial chemicals (e.g., polychlorinated biphenyls). Currently, PAM I Appendix I lists approximately 160 chemicals that are partially or completely recovered by the Mills fatty food method and approximately 215 by the MOG.

In 1987, of the 15,592 food and feed samples (21) analyzed by FDA laboratories, approximately 18 percent (2,827) were analyzed by one of these two methods. Usage and expansion are expected to continue, particularly with feed materials and fatty foods. These methods, originally designed for nonpolar OC compounds, do not recover many of the currently used pesticides and their metabolites. This limitation led to development of the Storherr method for the OP class of pesticides.

Storherr Method

As noted earlier, some of the OP class of pesticides are recovered quantitatively by the MOG method. However, many are polar or reactive and consequently are not recovered through the partitioning and/or Florisil cleanup steps of that procedure. Also, because of their polar or reactive nature, the OP pesticides are more difficult to determine by GC than the nonpolar OC pesticides.

The Storherr method is applicable to low and high moisture nonfatty foods (e.g., fruits, vegetables, grains) and, like the MOG method, it evolved from previous procedures designed for fly bioassay, paper chromatographic, and TLC determinative steps. Although method development for OP pesticides was being conducted concurrent with that for OC pesticides, researchers lacked selective GC detectors that were available for OC pesticides in the early 1960s. In 1964, Giuffrida (22) introduced the KC1TD, which was both sensitive and selective to OP chemicals. In the same year, Storherr et al. (23) published a method for OP determinations using this detector. The method demonstrated the detector's utility, but it did not extend recoverability to any chemicals beyond that achievable by the MOG procedure. Consequently, the detector was connected with the EC detectors used for OC analysis so simultaneous determination of some OP pesticides could be made. Thus, used in this way, the early Storherr method was an extension of the MOG method.

As Storherr et al. (23) noted, GC determination of the more polar OP pesticides was not possible at that time without development of different types of GC columns. In two separate studies in 1966 (24) and 1968 (25), GC columns containing diethylene glycol succinate (DEGS) were demonstrated to be compatible with polar OP pesticides. Storherr and Watts (26) investigated chromatographic properties of more than 60 OP and metabolite chemicals with DEGS and the commonly used silicone liquid phase columns. In a companion paper (27), the DEGS column was described for determining recoveries of highly polar OP chemicals in a method that used an ethyl acetate extractant and a charcoal column cleanup.

In 1971 (28) Storherr et al. changed the extraction step of the previous method so that it was identical to that used with the MOG. This improved overall analytical efficiency by enabling analysis for a wider variety of OP pesticides from a portion of the same extract prepared for MOG analysis. This method was collaboratively studied in 1974 (29) and is published in the OMA. The collaborative study also demonstrated equivalent performance of KC1TDs

and the newer FPDs that have been introduced for phosphorus selective detection in 1966 by Brody and Chaney (30). Unfortunately, determinations with DEGS columns could not be included in the collaborative test of the method because this material was not manufactured in a uniform manner; consequently its chromatographic performance proved extremely variable.

Prior to development of this method, other developments occurred in OP methodology that are still of interest. A study of the variation in different charcoals (27) set precedence for the cleanup step used in the Krause (31) method for N-methyl carbamates and an ancillary cleanup step in the Luke et al. (32) method. A distillation method of sample cleanup (sweep-codistillation), was developed (33) and collaboratively studied (34). The method was also investigated for use with OC pesticides (35, 36) and is of current interest because of recent commercial development and claimed efficiency (37). The commercial system, Unitrex®, is undergoing evaluation for FDA applications in multiresidue analyses.

The Storherr method had its most extensive use in FDA's Total Diet Program after modifications (38) were made to achieve lower limits of quantitation. Its application in the Total Diet Program and other FDA pesticide programs for high moisture products has now been essentially replaced by the Luke method. The method was referenced for use in only 13 analyses by FDA in 1987. The Luke method has also essentially replaced use of the MOG procedure for analysis of fresh fruits and vegetables.

Luke Method

This method, in one variation or another, was used in approximately 80 percent (11,922) of the 15,592 1987 FDA pesticide residue analyses. The evolution of this method's applicability and general acceptance has been in direct relationship to advances in GC technology since 1975.

The method (32) was proposed by FDA's Los Angeles pesticide analytical group and was designed to recover essentially all nonionic pesticides in the OC, OP, organonitrogen (ON) and hydrocarbon (HC) classes. The approach uses an acetone extractant, minimal cleanup and various GC systems with element-selective and element-specific detectors. The initial method determined residues of the OP and ON classes in a crude extract obtained after a solvent transfer step. These classes were to be determined with the KC1TD detector and use of two GC columns with methyl silicone and DEGS liquid phases. Separate portions of the extract were cleaned up with a modified MOG Florisil step prior to OC and HC determinations by GC with EC and flame ionization detectors, respectively. This approach could recover 15 OP, 9 OC, 5 ON, and 2 HC pesticides.

The major advantage of the Luke method when it was first proposed was an increase in efficiency of sample work up. Most chemicals initially studied could be recovered by existing multiresidue methods of Storherr, MOG, and Holden (39). The improvement in efficiency resulted from the modified MOG Florisil cleanup and substitution of acetone for acetonitrile (common to Storherr and MOG methods) as the extractant. Acetone eliminated the exhaustive concentration steps necessary for removing traces of acetonitrile if a KC1TD (acetonitrile sensitive) was used.

The Luke method was not immediately adopted outside the Los Angeles laboratory, however. Since FPDs were replacing KC1TDs in general use for OP determinations, residual acetonitrile was of diminishing concern, and efficiency claimed for the method seemed minimal. There also was an initial reluctance among chemists to subject GC systems to the crude sample extracts obtained by the method.

By 1977, several FDA laboratories realized the potential of this approach, and in 1978 the method was published in PAM I. However, the GC determinative steps were not well defined or rugged. Later in 1978, the first of several interlaboratory studies was initiated to standardize GTC conditions for use with this procedure. The first study addressed the troublesome DEGS chromatography (discussed in the Storherr method) with FPD detection. Satisfactory reproducibility was obtained with an improved quality of commercially available DEGS. Other studies with fortified samples in 1979, 1980, and 1981 showed that overall interlaboratory performance of the procedure was acceptable.

This method was further refined in 1981 when Luke et al. (40) reported that a satisfactory substitution of the EC detector could be accomplished with a newly designed Hall electrolytic conductivity detector for OC pesticide determinations. This refinement eliminated the need for Florisil cleanup and further increased the efficiency of analysis along with the potential for expanding recovery to additional compounds. After a successful interlaboratory study (41) of this detector's performance was completed, the method was successfully collaborated in 1983 (42) and was published in the OMA. This AOAC study included six pesticides that represented both OC and OP classes of pesticides. These are the only broad classes of chemicals for which the GC determination has AOAC official status, but the method is adaptable to any number of specialized determinative steps. The extraction and cleanup steps of this method have recently been proven adaptable to the multicarbamate detection of the Krause method (31).

Krause Method

This method is unique among the other multiresidue methods mentioned. It introduced high performance liquid chromatography (HPLC) for separation and fluorescence spectroscopy for detection. The HPLC method was developed after several GC approaches were investigated and considered inadequate for analysis for this class of pesticide chemicals.

FDA began monitoring for residues of one highly used carbamated insecticide (carbaryl) in the mid-1960s. The method was a semiquantitative TLC procedure (43) that also determined one carbaryl metabolite. In 1973, Holden (39) published a multiresidue method with a GC determinative step that recovered 13 chemicals of the carbamate class. It used the same extraction step as the MOG procedure, and GC conditions were basically those used for OC pesticide determinations; however, it required that residues be derivatized in order to be detected by the GC system. The method was officially collaborated in 1974 (44) and published in the OMA. For the most part, method performance was satisfactory. However, it was lengthy and interferences were common. A purified derivatization reagent was needed, and proper GC conditions were difficult to maintain. It also failed to recover some metabolites and two of the most widely used pesticides of this class, benomyl and methomyl. These two pesticides are thermally unstable and not amenable to GC analysis.

To overcome these inherent problems, Krause (31) adapted the HPLC approach pioneered by Moye et al. (45) for the determinative step. Besides HPLC separation and fluorescence detection, this approach featured a unique two step, in-line chemical reaction and derivation process. In developing the total method, a modification of a partitioning step used in Holden's procedure and a charcoal column cleanup based on the Storherr method were included. The extraction step was extensively studied and validated (46, 47) with ^{14}C labeled carbamate pesticides that were field-incurred. Another feature of the method is a refrigerated rotary evaporation step, which minimized losses attributable to thermal degradation.

After this method became generally available, it was 3 years before the method could be collaboratively studied. This time was needed so that a sufficient number of laboratories could obtain needed equipment and develop necessary expertise. The collaborative study was completed in 1984 (48) and the method is in the OMA.

This method is capable of recovering approximately 16 parent and metabolite chemicals of the N-methyl carbamate class. It also has shown the ability to recover certain other chemicals (49). In 1987, FDA analyzed only 34 samples by this method in its entirety, but the HPLC detection step was used with 588 other samples. Currently, the faster Luke sample work up is usually used in place of that initially researched and collaborated. A recovery study that supports the validity of this combination of methods has been completed (50). The primary use of the complete Krause method is to confirm levels of regulatory significance when found by the rapid approach.

Multiresidue Method Development: Summary

These necessarily brief discussions of the most widely used FDA multiresidue methods exemplify the constant evolution that has occurred, and is occurring, as new technologies are made available and experience with method performance is gained. They also illustrate the historical time that has elapsed from the first proposal of a method to completion of a successfully collaborated official method, about 10 years. By the time the Storherr, Holden, and Krause methods had gained official status, they were already being modified or preferentially replaced by more efficient procedures. The popular Luke method has been modified for use in FDA's Total Diet Program (51). [Note: Total Diet multiresidue methodology development and evolution have roughly followed those of the general methods, but this methodology is specialized enough that it warrants a separate discussion, which is not included here. The previously referenced (2) review article of the 26-year history of this program should be consulted for further details.]

Expanding the number of compounds recovered by multiresidue methods provides FDA with improved coverage of potential residues within existing monitoring programs. For this reason, FDA has committed resources every year to testing additional chemicals through existing methods. A computerized system, called Pestrak, has been developed to track the current status of data about compounds known to be recovered through each of the methods discussed here (10).

The constant hybridization of methods has made it difficult to describe which chemicals are recovered through any particular methods. Certain variations in all the basic methods can be, and are, employed to address particularly difficult analyte/food combinations. This may be accomplished through variation in any of the steps of the method, such as changing the extraction, modifying the cleanup, use of special GC columns or detectors, etc. Validation of the resulting method variation is an integral part of the process. FDA currently defines analytical method codes for 59 individual extraction/cleanup variations and 23 determinative steps for recording multiresidue method analysis results in its residue data system. Up to 20 of the extraction/cleanup codes apply to the MOG procedure alone. Specific knowledge of the capabilities of each of these steps and of exactly how they were applied determines the recovery capability of an analysis, not of a method per se.

Multiresidue methods are often criticized for their inability to produce rapid regulatory answers for samples collected for monitoring purposes. In reality, these methods, with modifications, are readily adaptable to provide this type of information when a specific pesticide/commodity problem has been identified or is suspected. In these situations, it is also not uncommon to utilize less formalized methods such as those found in FDA's Laboratory Information Bulletins or the scientific literature to facilitate rapid analyses. Much of the analytical data generated under these circumstances is semiquantitative. Examples of such rapid testing occurred in two recent widely publicized misuse situations: aldicarb in California watermelons and heptachlor metabolites in milk from an Arkansas dairy shed.

Application of such techniques, as used by FDA laboratories in the above instances, greatly increased sample throughput. However, this practice fails to detect other potential residues present in legal or illegal amounts. Since illegal residues occur in only a small percentage of samples, and other residues are routinely detected, classical multiresidue analytical approaches provide a better measure of the total pesticide residue burden in the food supply. Usage of such methods is applicable for those specific pesticide/commodity situations in which there is an identified need for rapid analysis and such analyses are carried out on a planned and coordinated basis to allow proper interpretation of the findings.

Multiresidue Method Development: The Future

Method development for pesticide residues is expected to continue evolving as it has in the past; researchers will apply and adapt technology, as it becomes available, to meet the needs resulting from pesticide usage and environmental contamination. Multiresidue methods are still the most effective way to examine food samples of unknown treatment history and so they will be used where applicable. Existing methods will continue to be used and expanded wherever practical. Special attention will be given to use of new determinative techniques.

However, new methods for residues not amenable to existing methods must be developed, and these will be multiresidue methods wherever possible. The method proposal by Clower for determination of a number of volatile fumigants (52) is an example.

New methods will be applicable to fewer residues than most of those described here because they involve chemicals whose structures vary widely and preclude easy separation and detection by today's technology. Method development for chemicals not recovered by existing methods may well follow the approach taken in developing the Krause method, in which a very selective determinative step was developed to focus on a relatively small group of chemically related residues.

Current examples of this approach include the Hopper method for chlorophenoxy acetic acid residues (53), the Luchtefeld method for phenylurea herbicides (54), and an ongoing effort within FDA's Pesticides and Industrial Chemicals Research Center to develop methods for compounds with benzimidazole structures, for the "quat" family (paraquat, etc.), and for organic tin compounds. Within the Division of Contaminants Chemistry, work continues to develop methods for residues with substitute aniline and nitro aromatic structures.

Technologies currently available and being tested for adaptability in multiresidue methodology include selective HPLC detection using photoconductivity and electrochemical detectors, capillary column chromatography, and simplified cleanup steps such as solid phase extraction and distillation (Unitrex®) techniques. Attempts continue to find a stable and reproducible GC detector that is selective for ON compounds. Other technologies yet to be applied broadly in residue monitoring include supercritical fluid chromatography and immunoassay techniques.

Certain analytical techniques that have been available for many years are still not used routinely in residue analysis. Mass spectrometry is used extensively for identification and confirmation of residue identity, but it has not been adapted to routine analysis because of its cost and the degree of expertise required to maintain the system. More routine use of mass spectrometry is expected in the future, however.

Portions of methods can be routinely automated. Equipment that is manufactured with microprocessor control units, such as automated injectors for chromatographs, is one example. The likelihood that complete methods will be automated within the next 10 years is small because of the diverse sample types that are encountered and the individual challenges that each poses.

A commonly acknowledged disadvantage of existing multiresidue methods is their "macro" design, which is based on analysis of a 100 g portion of sample. This analytical portion is larger than those used in recently developed methods and results in increased analytical expense from greater volumes of solvents required. This macro scale approach was initially validated with the MOG procedure and subsequently copied in other methods to assure that the size of the analytical portion would be representative of the amount of food collected (10-20 lbs.). A current FDA study is statistically addressing analytical sample size and homogeneity issues to establish a basis for reduction in sample and solvent volumes. Findings of this study should have a major impact on future method development efforts as well as future usage of current methods in "scaled down" versions. The ultimate goal is to achieve more rapid and efficient methodology without sacrificing analytical integrity.

The cleanup step is often a limitation in residue methods because it generally consumes a large amount of the total analysis time and restricts the number of pesticides that are recovered. Development of new, more effective or efficient approaches to removing unwanted materials in sample extracts, while minimizing the restrictions on number of residues recovered, would significantly improve analytical capability. Automation of cleanup procedures offers a partial solution in that it frees the analyst for other tasks. Application of automated cleanup procedures is itself severely limited however, since efficient use of automation requires that a large number of predictable analyses be planned for similar samples. As noted throughout this paper, development of determinative procedures that can tolerate extracts with less stringent cleanups will be a dominant factor in considering the cleanup issue.

Most of the above focuses on enhancement and adaptation of the type of methodology most widely employed in residue monitoring. Screening methods, e.g., immunoassay methods, may provide a useful extension to residue monitoring activities in the future. Although the concept of screening is not new, screening is defined and used in a number of different ways by regulatory agencies and others. One type of screening is aimed at providing rapid "yes/no" answers for one or more selected residues at specified levels, usually levels of regulatory interest in a compliance situation. A positive result would trigger reanalysis by more conventional and time-consuming quantitative methods. Although this screening would permit analyses of more samples, the time savings could be reduced or eliminated if followup analyses had to be conducted on a large proportion of the samples. The real gain in efficiency will thus need to be considered before screening analyses are applied.

Coverage for certain selected residues might increase with addition of screening methods. However, designing the monitoring program to incorporate these methods will require careful planning. The need to be able to summarize and evaluate data from diverse methods will remain a dominant factor.

Because residue analysis is so challenging and its successful application relies so heavily on the expertise of the analyst, development of new personnel is of critical importance to FDA. Within the next 10 years, the majority of today's FDA pesticide experts will have become eligible for retirement; recruitment and training of their replacements are vital considerations to the agency.

Impacts of Laws and Regulations

The laws and regulations governing the use of pesticides on foods in the United States have had a necessary impact on the development of the analytical methods used to enforce those laws. In turn, the capabilities and limitations of the methods have sometimes indirectly caused changes to be made in the regulations.

Two amendments to the Food, Drug and Cosmetics Act originally provided the basis on which the requirements for pesticide residue analytical methods depend: the Miller Pesticide Residue Amendment of 1954 and Food Additives Amendment of 1958. These laws established the concept of toler-

ances to describe the maximum residue limits of individual chemicals that would be permitted on specified foods. These limits in turn established the analyte concentration levels at which analytical methods would be required to function reliably.

The practical imperative for multiresidue analytical methods was also provided by these two amendments because they permitted more than one pesticide on a single food commodity. (Unknown spray histories for most foods and inadvertent pesticide contamination of nontarget foods provide other reasons for the reliance on multiresidue methods.)

Early laws established zero tolerances for certain pesticides in certain commodities. The abandonment of this concept was dictated by advancements in analytical methodologym which permitted determination of ever-diminishing quantities of residue and made the zero tolerance concept impractical. In a similar way, practical analytical capabilities are taken into account when reducing tolerances or action levels for pesticides whose uses have been suspended, and in setting action levels for unavoidable contamination from environmental sources.

In actual practice, FDA's analytical methods are applied at limits of quantitation sufficiently below the tolerance levels to provide data on incidence and levels of residues (both above and below tolerances) in the food supply, while still being realistic in terms of the effort required for each analysis. These data are vital for evaluation of pesticide regulations. Typical examples are the following: (1) FDA data for DDT findings from 1964 to 1969 were used in 1970 to reassess tolerances and resulted in cancellation of registration for certain uses and lower tolerances for other uses; (2) FDA's historic findings of aldrin and dieldrin were pertinent in the cancellation hearings of these pesticides; (3) FDA's lindane findings from 1964 to 1980 were used by EPA in its Special Review (56) to calculate the changing dietary exposure to lindane residues; (4) FDA data on methomyl residues from 1978 to 1987 are being used by EPA in its tolerance reassessment for re-registration of this pesticide; and (5) FDA data are used to assist in setting action levels for a pesticide when its use is suspended and the corresponding tolerance is no longer applicable.

FDA's monitoring program also directs agency laboratories to maintain uniform limits of quantitation below tolerance levels since levels for a given pesticide are not the same for all commodities. Tolerances for permethrin, chlorpyrifos and dimethoate in apples and peaches illustrate this complexity. Tolerances for these pesticides on apples are 0.05, 1.5, and 2.0 ppm. respectively. The corresponding tolerances on peaches are 5.0, 0.05, and none since dimethoate is not registered for use on peaches. Analytical procedures for both sample types are identical and cannot be readily adjusted for a given tolerance/commodity combination. In most cases, such adjustment would not result in significant savings in analytical cost or time.

EPA regulations have long required that registrants provide an enforcement method for each tolerance being requested. As mentioned earlier, these methods constitute the bulk of PAM II. Since PAM II is the reference of first choice when a single residue method is needed, it is important that the methods be reliable. Registrants must be encouraged to adhere to the spirit of this requirement and provide methods usable by regulatory laboratories without excessive adaptation.

A more recent EPA requirement (56) has permitted the expansion of FDA multiresidue methods to newly introduced pesticides. Registrants must determine analytical behavior of a new pesticide through these methods. This additional information provides FDA, state governments, and the food industry with better tools to inform consumers about pesticide residues in food. Availability of this information also frees research resources of these institutions to concentrate on development of methods for the more difficult compounds.

Certain recent situations have demonstrated that establishment of different acceptable residue levels by different government bodies have a profound impact on regulatory decisions, which in turn affect the development and application of residue methodology. The international organization, Codex, is seeking to remedy the international level of this dilemma by proposing pesticide maximum residue limits for adoption by member countries. This effort is expected to become more important as the level of international trade increases.

The Food and Agriculture Organization (FAO) of the United Nations and the World Health Organization (WHO) cooperate in a program that collects information from 34 countries on levels of pollutants in foods and other environmental samples. This Food Contamination Monitoring Programme is designed to assess human exposure and allow estimates of health threats caused by such pollutants. One of the main objectives of this portion of the Global Environment Monitoring System is to provide Codex with levels of pesticide residues in food to assist that organization in its determination of maximum residue limits. FDA's data base of quantitative residue data has permitted the United States to contribute requested data to this program throughout its history.

References

1. Gunderson, E.L. and Reed, D.V., FDA, personal communications, April 1988.
2. Pennington, J.A.T. and Gunderson, E.L., *J. Assoc. Off. Anal. Chem.* 70:772-782, 1987.
3. Lombardo, P., *Environmental Epidemiology*, 141-148, (1986).
4. Reed, D.V., Lombardo, P., Wessel, J.R., et al., *J. Assoc. Off. Anal. Chem.* 70:591-595, 1987.
5. Pesticide Analytical Manual (1987) Vol. I and II, Food and Drug Administration, Washington, DC.
6. Official Methods of Analysis (1984) 14th ed. (including annual supplements), Association of Official Chemists, Arlington, VA, Chapter 29, General Multiresidue Methods.
7. Hill, K.R. and Corneliussen, P.E., *Analytical Methods for Pesticides and Plant Growth Regulators XV*, 111-132, 1986.
8. 21 *CFR* 1987 ed. 2.19.
9. 40 *CFR* 1987 ed. 180.101(c).
10. McMahon, B.M. and Burke, J.A. *J. Assoc. Off. Anal. Chem.* 70:1072-1081, 1987.
11. Dewey, J.E., *J. Agric. Food Chem.* 6:274-281, 1958.
12. Jones, H.A., Gersdorff, W.A., Gooden, E.L., et al., *J. Econ. Entom.* 26:451-470, 1933.
13. Mills, P.A., *J. Assoc. Off. Agric. Chem.* 42:734-740, 1959.
14. Mills, P.A., Onley, J.J., and Gaither, R.A., *J. Assoc. Offic. Agric. Chem.* 46:186-191, 1963.
15. Burke, J.A., *Residue Reviews* 34:59-90, 1971.
16. Krause, R.T., *J. Assoc. Off. Anal. Chem.* 56:721-727, 1973.
17. Sawyer, L.D., *J. Assoc. Off. Anal. Chem.* 56:1015-1023, 1973.
18. Finsterwalder, C.E., *J. Assoc. Off. Anal. Chem.* 59:169-171, 1976.
19. Mitchell, L.R., *J. Assoc. Off. Anal. Chem.* 59: 209-212, 1976.
20. Sawyer, L.D., *J. Assoc. Off. Anal. Chem.* 61:282-291, 1978.
21. Gartrell, M.J., Food and Drug Administration, personal communication, February 1988.
22. Giuffrida, L., *J. Assoc. Off. Agric. Chem.* 47:293-300, 1964.
23. Storherr, R.W., Getz, M. E., Watts, R.R., et al., *J. Assoc. Off. Agric. Chem.* 47:1087-1093, 1964.
24. Takehara, A. and Takeshita, T., *J. Agric. Chem. Soc. Japan* 40:394-400, 1966.
25. Beroza, M. and Bowman, M.C., *Environ. Sci. Technol.* 2:450-457, 1968.
26. Watts, R.R. and Storherr, R.W., *J. Assoc. Off. Anal. Chem.* 52:513-521, 1969.

27. Watts, R.R., Storherr, R.R., and Pardue, J.R., *J. Assoc. Off. Anal. Chem.* 54:522-525, 1969.

28. Storherr, R.W., Ott, P., and Watts, R.R., *J. Assoc. Off. Anal. Chem.* 54:513-516, 1971.

29. Laski, R.R., *J. Assoc. Off. Anal. Chem.* 57:930-933, 1974.

30. Brody, S.S. and Chaney, J.E., *J. Gas Chromatog.* 4:42-46, 1966.

31. Krause, R.T., *J. Assoc. Off. Anal. Chem.* 63:1114-1124, 1980.

32. Luke, M.A., Froberg, J.E., and Masumoto, H.T., *J. Assoc. Off. Anal. Chem.* 58:1020-1026, 1975.

33. Storherr, R.W. and Watts, R.R., *J. Assoc. Off. Anal. Chem.* 48:1154-1158, 1965.

34. Storherr, R. W. and Watts, R.R., *J. Assoc. Off. Anal. Chem.* 51:662-665, 1968.

35. Storherr, R.W., Murray, E.J., Klein, I., et al., *J. Assoc. Off. Anal. Chem.* 50:605-615, 1967.

36. Malone, B. and Burke, J.A., *J. Assoc. Off. Anal. Chem.* 52:790-797, 1970.

37. Luke, B.G., Richards, J.C., and Dawes, E.F. *J. Assoc. Off. Anal. Chem.* 67:295-298, 1984.

38. Carson, L.J., *J. Assoc. Off. Anal. Chem.* 64:714-719, 1981.

39. Holden, E.R., *J. Assoc. Off. Anal. Chem.* 56:713-717, 1973.

40. Luke, M.A., Froberg, J.E. and Masumoto, H.T., *J. Assoc. Off. Anal. Chem.* 64:1187-1195, 1981.

41. Carson, L.J., *J. Assoc. Off. Anal. Chem.* 66:1344-1355, 1983.

42. Sawyer, L.D., *J. Assoc. Off. Anal. Chem.* 68:64-71, 1985.

43. Finocchiaro, J.M. and Benson, W.R., *J. Assoc. Off. Agric. Chem.* 48:736-738, 1965.

44. Holden, E.R., *J. Assoc. Off. Anal. Chem.* 58:562-565, 1975.

45. Moye, H.A., Scherer, S.J. and St. John, P. A., *Anal. Lett.* 10: 1049-1073, 1977.

46. Wheeler, W.B., FDA Contract 223-74-2223 (1974) University of Florida, Gainesville, FL.

47. Wheeler, W.B., FDA Contract 223-76-2220 (1976) University of Florida, Gainesville, FL.

48. Krause, R.T., *J. Assoc. Off. Anal. Chem.* 68:726-733, 1985.

49. Krause, R.T., *J. Assoc. Off. Anal. Chem.* 66:234-240, 1983.

50. Pardue, J.R., *FDA Laboratory Information Bulletin 3138,* 1987.

51. Hopper, M.L., *J. Assoc. Off. Anal. Chem.* (in press).

52. Clower, M.G., *J. Assoc. Off. Anal. Chem.* 63:539-545, 1980.

53. Hopper, M. L., *J. Agric. Food Chem.* 35:256-269, 1987.

54. Luchtefeld, R.G., *J. Assoc. Off. Anal. Chem.* 70:740-745, 1987.

55. *Fed. Regist.* (Oct. 19, 1983), 48 (203), 48,516.

56. *Fed. Regist.* (Sept. 26, 1986), 51 (187), 34,249-34, 250.

Pesticide Design: Outlook for the Future

Jack R. Plimmer, and Kenneth R. Hill, Environmental Chemistry Laboratory, Natural Resources Institute

Julius J. Menn, Plant Sciences Institute, Agricultural Research Center, Agricultural Research Service, U.S. Department of Agriculture, Beltsville, MD 20705

Contents

	Page
Abstract	123
Introduction	124
Economics	124
Screening	125
Safety	126
Resistance	126
Design of New Pesticides	127
Emerging Classes of Compounds: Examples of Specific Analytical Problems	129
The Utility of Pesticide/Pest Chemical Interactions	131
Conclusions	132
References	134

Figures

Figure	Page
1. Structures of Representative Synthetic Pyrethroids	126
2. Biphenylmethylpyrethroid Series (Plummer)	128
3. Sulfonyl Ureas	129
4. Separation of Pyrethroids on GLC	131

Tables

Table	Page
1. Ten Most Widely Used Herbicides and Insecticides in the USA	125
2. The Quantitative Structure Activity Relationships of Some Benzoyl Phenyl Urea Larvicides	128
3. Recommended Application Rates of Selected Pyrethroids	130
4. Relative Mammalian Toxicities of Selected Pyrethroids	131

Abstract

The need to analyze pesticide residues in food and drinking water for regulatory purposes creates increasingly complex analytical problems because so many diverse molecular types must be determined in a large variety of crops or foods. Multiresidue procedures (MRPs) are important because a method must detect as many pesticides as possible and it must be applicable to samples of unknown treatment history.

For a number of reasons, including the high costs of development and safety tests, reduced success in screening programs, and pest resistance, the number of pesticides entering the U.S. market has decreased in recent years. However, there continues to be a strong demand for pesticides, particularly herbicides, and this is likely to continue into the future. Despite rapid progress in fundamental aspects of biotechnology, its widespread application to pest control technology will proceed at a steady pace because many questions of safety must be answered.

New biochemical and biological knowledge is important in developing new leads for synthesis, and quantitative structure activity relationships are guiding the optimization of promising, active molecules. Complexity may increase as products of microbial metabolism (such as the avermectins) are found to be pest control agents.

Extremely low rates of application result in low residue levels, and the detection and quantitation of such low levels presents a considerable challenge to analytical chemists and designers of instrumentation. The sulfonylureas and the pyrethroids are two examples of classes of pesticides that may be used at very low rates of application and, in consequence, require analytical methods capable of determining residues at the parts-per-billion level.

Novel methods of analysis (such as biosensors) are being developed, and immunoassay techniques are increasing their range of applicability and sensitivity. The latter are beginning to meet the need for simple and rapid screening procedures that may simplify the task of the analyst.

A consequence of the increased complexity and the potent biological activity of new pesticide molecules is the need for more sensitive methods of detection and improved methods of separation. Multiresidue methods will continue to be adaptable to many new compounds. It is recommended that information concerning their applicability to new compounds be made readily available.

Introduction

There is increasing awareness among consumers of the potential of man-made chemicals to contaminate sources of food and drinking water. There is particular concern over the implications of food contamination by pesticide residues. The capability of analytical techniques to detect extremely low levels of trace contaminants has continually expanded. However, knowledge of the toxicological significance of such contaminants has not progressed at the same rate. It is also important to bear in mind that the study of the effects of individual compounds on biological organisms does not provide satisfactory information concerning the biological effects of several interacting compounds.

Residue analysis may be conducted for several purposes. The registration and use of a pesticide is preceded by supervised trials to determine the rate of disappearance. Residues on raw agricultural commodities must also be determined.

For regulatory and monitoring purposes, residues in food for human consumption and residues in environmental samples must be determined in samples that do not have a known treatment history. Therefore, procedures must be employed that can detect as many pesticides as possible in the most economical way. Multiresidue procedures (MRPs) are used for this purpose, and these are usually limited to the parent compound and closely related compounds. An excellent survey of the scope and capabilities of MRPs appeared in a recent International Union of Pure and Applied Chemistry report (3).

Rapid developments in analytical technology contribute to, but cannot be equated with, improved ability to determine the presence and amounts of contaminants in food. Much progress has been limited to the analysis of specific analytes or groups of analytes. Before beginning an overview of developments in agricultural chemicals, it should be stressed that the problem of analysis requires for its solution that we consider both *analyte and matrix*. The former is the compound of interest, a definition that is often extended to cover not only the parent compound but also its metabolites and transformation products; the latter refers to the particular crop or food type for which the information is desired.

The magnitude of this problem can be gauged by considering the efforts of the Codex Alimentarius Committee on Pesticide Residues (CCPR), which has established minimum residue levels for 150 compounds and more than 2,500 pesticide/commodity combinations over a period of 20 years (10). Multiresidue procedures are essential if it is necessary to determine as many pesticides as possible in various types of matrices. The complexity of the problem will increase in future years as new classes and types of pest control agents are introduced in response to a variety of constraints.

Economics

There is little likelihood that agricultural production and pest control will abandon their prime reliance on chemical methods of pest control in the coming decades, although there will be greater emphasis on the use of biological controls and technology that will contribute to the reduction of pesticide use. The market for agrochemicals continues to grow but more slowly than in the past. In the United States, there was an 8 percent decline in cropland from 1986 to 1987, and it was predicted that pesticide use would decrease 9 percent during that period (30). A market study predicted that herbicide growth would be most rapid primarily for corn and soybeans with a growth of about 5.3 percent per annum to a value of $3.47 billion. Expansion would emphasize new compounds (such as the imidazolinone and sulfonyl urea herbicides) that possess new modes of action and are used at extremely low rates. The synthetic pyrethroids that now account for about one-third of world insecticide use (27) would lead the way in insect control, and new fungicides, primarily the ergosterol biosynthesis inhibitors, would be emphasized. Table 1 indicates the herbicides and insecticides that are currently most widely used in the United States.

Economics of pesticide production is a major factor in change. The end of patent protection for a number of compounds of major importance means that there will be a shift to a commodity market with a more competitive approach. Pesticide manufacture is also becoming consolidated. Foreign buyers have now acquired many U.S. businesses. The agrochemical market is international, but the developing countries' market has not materialized to the extent anticipated. New compounds are slow to appear on the market. Successful introductions have dropped from 60 new compounds between the 1950s and '60s to 21 between the 1970s and '80s. Because the costs of research, development, and market introduction have increased to about $40 million per compound according to data developed in 1982 (22), the market will be largely restricted to major international companies who will emphasize the needs of major world crop markets. Profitability continues to be limited by the time that elapses between discovery, market introduction, and patent expiration. About 13 years is needed to reach a break-even point after discovery.

The food producer must also cope with major constraints because the cost of pesticide development is passed on unaccompanied by any increase in farm prices. Thus, the farmer must continually review the cost of all chemical inputs to adjust pesticide and fertilizer use to maximize his return. To attain this goal in part may be practicable if substantially lower rates of application can be achieved by using pesticides of greater biological effectiveness and by using better application technology.

Screening

Although there is little doubt that synthetic chemical pesticides will continue to be the main weapon in our crop protection arsenal in the next 10 to 20 years, the rate of new compound introductions has dramatically decreased in recent years. This decrease is largely due to the reduced number of companies engaged in agrochemical research and development, to the difficulty in discovering viable new pesticides by the process of empirical synthesis and screening, and to cost and safety considerations.

The rate of commercial success from screening to market development has fallen from 1 in 1,800 in 1956 to 1 in 15,000 in 1979 (21), and this adverse ratio is expected to increase in the coming years. From the 1950s through the 1970s, the majority of insecticides were neurotoxicants represented by chlorinated hydrocarbons, carbamates, and organophosphorus esters. These pesticides have similar modes of action in insects and vertebrate species, including humans. Today, the largest class of insecticides in use are the synthetic pyrethroids, which are also neurotoxicants. Representatives of this class are shown in figure 1.

At present, the major agrochemical companies are directing greater efforts and resources toward more fundamental research to discover novel classes of pesticides. Morrod (23) discussed approaches to current and future directions for discovery involving the following: novel synthesis, speculative biological chemistry, directed synthesis, natural product ana-

Table 1.—Ten Most Widely Used Herbicides and Insecticides in the USA

Herbicides		Insecticides	
Common name	Trade name	Common name	Trade name
alachlor	Lasso	aldicarb	Temik
atrazine	Aatrex	carbaryl	Sevin
butylate	Sutan	carbofuran	Furadan
cyanazine	Bladex	chlorpyrifos	Dursban
2,4-D	many	malathion	Cythion
glyphosate	Roundup	methyl parathion	Penncap
metolachlor	Dual	parathion	Folidol
metribuzin	Sencor	phorate	Thimet
propanil	Stam	synthetic pyrethroids	many
trifluralin	Treflan	terbufos	Counter

SOURCE: P.C. Kearney, A.R. Isensee, and J.R. Plimmer, "Contribution of Agricultural Pesticides to Worldwide Chemical Distribution," *Toxic Contamination in Large Lakes*, vol. III, N.W. Schmidke, Lewis, Chelsea, MI, 1988.

Figure 1.—Structures of Representative Synthetic Pyrethroids

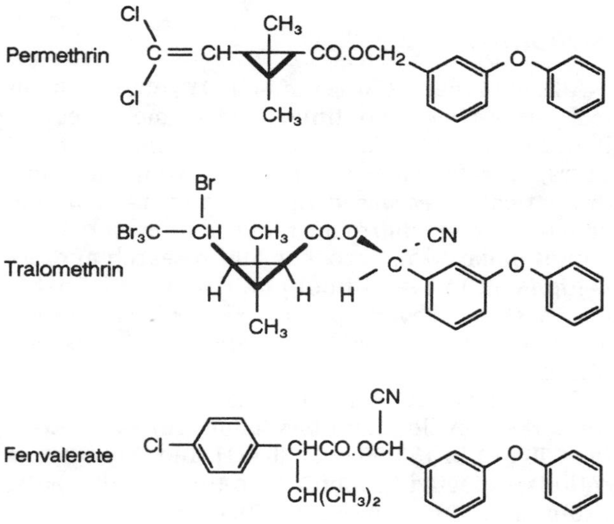

Permethrin

Tralomethrin

Fenvalerate

SOURCE: C.R. Worthing ed., *Pesticide Manual*, 8th edition, British Crop Protection Council, Thornton Heath, U.K., 1987.

log synthesis, and greater reliance on quantitative structure-activity relationship (QSAR) methods.

Safety

An important part of the high cost of a pesticide is the continual increase in the cost of safety tests. Environmental consequences and health effects of pesticide use continue to be major topics of public and regulatory concern. Testing for acute and latent toxicity is a substantial portion of the cost of pesticide development. These costs and the regulatory implications of such factors as the production of oncogenic responses in test animals substantially influence the current directions of chemical innovation. A recent National Academy of Sciences study on the issue of pesticide residues in food has addressed some controversial issues involved in pesticide regulation, especially as they pertain to the Delaney Clause (26).

Because the environmental behavior of a pesticide is largely determined by its chemical structure, the constraints on the selection of structural classes continue to be more pressing. For example, the contamination of groundwater by pesticides may result from agricultural use under certain conditions depending on soil, crop, method of application, etc. Although the amounts reaching groundwater may be well below the limits deemed as potentially harmful to human health, the fact that such trace amounts

are present was not predicted on the basis of existing knowledge at the time of registration. Aldicarb, alachlor and atrazine are among the compounds detected in groundwater, and a number of survey programs are planned or in progress to determine the scope of the problem.

Studies are being undertaken to detect precise conditions under which contamination occurs and to limit its occurrence by changes in pest management practice. However, the recognition that the major contributing factors are the soil environment (e.g., soil fractives; channels; agricultural practices; microbial activity; moisture; clay, mineral, and organic matter content; etc.) and the structure and physical properties of the pesticide molecule (e.g., rate of degradation in soil, water solubility, vapor pressure, partition coefficient between water and soil, organic matter, etc.) lead to the conclusion that pesticide design must take into account leachability or the potential for biologically active materials to move vertically in soil to groundwater.

The regulatory foundation for safety issues will continue as a major factor in the design of chemicals. The emerging issues include the U.S. Environmental Protection Agency (EPA) actions to bring the Federal Insecticide, Fungicide and Rodenticide Act (FIFRA) into compliance with the Endangered Species Act in the United States, beginning in 1988. This action will prohibit pesticide use in specified areas that are the habitats of endangered species. The issues of health and safety are not only of concern to the consumer. Farmers, formulators, applicators, and field workers are by their occupations exposed to pesticides. Home and garden use is also an important safety consideration. Thus, the scope of regulation extends over a wide range of activities.

Thus, only a limited number of structural types will be considered for development as they emerge from the elaborate program of safety testing. Analytical considerations will follow these dictates in so far as they are part of the accountability needs during the process.

Resistance

A further constraint on molecular design is the problem of pest resistance to pesticides. Insecticides are particularly susceptible, and reliance on chemical classes that possess closely related modes of action or similar target sites hastens the obsolescence of particular classes of compounds. The response of the manufacturer is to broaden the chemical screen to search for new modes of action, and several classes of insecticides and herbicides introduced in recent years reflect this consideration. As an example, diflubenzuron may be considered the first of the commercially introduced chitin synthesis inhibitors. Chitin, the skeletal material of insects, is absent in man and vertebrates. Innovative pesticide design and the search for alternatives will continue to challenge the potential development of resistance.

In summary, many factors have combined to create pressure to reduce the use of pesticides in food production. These include economic and regulatory pressures at the producer and farm level. In addition, changes in agricultural management (for example, adoption of conservation tillage, change in land use, and new irrigation and application systems) and formulations have contributed to the evolution of new agrochemicals. Although biological control and developments in biotechnology will contribute to decreased reliance on chemicals, it is probable that at least a decade will elapse before a substantial contribution can be expected from such sources. These changes will then be accompanied by shifts in regulatory emphasis. The current problem of analysis of pesticides may be relatively less complex than the problem of satisfying the safety concerns arising from new technologies.

Design of New Pesticides

As discussed previously, more rational approaches are needed to improve the odds for developing a successful, marketable pesticide chemical.

In recent years, there have been considerable advances in the understanding of basic biology, biochemistry, and the physiology of host and target species. In addition, there is improved understanding about the site of action and effects of pesticides at the molecular, cellular, and whole organism levels. These have contributed substantially to rationalization of approaches to molecular design of pesticides. Research discoveries as related to bioactivity have been greatly aided by the development of regression functions that form the basis of QSAR.

QSAR combines elements of quantum chemistry, biodata, and computerization to fit parameters predefined by biochemical processes. Knowledge derived from this methodology should provide a better foundation for the rational design of novel, highly active, and environmentally sound crop and livestock protection chemicals. More detailed aspects of QSAR in pesticide design were reported in a symposium on this topic (17).

The following examples illustrate the utility of QSAR in optimizing synthesis and bioactivity.

Nakagawa et al. (24) described the optimization of quantitative structure-activity of benzoylphenylurea larvicides with reference to substituents at the aniline moiety against the major rice insect pest, the rice stem borer (*Chilo suppressalis* Walker).

Table 2 shows the empirical formula for a series of N-2,6-difluoro and N-2,6-dichlorobenzoyl-N'-(4-substituted phenyl)ureas and the regression equation parameters used in the QSAR analysis to predict optimal insect (chitin synthesis inhibition) activity. The analysis was performed with each compound synergized with piperonyl butoxide (PB) to reduce metabolic degradative effects in the insect.

Also included in table 2 is the resultant analysis for four compounds in the series. Activity is enhanced by electron withdrawing (σp) and hydrophobic substituents (π) and reduced by bulky groups (ΔB).

Plummer (28) succeeded in designing a novel series of highly active biphenylmethylpyrethroids through the QSAR approach. His success was specially significant since it came when the field appeared to be already saturated with synthetic pyrethroids.

From these studies, Plummer concluded that where X = F or CH3, activity was optimal resulting from the conformational preference of these compounds for a twist angle at about 50° involving ring B. The latter is most likely involved as a ligand of the active site, involving a specific fit (figure 2).

In a comprehensive QSAR study of terpenoid and non-terpenoid insect juvenile hormone mimetic compounds (juvenoids), Nakagawa et al. (24), through regression analysis and correlation equations formulated for 85 compounds on two insect species, developed hypothetical "mode of action" models involving overall similarity as well as species differences at the receptor site showing structural conditions necessary for activity. Without such quantitative calculations, it would have been difficult to predict similarity in the mode of action of such diverse compounds as terpenoids and N-alkyl-N,N-ethylenebis (thiocarbamates).

The QSAR approach to design of candidate compounds offers a great deal to the analytical chemist who shares the need for much of the physicochemical data, such as the octanol/water partition coefficients that must be generated for the calculation of regression functions. Analytical schemes could benefit by close cooperation at the pesticide design stage.

Undoubtedly, greater structural diversity is in store for the future as biochemically inspired targets in insects, weeds, and fungi are better understood and exploited.

Such new bioactive models include insect neuropeptides (15, 22), which provide potential new vistas in insect control by which insects' native

Table 2.—The Quantitative Structure Activity Relationships of Some Benzoyl Phenyl Urea Larvicides

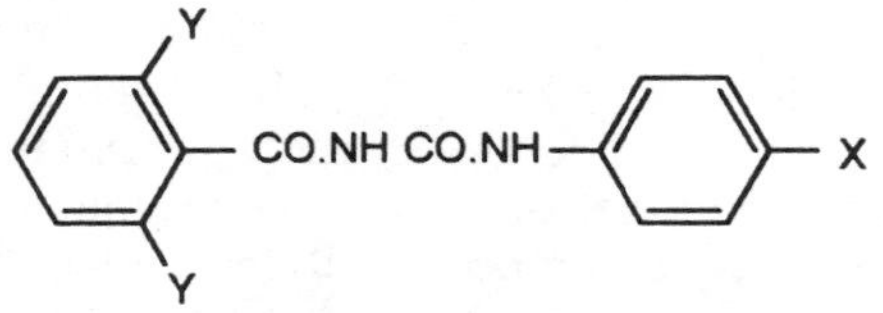

	X	Calcd pLD_{50}	Obsvd pLD_{50}	σ	ΔB_5	$\Sigma \pi$	$1.695 \Sigma \pi$ $-0.179 (\Sigma \pi)^2$
IA	Cl	6.32	6.64	0.23	0.80	0.49	0.79
IIB	CF	6.86	6.92	0.54	1.60	0.93	1.42
III	CH_3	5.10	4.60	−0.17	1.04	−0.02	−0.03
IV	CH_3	3.47	4.30	−0.27	2.07	−0.41	−0.73

Y = 2, 6–D (Iy = 0).   A. Diflubenzuron   B. Penfluron

Larvicidal activity of piperonyl butoxide (PB) synergized compound against larvae of rice stem borer (*Chilo suppressalis* Walker)

$$pLD(PB) = 5.690 + 0.748^{\sigma\varrho}$$
$$-0.398 \,\Delta B_5 + 1.695 \,\Sigma \pi$$
$$-0.179 (\Sigma \pi)^2 - 1.172 \text{ Iy}$$

$\sigma\rho =$ Hammett sigma factor for parasubstituent (inductive component of electronic effects of substituents). Strong electron-withdrawing groups increase activity. Electron donating groups ineffective, e.g., III and IV.

$\Delta\beta_5 =$ Volume factor (Verloop's STERIMOL parameters). Activity increases as bulk decreases.

$\pi =$ Hansch's constant. Hydrophobicity (solubility) parameter of the anilide constituent, derived from partition coefficient of substituted anilides in octanol/water system. Activity increases as hydrophobic character increases.

$\Sigma \pi =$ Sum of π values.

$pLD_{50} =$ -Log LD_{50} (Larvicidal activity).

$\text{I}\gamma =$ Indicator variable represents effects of structural modifications in the benzoyl moiety.

SOURCE: Nakagawa *et al.*, "Quantitative Structure-Activity Studies of Benzoylphenylurea Larvicides," *Pestic. Biochem. & Physiol.*, 21:309–325, 1984.

Figure 2.—Biphenylmethylpyrethroid Series (Plummer)

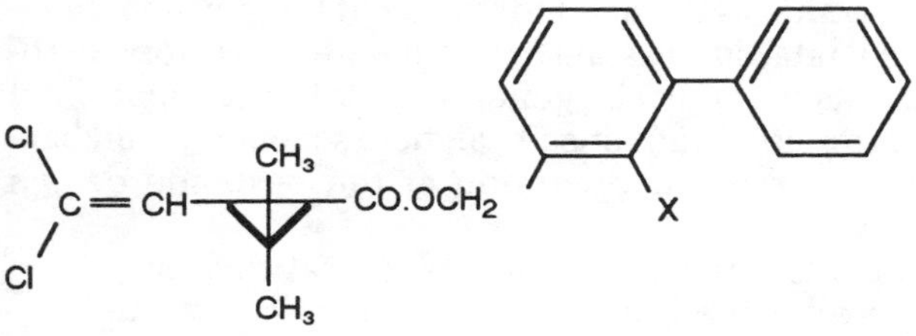

X = F or CH_3

SOURCE: C.R. Worthing ed., *Pesticide Manual*, 8th edition, British Crop Protection Council, Thornton Heath, U.K., 1987.

biochemicals serve as prototypes for lethal peptide agonists and antagonists (19).

It is likely that in the next two decades, increasing resources will be directed toward pest management technologies that involve the use of microbiologicals, natural products, genetic and behavioral biochemicals, and transgenic plants (20).

The question of the impact of biotechnology on pest control presents difficulties because the future direction of expansion is not clear and techniques are in the exploratory stage at present. For example, a technique that appears promising is the potential control of insects that attack corn roots by infecting corn with a vascular, endophytic microorganism that carries the gene capable of expressing the bacillus thuringiensis endotoxin. This technique and some others that rely on gene transfer to plants or microorganisms depend on the expression of toxins to achieve insect control. Safety considerations in biotechnology are viewed quite differently from considerations of food contamination by residues of synthetic pesticides, although some of the same questions must ultimately be asked, and it seems likely that the analysis of bacterial toxins or other complex molecules of biological origin will become more important in future. Because MRPs exclude biological macromolecules during the cleanup stage, methods of study or assay that have been developed for biological or clinical studies will probably be more appropriate in this field and immunoassay would appear to be a logical technique.

These new developments will pose increasingly more difficult challenges to the analytical chemist in the quest of accessible and practical residue analytical methods.

Emerging Classes of Compounds: Examples of Specific Analytical Problems

A number of newer herbicides are active at extremely low rates of application. For example, fluazifop applied at 4 to 8 oz. per acre will control annual grasses and perennial weeds. Sethoxydim is active at 3 to 7.5 oz. per acre, chlorsulfuron at 0.17 to 0.5 oz. per acre, and chlormeturon at 1 to 5 oz. per acre.

Several manufacturers are involved in the development of these compounds. Chlorsulfuron and sulfometuron (figure 3) are the active ingredients of GleanR and OustR, respectively, both introduced by DuPont. Other manufacturers have introduced similar herbicides. The activity of these and other new herbicides currently being developed is extremely high, and as application rates will be low, the residue levels in soils and plants will also be extremely low.

Residue levels in agricultural products will be so low as to challenge the ingenuity of the analyst. Since chlorsulfuron and sulfometuron are both thermally unstable, they cannot be directly determined by GLC. Chlorsulfuron was analyzed by gas chromatography after conversion to the methyl derivative. Residues in agricultural runoff water were determined at the parts-per-trillion level (2). The earliest method for analysis in soil at the parts-per-billion level relied on HPLC separation combined

Figure 3. — Sulfonyl Ureas

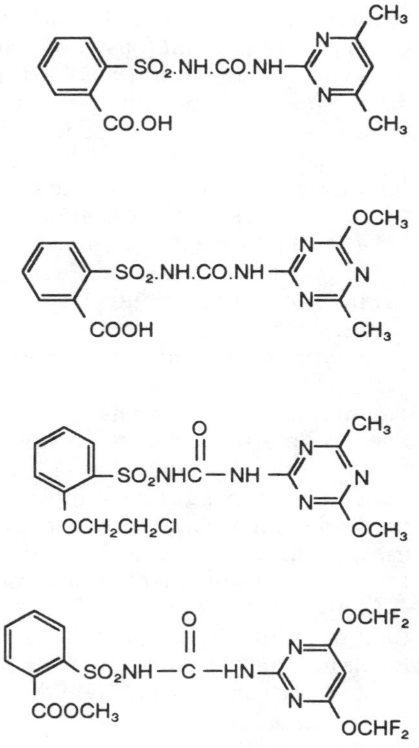

SOURCE: C.R. Worthing ed., *Pesticide Manual*, 8th edition, British Crop Protection Council, Thornton Heath, U.K., 1987.

with photoconductivity detection. Because extraction procedures normally used for soil liberate quantities of ultraviolet-absorbing material, there is considerable interference with the operation of the UV detector (33). The procedure was used because no chemical methods were available when field evaluation was conducted. A 5-day incubation period gave the most satisfactory data. Groves and Foster (11) described a bioassay for chlorsulfuron in soils that was based on the inhibition of corn root growth after a 7-day period of development in soil containing chlorsulfuron. The benefit of such bioassays is their reliance on simple techniques and their potential accuracy. For such highly active herbicides, simple bioassays may offer some advantages. Disadvantages are the length of time needed to conduct the bioassay and the need to conduct the test in a greenhouse or growth chamber.

Chlorsulfuron is a water-soluble compound, and a scheme for extraction and separation of the compound and its metabolites from treated plants was proposed by Bestman et al. (5) using aqueous extraction of plant tissue. Subsequent chromatography on a reverse-phase column and elution with aqueous formic acid/methanol gave an average recovery of 94 percent (based on 14C data). The use of reverse-phase solid-phase extraction for analysis of aqueous environmental samples has been advocated as a general method for trace organics, and this appears to work well in the case of the sulfonylurea herbicides (31). The paper contains useful suggestions for the development of procedures for a solid-phase extraction method and discussion of the potential value of this technology for extracting of organic compounds from aqueous solutions. Confirmatory procedures for the identification of sulfonylureas include combinations of gas chromatography with liquid chromatography (29, 18). An immunoassay analysis for chlorsulfuron can be used to determine chlorsulfuron in unfiltered soil samples at nanogram levels (16) and the technique appears promising. The authors comment that the method is relatively specific in contrast to the bioassay method, and interferences with the HPLC method may raise detection limits considerably.

Analytical methods for the new herbicides are thus in an evolutionary stage. The extremely low levels at which residues are to be expected contribute to the analytical problem, but these low levels represent a desirable factor in future pesticide design.

Bioassay is useful for the determination of chlorsulfuron, as well as for dichlofop acid and sethoxydim residues in soil at very low levels. The test involves measurement of the root length of pregerminated oat or corn seedlings (13).

An example of the trend in insecticide development can be found in the class of compounds known as synthetic pyrethroids. The synthetic pyrethroids are derived from the structures of natural pyrethrins, a series of chrysanthemic acid esters extracted from chrysanthemum flowers. Beginning with allethrin in 1949, both the acid and alcohol moieties of the ester have been replaced, modified, or substituted to produce a family of insecticides having greatly enhanced activity and stability. The original pyrethroids could only be used indoors as sprays in homes and greenhouses due to short residual activity. However, the discovery that halogenation of the vinyl moiety of the chrysanthemic acid increased photostability and enhanced insecticidal activity led to the modern pyrethroids that can be used as field insecticides on crops.

The application rates of some of the current products are measured in grams/acre instead of the traditional pounds/acre of other pesticides (table 3). Relative mammalian toxicities are shown in table 4. The lower application rates of the synthetic pyrethroids are due to their greater toxicity to insects, but not to mammals. For example, permethrin and carbaryl have about the same mammalian toxicity, but permethrin can be used at rates about 10 to 20 times lower than carbaryl (tables 3 and 4). Similarly, deltamethrin and chlorpyrifos have similar mammalian toxicities, but deltamethrin rates average about 100 times less than chlorpyrifos. Therefore these lower application rates also imply that the potential health hazard is reduced. Low application rates and consequent low residues and the lipophilicity imparted by the halogen functional groups determine the approaches used in developing multiresidue methods of analysis. Residues can be extracted by methods already developed for the organochlorine insecticides such as DDT, etc. Fortunately, the group is characterized by fairly high melting and/or boiling points, which permit their separation from other halogenated compounds by high-temperature gas chromatography and sensitive electron-capture detection. The lipophilic properties also result in accumulation in animal fat when treated grains, forage, and other crop products are fed to animals.

However, the general structure of this family of compounds results in both cis/trans isomers and optical isomers, which complicate the chromatographic

Table 3.—Recommended Application Rates of Selected Pyrethroids

Fenpropathrin decreasing Compound		Rate, lb./Acre
Permethrin		0.050-0.200
Fenvalerate		0.050-0.200
Fluvalinate		0.025-0.100
Flucythrinate		0.025-0.080
Cypermethrin		0.020-0.075
Tralomethrin		0.013-0.024
Cycloprothrin		0.009-0.180
Cyfluthrin		0.009-0.045
Deltamethrin		0.008-0.024
Alphamethrin		0.0045-0.027
Karate		0.0045-0.027
Phenothrin		0.004-0.016
Fenpropathrin		0.002-0.010
Other insecticides for comparison:		
Chlordane	OC	1.0-10.0
Aldicarb	carbamate	0.5-10.0
Carbaryl	carbamate	0.5-4.0
Malathion	OP	0.5-3.0
Diazinon	OP	0.25-2.0
Chlorpyrifos	OP	0.10-5.0
Parathion	OP	0.10-1.0
Diflubenzuron	IGR	0.02-0.14

SOURCE: Agricultural Chemicals, Book I, Insecticides, W.T. Thomson, (ed.) (Fresno, CA: Thomson Publications, 1986).

Table 4.—Relative Mammalian Toxicities of Selected Pyrethroids

Compound		Increasing Toxicity LD (rat, oral), mg/kg body wt.
Phenothrin		10,000
Cycloprothrin		5,000
Tralomethrin		1,070
Cyfluthrin		500
Fenvalerate		451
Permethrin		450
Fluvalinate		261
Cypermethrin		200
Deltamethrin		128
Alphamethrin		79
Flucythrinate		67
Karate		56
Fenpropathrin		54

Other insecticides for comparison:

	Class	
Diflubenzuron	IGR	4640
Malathion	OP	1375
Carbaryl	carbamate	500
Diazinon	OP	300
Chlordane	OC	250
Chlorpyrifos	OP	135
Dichlorvos	OP	56
Parathion	OP	3
Aldicarb	carbamate	0.79

SOURCE: Agricultural Chemicals, Book 1, Insecticides, W.T. Thomson, (ed.) (Fresno, CA: Thomson Publications, 1986).

Figure 4.—Separation of Pyrethroids on GLC

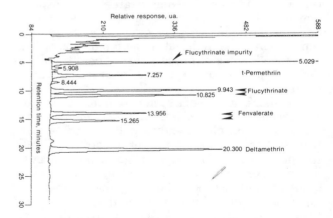

SOURCE: Hill, Kenneth, Agriculture Research Service, U.S. Department of Agriculture, Beltsville, MD.

determination step. If resolution of the isomers is desired, then high-quality capillary column GC must be used. Some success along this line has already been achieved with special large-bore capillary columns as demonstrated by a typical gas chromatogram showing the separation of four pyrethroids in a fortified animal-fat extract (12). The success of the pyrethroids as agricultural insecticides will likely lead to new structural variations in the future with even more enhanced stability and activity (figure 4).

The Utility of Pesticide/Pest Chemical Interactions

Many pesticides act by inhibition of an important enzyme system. In those cases where the mode of action is well defined and the activity of the enzyme can easily be determined, a method of analysis based on enzyme inhibition may be very useful as a screening technique. For example, organophosphate esters or carbamates inhibit the enzyme cholinesterase, which is responsible for the hydrolysis of the neurotransmitter acetylcholine. Rapid assays have been based on colorimetry or radioac-

tivity as a measurement of the extent of reaction. For assay, acetylcholine chloride is used as a substrate to determine the activity of cholinesterase in a sample (blood, tissue, etc.) The reaction produces acetic acid, which can be detected by an indicator dye or, using 14C-acetylcholine chloride, by determining residual radioactivity in the sample after removing acetic acid by evaporation. Indicator papers are commercially available for field tests of insecticides that inhibit cholinesterase. Such tests are useful for screening and indicate the presence of one or more compounds of the general class. Although other types of enzyme inhibition may be common to classes of pesticides, and methods of analysis based on these reactions are feasible, they have not been widely exploited or passed into regular analytical use for pesticide determination.

A method of analysis for chemicals affecting insect behavior involves the detection of pheromones by isolated insect antennae. Since this method offers unique selectivity, it has been used as the basis of gas chromatographic detection (4). The method depends on specific recognition of a complex organic compound by a biological receptor site. Recognition of an organic molecule by a specific receptor is also the basis for the immunoassay techniques, which depend on the interaction between a pesticide and a complex antibody. The production of antibodies capable of recognizing individual pesticides or groups of pesticides is being rapidly exploited, and immunoassay techniques are currently available for qualitative analysis and quantitative determination of pesticides. The ability to recognize a class of pesticides renders this technique extremely suitable for screening. Its advantage is that it relies on some degree of correspondence between the biological site (on the antibody) and the pesticide, whereas many enzyme systems function *in situ* and the site of action of a pesticide in a linked series of processes may be difficult to define or isolate for use as a basis for an analytical technique.

A further example of a system that may be useful for screening purposes is the ability of many herbicides to inhibit photosynthesis. This activity may be correlated with inhibition of the ability of cell-free plant extracts to catalyze a light-dependent evolution of oxygen in the presence of an acceptor such as ferricyanide, a process known as the Hill reaction (8). A variety of herbicides inhibit the Hill reaction (ureas, triazines, uracils, dinitrophenols, diphenylethers, pyrimidones, carbamates, anilides, etc.), and such a reaction may have analytical utility as a screening tool.

Pesticide/pest chemical reactions may be useful in the future as part of a screening system to indicate the presence or absence of one or more of group of analytes. A procedure that demonstrates the presence of one or more of a very wide range of compounds could provide a useful screen to indicate which samples should be selected for further analysis.

The value of cholinesterase inhibition as a rapid field method is well accepted, but new approaches are needed to combine biochemical and analytical thinking in devising procedures that will provide potential for both broad screening and quantitative, specific detection of analytes. There is an indication that some biosensor techniques can meet the latter need, but at present, biosensors are primarily developed to address specific problems of substrate analysis. A sensor that could respond to each individual member of a group of analytes still remains beyond practical limits.

Methods based on biological properties (immunoassays and enzyme inhibition) are likely to find application in rapid screening of samples in order to eliminate negative samples prior to instrumental analysis in a laboratory. Biological methods will be unlikely to provide satisfactory multiresidue methods for the following reasons: 1) They are not sufficiently selective to distinguish members of family groups (enzymatic methods); or 2) They may be too selective (immunoassays) and therefore will require a separate reagent for each of the thousands of possible pesticides, degradation products, and metabolites. However, highly automated procedures would permit rapid screening for perhaps a few hundred selected compounds.

Conclusions

A number of major concerns have dominated the design of new pest-control chemicals. Predominant among these is the combination of optimized biological activity against target species with minimal acute or latent toxicity toward other organisms. To accomplish this and reduce the possibility that pest resistance may rapidly render the product worthless, approaches to the discovery of pest control chemicals now proceed with a greater understanding and regard for modes of action and metabolism. In recent years, the major advances in techniques by which structure-activity relationships are investigated and interpreted have also been reflected in product chemistry, where the producers now offer new chemicals that may be pure isomeric or optically active forms. Progression from the use of relatively crude materials containing many isomers or related impurities (e.g., toxaphene) applied at rates of several pounds per acre to chemicals that are highly purified and are active at a few ounces per acre has significant impact on the work of the analyst because, in the future, residues from field use will generally be much lower.

Initially, the major problem for the regulatory analyst is the question of tolerance, and it is to be expected that reductions in rate of use will be beneficial if corresponding median lethal dose (LD50) values remain high. Although absolute sensitivity is not a factor in the analysis, it is to be expected that tolerances will be reduced as methods improve.

There are many new approaches to control of pests, and these will continue to gain ground at the expense of chemical control. However, pest-control chemicals are significant in an international market. Their use will continue, and there will be increasing diversity of chemical structures as molecular architecture is varied and refined to combine biological activity with the reduction of adverse effects on nontarget organisms and the environment. Although the range of structural types is increasing, compounds currently being developed do not appear to present insuperable analytical difficulties. The major problem is the increase in number and variety and the proliferation of structures that differ only in detail (for example, the pyrethroids), thus calling for more sophisticated separation techniques.

Multiresidue procedures appear to be adaptable to many new chemicals, and it is now required that the performance of new chemicals in standard MRPs be investigated as part of the registration process. This information is of great assistance to the regulatory analyst and it is important that it be made readily available. However, as the number of potential matrix/compound interactions increases, so the difficulties of the regulatory analyst will also increase. The parent compounds can usually be recognized by MRPs, but the type and variety of metabolic products from a single pesticide may obviate their determination in a single MRP, or even in any MRP. To simplify this problem, Frehse (10) has proposed that a single indicator compound should be selected to represent the residue of a certain pesticide and its metabolites. It was suggested that the concentration of the indicator compound should bear a known relationship to the concentration of the toxicologically significant residue; in addition, the indicator compound should be available as a standard, be recoverable in MRPs, and sufficiently stable for reproducible analysis. The concept of indicator compounds is a useful one and is one that could be included in the framework of efforts to bring about international harmonization of maximum residue limits.

The simplification of approaches to the problems of the regulatory analytical chemist was also advocated by Frehse (10), who described a three-step system proposed by Westlake and Gunther (32). The first stage involves screening for given constituents to previously established limits of detectability. The second stage consists of screening to discriminate samples that are above tolerance from those below. The third stage is that of quantitative analysis. Clearly, current screening methods for groups of compounds, such as immunoassays, are capable of providing much information and could form part of a tiered analytical procedure.

The major obstacle to improved multiresidue methods is still the labor intensive extraction and cleanup procedures required. The initial stages of analysis involving the selection of a representative sample, extraction, and cleanup of the extract are critical and also time-consuming. Much more research is needed in automation and robotics to increase throughput and reduce per-sample costs for the conventional approaches. Not much research effort has yet been expended on techniques for eliminating cleanup steps, although direct injection of extracts without extensive cleanup was reported as long as 17 years ago for organophosphorus compounds (6, 7).

The introduction of synthetic organic pesticides was followed closely by the rapid development of gas chromatography in the early 1960s. Element specific detectors simplified residue determination for such compounds as the organochlorine, organophosphorus ester, and carbamate insecticides. Procedures for extraction, solvent partitioning, purification, and determination have evolved, but in the past two decades there have been remarkable advances in the performance of columns for gas or liquid chromatography. Identification of specific residues has been made easier by combination of liquid or gas chromatography with mass spectrometric detection. Nevertheless, a variety of compounds remain outside the capability of MRPs and the analyst must resort to special procedures. Highly polar or water-soluble materials often present difficulties and must be converted to lipid-soluble derivatives. Unfortunately, many metabolites belong to this category and cannot be included in general MRP procedures. There is no simple generalization to describe new compounds appearing on the market, and there may be difficulties if polar or thermally unstable compounds must be analyzed. Lower rates of application are to be expected in the future because the design of biologically active molecules can more readily be optimized. If toxicity is extremely low, there may be fewer residues of significance, but analytical needs will still exist. Simple, rapid, and sensitive screening methods will be essential to indicate whether further analysis of samples should be undertaken. There is a critical need for such methods to reduce the burden on the regulatory analyst.

There is little reason to believe that the necessity to continue to develop and apply MRPs will decrease in the next two decades. Agricultural chemicals will continue to be used worldwide and it is important to protect the quality of produce reaching the consumer. However, it is important to increase effectiveness and reduce costs of current methods and some priorities should be allocated; among these the following may be considered:

1. Current MRPs will probably be adaptable to many new chemicals entering the market. However, analysis of closely related isomers will require improved separation techniques, and the potential requirement to determine residues at the parts-per-billion level will demand more sensitive detectors.

2. Sampling, extraction, and cleanup procedures are generally time-consuming and expensive in terms of solvents, etc. The application of automated techniques may avoid some labor costs, but new technology is needed.

3. Rapid methods for screening that require no processing or minimal processing of the sample would be extremely valuable, particularly if they were applicable in the field.
4. Methodology is needed that is applicable to separation and analysis of macromolecules or complex molecules of biological origin that might be involved as new active principles in future pest-control technology.

References

1. *Agricultural Chemicals, Book 1, Insecticides*, W.T. Thomson (ed.) (Fresno, CA: Thomson Publications, 1986).
2. Ahmad, I., "Capillary Column Gas Chromatographic Determination of Trace Residues of the Herbicide Chlorsulfuron in Agricultural Runoff Water," *J. Assoc. Off. Anal. Chem.* 70:745-748, 1987.
3. Ambrus, A. and Thier, H.P., "Applications of Multiresidue Procedures in Pesticides Residues Analysis," *Pure and Appl. Chem.* 58:1035-62, 1986.
4. Arn, H., Stradler, E., and Rauschler, S., "The Electroantennographic Detector—A Selective and Sensitive Tool in the Gas Chromatographic Analysis of Insect Pheromones," *Z. Naturforsch. Teil C* 30:722-725, 1975.
5. Bestman, H.D., Devine M.D., and Vanden Born, W.H., "Extraction and Separation of Chlorsulfuron and Its Metabolites from Treated Plants," *Weed Sci.* 35:22-26, 1987.
6. Bowman, M.C. and Beroza, M., *J. Assoc. Off. Anal. Chem.* 53:499-508, 1970.
7. Bowman, M.C., Beroza, M., and Hill, K.R., *J. Assoc. Off. Anal. Chem.* 54:346-358, 1971.
8. Corbett, J.R., *The Biochemical Mode of Action of Pesticides* (New York: Academic Press, 1974).
9. *Farm Chemicals Handbook* (Willoughby, OH: Meister Publishing Company, 1988).
10. Frehse, H., "Trends in Pesticide Residue Methodology," *Pesticide Science and Biotechnology*, R. Greenhalgh and T.R. Roberts (eds.) (Oxford, UK: Blackwell Scientific Publications, 1983), pp. 293-300.
11. Groves, K.E.M. and Foster, R.K., "A Corn (Zea mays L.) Bioassay Technique for Measuring Chlorsulfuron Levels in Three Saskatchewan Soils," *Weed Science* 33:825-828, 1985.
12. Hill, K.R., personal communications, 1988.
13. Hsiao, A.I. and Smith, A.E., "A Root-Bioassay Procedure for the Redetermination of Chlorsulfuron Diclofop Acid and Sethoxydim Residues in Soils," *Weed Research* 23:231-236, 1983.
14. Kearney, P.C., Isensee, A.R., and Plimmer, J.R., "Contribution of Agricultural Pesticides to Worldwide Chemical Distribution," In: *Toxic Contamination in Large Lakes*, vol. III, N.W. Schmidke, Lewis, Chelsea, MI, 1988, pp. 49-60.
15. Keeley, L.L. and Hayes, T.K., "Speculations on Biotechnology Applications for Insect Research," *Insect Biochem.* 17(5):639-657, 1987.
16. Kelley, M.M., Zahnow, E.W., Petersen, W.C., et al., "Chlorosulfuron Determination in Soil Extracts by Enzyme Immunoassay," *J. Agric. Food Chem.* 33:962-965, 1985.
17. Magee, P.S., Kohn, G.K., and Menn, J.J., *Pesticide Synthesis Through Rational Approaches* (Washington, DC: ?, 1984).
18. McFadden, W.H. and Lammert, S.A., "Techniques for Increased Use of Thermospray Liquid Chromatography—Mass Spectrometry," *J. Chromatog.* 385:201-211, 1987.
19. Menn, J.J. and Borkovec, A.B., "Insect Neuropeptides: Potential New Insect Control Agents," *Jour. All Union Chem. Soc.* in press.
20. Menn, J.J. and Christy, A.L., "New Directions in Pest Management," *Proceedings US/USSR Symposium on Fate of Pesticides and Chemicals in the Environment*, J. Schnoor (ed.) (Iowa City: Univ. of Iowa, 1988).
21. Menn, J.J. and Henrick, C.A., "Rational and Biorational Design of Pesticides," *Phil. Trans. R. Soc. Lond. B* 295:57-71, 1981.
22. Menn, J.J. and Henrick, C.A., "Newer Chemicals for Insect Control," In: *Agricultural Chemicals of the Future*, BARC Symposium 8, J.L. Hilton (ed.) (Ottowa: Rowman and Allanheld, 1984), pp. 247-265.
23. Morrod, R.S., "Lead Generation: Designing the Right Approach," *Phil. Trans. R. Soc. Lond. B* 295:35-44, 1981.
24. Nakagawa, A., Iwamura, H., and Fujita, T., "Quantitative Structure Activity Relationship of Insect Juvenile Hormone Mimetic Compounds," *J. Med. Chem.* 27:1493-1502, 1984.
25. Nakagawa, Y., Kitahara, K., Nishioka, T., et al., "Quantitative Structure-Activity Studies of Benzoylphenylurea Larvicides," *Pestic. Biochem. & Physiol.* 21:309-325, 1984.
26. National Research Council, Board on Agriculture, *Regulating Pesticides in Food: The Delaney Paradox* (Washington, DC: National Academy Press, 1987).
27. Pickett, J.A., "Chemical Pest Control—The New

Philosophy," *Chemistry in Britain* 24:137-142, 1988.

28. Plummer, E.L., "Biphenylmethylpyrethroids: A Quantitative Structure Activity Relationship Approach to Pesticide Design," In: *Synthesis through Rational Approaches*, 1984.

29. Shalaby, L.M., "Liquid Chromatography/Mass Spectrometry of the Thermally Labile Herbicides, Chlorsulfuron and Sulfometuron Methyl," *Biomed. Mass Spectrom.* 12:261-268, 1985.

30. Storck, W.J., "Pesticide Growth Slows," *Chem. & Eng. News* 65 (46):35, Nov. 16, 1987.

31. Wells, M.J.M. and Michael, J.L., "Revised-Phase Solid-Phase Extraction Aqueous Environmental Sample Preparation in Herbicide Residue Analysis," *J. Chromatog. Sci.* 25:345-350, 1987.

32. Westlake, W.E. and Gunther, F.A., *Residue Reviews* 18:175-217, 1967.

33. Zahnow, E.W., "Analysis of the Herbicide Chlorsulfuron in Soil by Liquid Chromatography," *J. Agric. Food Chem.* 30:854, 1982.

Validation of Analytical Methods for Pesticide Residues and Confirmation of Results

Henry B.S. Conacher, Food Research Division, Bureau of Chemical Safety, Food Directorate, Health Protection Branch, Health and Welfare Canada

Contents

	Page
Abstract	136
Development of Validated Analytical Methods	137
Quality Assurance Of Data	140
References	141

Figure

Figure	Page
1. Stages in Method Development and Validation	137

Tables

Table	Page
1. FICP Check Sample Program Outline	139
2. Confirmation Techniques and Reporting Limits for HPB Surveillance and Compliance Programs	140

Abstract

Decisions by governmental agencies based on analytical data on pesticide residues in food can have a significant impact on public health and other socioeconomic factors. It is therefore essential that this data be of the highest quality and generated through the application of validated methods in conjunction with a well-designed quality assurance (QA) program.

Details are given of the varying degrees of validity achievable for analytical methods. These can range from validation within a single laboratory up to the demonstration of satisfactory performance in a collaborative study conducted and evaluated according to the guidelines established by international standards-setting organizations such as the AOAC.

The main problems associated with the development and utilization of collaboratively studied methods in pesticide surveillance and compliance activities relate to the plethora of possible pesticide/commodity combinations and the daunting task of devising and conducting collaborative studies of methods to handle such situations. Some details of the QA program in effect in the Canadian Health Protection Branch to ensure the production of valid analytical data are also presented.

Among a variety of other responsibilities, the Health Protection Branch, Health and Welfare Canada, is accountable for ensuring the safety of the Canadian food supply—one aspect of which is the control of pesticide residues in food. The branch fulfills this responsibility by (1) establishing maximum residue limits (MRLs) for pesticides (and their metabolites) in foods, and (2) establishing monitoring programs to ensure compliance with these MRLs and to assess the presence of pesticide residues for which no provision exists in the Canadian Food and Drug Regulations.

The analytical data generated in these programs form the basis of decisions regarding compliance that can have a considerable socioeconomic impact. It is therefore important that the data be of the highest quality. To this end, an intensive quality assurance (QA) program is in place for pesticide residue analysis throughout the branch (12). Similar QA programs are in place in other Federal agencies (Canadian Department of Agriculture, U.S. Department of Agriculture, and U.S. Food and Drug Administration) with responsibilities for ensuring the safety of the food supply in North America. The Association of Official Analytical Chemists (AOAC) has also recently published a handbook in this area (15) that has drawn extensively on the procedures and practices of the aforementioned and other organizations.

Although there are many critical elements in these QA programs, there are two that refer to the analytical aspects of the validation process:

1. Development and/or use of appropriate validated methods.
2. Use of appropriate quality control systems to ensure the production of valid data.

It is particularly important to note that the use of a validated method, although necessary, is not in itself sufficient to ensure the production of valid data. Quality assurance of the measurements on an ongoing basis is also required.

Development of Validated Analytical Methods

Validation has been defined (17) as the process of determining the suitability of methodology for providing useful analytical data.

There are several steps in the process of developing and of demonstrating the validity of an analytical method. These steps can be conveniently broken down into the three stages outlined in figure 1.

As one proceeds from stage 1 to stage 3, the degree of confidence that one can ascribe to the validity of a particular method increases. Stage 3 represents what is generally accepted (2, 3, 8, 16) to be the highest degree of method validation, i.e., successful performance in a collaborative study conducted according to the guidelines of recognized international standards-writing organizations, such as the AOAC (9).

Figure 1.—Stages in Method Development and Validation

Stage 1. Estimation of acceptable performance parameters within a laboratory.
Stage 2. Demonstration of successful performance in limited interlaboratory studies.
Stage 3. Demonstration of successful performance in recognized collaborative study.

The main parameters, referred to in stage 1, that should be taken into account have been identified in several papers (2, 8) and include accuracy, precision, specificity, limit of detection, limit of determination, linear range, and scope. While these parameters have also been thoroughly discussed in these publications, it is considered important to reiterate them here, particularly with reference to the determination of pesticide residues.

(i) **Accuracy**—a measure of how closely the determined value (generally expressed as the mean of several determinations) approximates the true value of the analyte. This is best supported by the analysis of standard reference materials; however, the availability of such materials, especially for pesticides in foods, is generally extremely limited. Normally the recovery of added analyte to "blank" samples of the commodity in question, over an appropriate range of concentrations, is taken as an indication of accuracy. For pesticide compliance work, the concentration range chosen should certainly bracket the MRL. It should also be recognized that analyte added to a field sample may behave differently (typically showing higher recovery) from field-incurred residues. For analysis at the ppb/ppm level, recoveries of 70 to 120 percent are generally considered acceptable.

(ii) **Precision**—the total interlaboratory precision, or reproducibility, is the most important aspect of precision because it is a measure of how much allowance should be made for between-laboratory variability in interpreting results produced by different laboratories. It is possible, however, to have a measure of one component of this, the within-laboratory precision, or repeatability, by multiple analyses of samples in the same laboratory over a short time-period. The reproducibility coefficients of variation (CVs) should fall within the range estimated by Horwitz et al. (7) with the repeatability components being somewhat lower, generally one-half to two-thirds of the former. For example, at a pesticide residue level of approximately 1 ppm, the expected reproducibility CV is approximately 16 percent and the repeatability CV, approximately 10 percent. Similar values have been found by Smart (16) in an examination of UK collaborative studies on pesticide residues.

(iii) **Specificity**—the ability of the method to measure only what it is intended to measure. In any method, it is absolutely essential to run reagent and field blanks to ensure no interfering compound, or indeed none of the analyte itself, is present. These blanks should be run for each commodity examined. To verify the identity and amount of an analyte, it has been suggested that the ideal approach is to utilize two entirely different analytical methods, based on different analytical principles (1). However, the availability as well as the characteristics of such methods often place a practical limitation on the application of this suggestion. Thus in the pesticide area, advantage has been usually taken of the following confirmatory techniques:

a) Mass spectrometric confirmation of identity.
b) Use of different detector, i.e., operating under different principles such as Coulson vs. Electron Capture.
c) Chromatography using different systems.
d) Chemical reaction followed by analysis.

More detailed descriptions of such techniques can be found in reviews by Cochrane (5) and by Lawrence (13).

In the past, these confirmatory techniques have been generally qualitative in nature and have been used by the analyst to give reassurance that the validated method was in fact measuring the residue that it was intended to measure. Since only the qualitative aspects were sought, such techniques were not required to be subjected to the same rigorous assessment as were the validated methods.

Now, with the availability of the smaller, more affordable benchtop-type mass spectrometers, the emphasis is moving toward quantitative mass spectrometric confirmation. This necessitates much more detailed study of the confirmatory technique.

(iv) Limit of Detection—the lowest concentration of an analyte that the analytical process can be reliably differentiated from background levels. This has been defined as the level (background level) measured in the field blank plus 3 standard deviations (2, 3).

(v) Limit of Quantitation (LOQ)—The lowest concentration of an analyte that can be measured with a stated degree of confidence. This has been defined as the level measured in a field blank plus 10 standard deviations; however, it is recommended that this value be established in the laboratory by repeated analysis of appropriate samples (spiked or endogenous). In collaborative studies, the LOQ of the method should be considered as the lowest level successfully analyzed in the study. Collaborative studies have in fact been used to establish the LOQ (14).

(vi) Linear Range—this is generally taken as the range over which the procedure has been demonstrated to give a linear response. A reproducible non-linear response, which is the case with certain immunological procedures, can also be acceptable.

(vii) Scope—the scope of a method refers to the number of substrates and the number of analytes to which the procedure can be successfully applied.

Which of these seven factors is the most important depends on the purpose for which the data will be used. In the Canadian Food and Drug Regulations, there is a general MRL of 0.1 ppm to cover pesticides for which MRLs have not been established. Thus, in the Health Protection Branch, in selecting methodology for surveillance and compliance programs, a major effort is directed toward the development and validation of methods with acceptable values for accuracy and precision down to the 0.05 ppm level.

A higher degree of validation (stage 2) for an analytical method can be obtained by participation in internal (to the organization) or external check sample programs.

Within the Health Protection branch, certain procedures have evolved over the years to validate the methodology. These have included the exchange and analysis of individual (generally violative) samples among branch laboratories, and the distribution and analysis of a variety of check samples. The latter have usually been distributed in connection with the emergence of certain contentious issues, such as the recent ethylene dibromide problem, but plans are underway to increase the frequency of check sample distribution during normal monitoring programs. For example, a check sample program underway at present involves the distribution of two commodities, each containing two different levels of 1,1-dimethylhydrazine (UDMH) to three Health Protection Branch laboratories. This study will serve to validate the methodology recently developed (18) for UDMH.

Undoubtedly the major external check sample program in which branch laboratories participate is the Federal Interdepartmental Committee on Pesticides check sample program, details of which have been given in a recent paper (6). The present program outline is shown in table 1.

As mentioned previously, the highest degree of validation (stage 3) for an analytical method is the demonstration of its performance in a successful collaborative study. Current AOAC guidelines (9) require the successful analysis of at least five samples in six laboratories. The collaborative study approach not only demonstrates that the method can be applied successfully in several laboratories but that it can also withstand an objective, rigorous peer-review process.

However, a collaborative study generally demonstrates validity for only those commodities and those analytes included in the study—a fact that presents a major problem in the area of pesticide residues because of the large number of pesticide/commodity combinations possible. This, together

Table 1.—FICP Check Sample Program Outline

Sub-Program	Substrates	Distribution[a]	Pesticides
Soils	Soil	3	2,4-D Picloram Atrazine
Foods	Tallow Strawberries Potatoes	4	Captan Iprodione Carbofuran Chlorophenols
Water	Standards Sediments, Water	3	Common OCs Phenoxy Acids
Fish	Fish, Eels, Cod Liver Oil	6	DDE, Mirex PCBs
Forest Substrates (Insecticides)	Fish, Soil Balsam Fir Needles	3	Pirimicarb Aminocarb Mexacarbate Carbaryl
Forest Substrates (Herbicides)	Soil	1	Hexazinone
Wildlife	Herring Gull Lipids and Homogenates	3	DDE, Mirex, PCBs Heptachlor Epoxide Chlordane Oxychlordane Dieldrin
Feeds	Grains	2	Triallate Malathion Carbathion Permethrin Lindane Chlorpyrifos

[a]Numbers of check sample projects conducted in last 5 years.

with the wide range of MRLs, would render the design and conduct of collaborative studies to cover all possible combinations a most formidable task that cost alone would surely doom to failure.

An excellent example of these difficulties and the approach taken to resolve them can be obtained from consideration of a recent AOAC collaborative study conducted by Krause (10) of a multiresidue method for the determination of N-methyl carbamate insecticides and related metabolites in crops, and a subsequent publication by the same author (11).

The collaborative study involved the determination of seven methyl carbamates and two carbamate metabolites at two levels in two crops: grapes and potatoes. This study proved extremely successful and was adopted Official First Action by AOAC. Nevertheless the collaborative study had only included two commodities and therefore the method was only validated for these commodities.

To extend the scope of an Official AOAC Method, a mini-collaborative study can be required demonstrating that the performance parameters generated in the main study can be met with the additional commodities and/or analytes. In Krause's study, the method had been initially studied successfully by four laboratories in an interlaboratory trial on lettuce, in effect a mini-collaborative study, thus permitting the scope to be extended to include lettuce.

The main question relates to what is required to extend the scope of the official carbamate method to include other carbamates and other commodities. In his subsequent publication (11), Krause describes recovery values obtained over a 3-year period in four FDA laboratories for seven parent carbamates and five carbamate metabolites added to 14 crops. These data were obtained as part of the in-laboratory quality assurance programs. In many cases, the recoveries obtained were similar to those obtained in the collaborative study. Whether this data is sufficient to further extend the scope of the Official Method depends on its evaluation by the relevant AOAC committee. In the author's opinion, some form of interlaboratory study would be preferable for this purpose.

Similar situations exist with the other multiresidue screening methods for pesticides.

The stage to which validation should be taken depends to a large extent on the use to which the data will be put, on the urgency with which the data is required and, indeed, on the operational structure and philosophy of the organization involved.

In general, regulatory agencies, when faced with important compliance decisions, wish to have data of the highest quality. There is therefore a preference for fully collaboratively studied methods (stage 3) or, at a minimum, methods that have been subjected to some form of interlaboratory study (stage 2).

However, if the objective of a survey is simply to assess if a problem exists, a method in the stage 1 category can readily be used. Even in such cases, agencies with several field laboratories involved in generating the data generally undertake limited interlaboratory assessment (2 or 3 check samples) prior to the survey.

The main drawback to the collaborative process is the length of time required from initiation of the study to the stage where the method is given official approval. At present, within AOAC, this takes a minimum of one year. Thus in situations where the data is required on an urgent basis, and collaboratively studied methods do not exist, many agencies resort to the use of methods validated to a lesser degree.

Quality Assurance of Data

It cannot be stressed enough that the adoption of, and strict adherence to, a sound quality assurance program is essential toward the production of valid analytical data. Within the Health Protection Branch, an important part of this whole QA program is the use of appropriate quality control systems in conjunction with validated methods to ensure the production of valid data. The quality control systems, which include the confirmation of results and the

reporting limits required, vary depending on the nature of the program. The national surveillance and compliance programs generally have the highest level of quality control.

The national surveillance program is designed to determine the state of compliance of selected food commodities in the marketplace with respect to specific pesticides. The pesticides are divided into high, medium and low priority groups, and emphasis is placed first on the high priority group. All laboratories involved must ensure that these pesticides can be determined by the general screening methodology, or by specific methods, (4) by analyzing samples spiked with a mixture of pesticides at a minimum frequency of 1 in every 20 samples. Commodities used as the spiked sample are required to be varied throughout the year, and all high priority pesticides must be included in the spiking mixtures at least once per year at, or below, the MRL. If these recoveries are less than 70 percent or if the limits of quantitation are greater than one tenth the MRL, or 0.05 ppm (in the case of the 0.1 ppm MRL), it is concluded that the particular chemical/commodity cannot be handled by the methodology and/or the laboratory in question, and steps are taken to investigate and correct the situation. The medium and low priority groups of pesticides are included as time permits.

The confirmation techniques and reporting limits for the surveillance program, together with the corresponding requirements for the compliance program for comparative purposes, are summarized in table 2.

Additional confidence in the quality of the data is obtained through continued (and, it is hoped, successful) participation in the internal and external check sample programs.

Table 2.—Confirmation Techniques and Reporting Limits for HPB Surveillance and Compliance Programs

Program	Concentration of residue (ppm)	Report	Confirmation technique
Surveillance	<.01 (or quantitation limit, whichever is higher)	no report required	
	≥.01 - <1/2 MRL	1 significant figure	1/10 of specimens by level 1* or by GC/MS
	≥1/2 MRL - MRL	2 significant figures	level 2** or GC/MS
	>MRL	2 significant figures	GC/MS
Compliance	<1/10 MRL	no report	
	≥ 1/10 MRL (or 0.0 ppm, whichever is higher	2 significant figures	GC/MS

*level 1 = quantitative agreement between 2 columns/2 detectors
**level 2 = level 1 plus an additional column or detector, derivative, or other technique

References

1. ACS AdHoc Subcommittee Dealing with the Scientific Aspects of Regulatory Measurements, *Chem. Eng. News*, 44: June 7, 1982.
2. ACS Committee on Environmental Improvement, *Anal. Chem.* 52:2242, 1980.
3. ACS Committee on Environmental Improvement, *Anal. Chem.* 55:2210, 1983.
4. *Analytical Methods for Pesticide Residues in Foods* (Ottawa, Canada: Canadian Government Publishing Centre, Supply and Services Canada, K1A 0S9, 1986).
5. Cochrane, W.P., "Chemical Derivatization in Pesticide Analysis," *Chemical Derivatization in Analytical Chemistry*, R.W. Frei and J.F. Lawrence (eds.) (New York: Plenum Press, 1981).
6. Conacher, H.B.S., *J. Assoc. Off. Anal. Chem.* 70:941, 1987.
7. Horwitz, W., Kamps, L.R., and Boyer, K.W., *J. Assoc. Off. Anal. Chem.* 63:1344, 1980.
8. Horwitz, W., *J. Assoc. Off. Anal. Chem.* 65:525, 1982.
9. Horwitz, W., *J. Assoc. Off. Anal. Chem.* 67:433, 1984.
10. Krause, R.T., *J. Assoc. Off. Anal. Chem.* 68:726, 1985.
11. Krause, R.T., *J. Assoc. Off. Anal. Chem* 68:734, 1985.
12. *Laboratory Quality Assurance Manual*, Field Operations Directorate (Ottawa, Ontario, Canada: Health Protection Branch, 1977).
13. Lawrence, J.F., "Confirmatory Tests," *Pesticide Analysis*, K.G. Das (ed.) (New York: Marcel Dekker, Inc., 1981).
14. Page, B.D., *J. Assoc. Off. Anal. Chem.* 68:776, 1985.
15. *Quality Assurance Principles for Analytical Laboratories*, F.M. Garfield (ed.) (Washington, DC: Association of Official Analytical Chemists, Inc., 1984).
16. Smart, N.A., *Analyst* 109:781, 1984.
17. Taylor, J.K., *Anal. Chem.* 55:600A, 1983.
18. Health and Welfare Canada, Health Protection Branch, Laboratory Procedure LPFC-147, 1987.

Conventional Pesticide Analytical Methods: Can They Be Improved?

James N. Seiber, Environmental Toxicology, University of California, Davis, CA

Contents

	Page
Abstract	142
Introduction	142
Pressure Points In Multiresidue Methods	144
Other Stages Of Pesticide Analyses	148
Putting It All Together	150
Conclusions	151
Who Should Do It?	151
References	152

Figures

Figure	Page
1. The Evolution of Analytical Methodology for Organic Toxicants in Environmental Samples	143
2. Tradeoffs in Multiresidue Methods	144
3. Mills Procedure (PAM)	145
4. Acetone Extraction Method (Luke)	147
5. CDFA Multiresidue Screen	149
6. Hypothetical MR Scheme	151

Abstract

Pesticide multiresidue analytical methods have been continually improved and expanded over the years. Further improvements are possible based upon recognition of the limitations of existing methods and their modification with new sample-handling and instrumental techniques. For example, the use of solid phase extraction (SPE) cartridges in place of liquid-liquid extraction and, perhaps, Florisil column fractionation might allow for miniaturization, smaller solvent volumes, extended breadth of applicability, and greater throughout when integrated into existing multiresidue schemes. Wide-bore capillary gas chromatography columns can eliminate the need for some derivatizations and, when interfaced with autoinjectors and integrating data systems, can improve throughput and data quality. High performance liquid chromatography can be used for fractionation and also for determination of compounds (including some new classes of pesticides) that can not be gas chromatographed without derivatization. Mass-selective detection (GC/MS), particularly in the selective ion mode, can improve detection limits and the accuracy of analytical results. These types of potential improvements will require coordinated research involving academic, industrial, and regulatory laboratories, including new levels of funding for the academic and regulatory sectors. The importance of academic involvement can not be overemphasized because of the need to attract a new cadre of well-trained young scientists into the residue analytical field.

Introduction

The field of trace analysis, including pesticide residue analysis, has made tremendous advances in terms of selectivity and detection limits (figure 1) (9). In the 1940s and early 1950s, gravimetric and bioassay techniques were the mainstays in "trace" analysis, extending detection limits to the then-frontier levels of about 1 ppm. These were time-consuming methods, lacking in compound selectivity but broad-based in terms of responding to whole classes of chemicals. Colorimetric and spectrophotometric methods held sway through the 1950s and early 1960s, providing improvements in both detection limits and specificity. Many of these,

Figure 1.—The Evolution of Analytical Methodology for Organic Toxicants in Environmental Samples

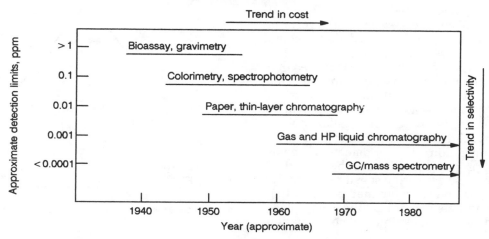

SOURCE: J.N. Seiber, *1982 Analysis of Toxicants in Agricultural Environments*, Genetic Toxicology, R.A. Fleck and A. Hollaender (eds.) Plenum, NY, pp. 219–234.

such as the Shecter-Haller method for DDT and Averill-Norris method for parathion, involved extensive derivatization because they required that a visibly colored product be formed even when the parent compound was colorless (as was the usual case). The inroads of chromatography began roughly in the 1950s with paper and thin layer chromatography (TLC), and for the first time, chemists were able to resolve in a given sample several individual chemicals using a single technique without extensive sample preparation-derivatization. Paper chromatography (PC) and TLC were essentially qualitative techniques, best used to screen samples for the presence or absence of specific compounds. Clinical chemists interested in drug analysis, natural-products chemists interested in plant secondary products, and pesticide residue chemists quickly adopted these chromatographic techniques. At present, gas liquid (GLC) and high performance liquid chromatography (HPLC) techniques have largely supplanted (but have not completely eliminated) PC and TLC. These are resolution techniques par excellence, with the added dimension of quite precise quantitation made possible by very sensitive and often highly selective detectors. A few of these, such as the thermionic detector, were developed by pesticide residue chemists while others (electron capture, microcoulometric) were popularized just for the field of pesticide analysis. The now common use of mass spectrometry (MS) coupled with GC provides detection limits to 1 ppb routinely, and it adds the dimension of near-absolute confirmation

of residue identity when somewhat higher residue levels are encountered. These achievements in sensitivity and selectivity have been costly, such that equipping a modern laboratory for a broad spectrum of trace analyses requires considerable capital—several GCs and LCs plus mass spectrometry capability. Figure 1 shows the interplay, trade-off, and trends in a very general way for the analytical transition from the 1950s to 1980s. Figure 1 omits the important point that many analyses are now possible that were not possible in the 1940s and 1950s, examples being provided by volatile halogenated organic compounds (VHOC) in drinking water and pesticide multiresidue analysis in foods.

While these sophisticated methods have revolutionized trace analysis in many respects, the analytical process itself has not changed materially in that all analyses conform to basic steps, or unit processes, which vary little regardless of the application. These steps include extraction to remove the analyte from the bulk matrix, cleanup of the extract to remove potentially interfering coextractives, modification or derivatization to change the analyte to a more readily determinable form (an optional step), and resolution to separate analyte or a derivative from other chemicals remaining in the prepared sample. The elements of concentration, removing a few micrograms of analyte from several grams or kilograms of sample substrate to a small volume of solvent, and purification, isolating one or a few specific compounds from the thousands present in the raw sample, run through these steps. The determination phase includes detection —obtaining a response related to the structural feature and amount of analyte; measurement—relating the response to a reference standard of the chemical of interest or a close relative; and confirmation— assuring that the measured response is indeed due to the analyte and not an artifact or imposter. This time-honored strategy takes advantage of physical and chemical properties unique to the analyte or analyte class: properties of solubility, polarity, volatility, reactivity, and interaction with electrochemical, optical, ionization, or other detectors. Generally, the more properties built in to the analytical scheme, the more selective and sensitive the analysis. A corollary is that short-cut methods are often less selective and sensitive, and thus they place more demands on the detection and confirmation instrumentation.

The tradeoffs involved in selecting methods can also be seen in the following types of analysis:

Qualitative (Screening)—What is present or absent.
vs.
Quantitative—How much is present.
Multiresidue—Capable of measuring many chemicals in a given sample.
vs.
Specific—Tailored to just one or a few chemicals (e.g., a single parent pesticide plus its major metabolites).

Regulatory agencies will require and routinely use multiresidue pesticide screening techniques because they need to ascertain the presence (or absence) of many chemicals in a given sample of unknown origin. Chemical companies, on the other hand, need specific and quantitative methods to determine the residue distribution and dissipation of their own specific pesticide products in a given sample set, in connection with EPA registration requirements or their own need to know.

The dilemma in multiresidue methods may be stated as follows: The method must cover a broad waterfront of chemical types and matrices. In so doing, however, the science of the method, reflected in the analysts' prime quality control characteristics—detection limits, precision (reproducibility), and accuracy—becomes diluted. Very often, costs (both capital and labor) increase as breadth increases. These tradeoffs, summarized in figure 2, occur with present-day methodology and thus are responsible, at least in part, for the compromise nature of existing multiresidue methods. But must it be this way? Are there approaches yet to be found that will combine low costs and broad applicability with good science? If so, will they involve modi-

Figure 2.—Tradeoffs in Multiresidue Methods

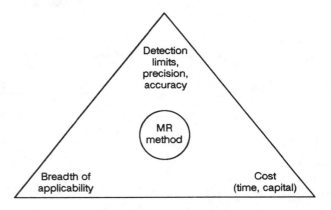

SOURCE: James Seiber, University of California, Davis, CA, 1988.

fying methods that now exist (based largely on GC and HPLC with selective detection) or instituting whole new technologies (MS-MS or immunoassay)?

In order to answer these questions it is useful to look at a few leading multiresidue methods in terms of their advantages and limitations; in essence, to find their "pressure points" that are amenable to incremental (or drastic) improvement.

Pressure Points in Multiresidue Methods

Every analytical method has inherent limitations that may or may not be amenable to manipulation. As an example, the PAM (Section 201) Mills procedure (figure 3) represents a "middle of the road" method optimized to provide quality data on pesticides of intermediate polarity and volatility. It has at least six points where losses of individual pesticides may occur. For example, paraquat is insoluble in acetonitrile and petroleum ether and is thus lost in the first step (#1). Aldrin has an unfavorable petroleum ether/acetonitrile partition coefficient and is thus partially lost in the discard of the petroleum ether when high fat samples are processed (#2). Very water-soluble pesticides, such as some organophosphates, may be lost in the back extraction from aqueous acetonitrile to petroleum ether (#3). Very nonpolar and very polar pesticides, which survive to the Florisil cleanup, are further lost because they elute prior to (#4) or after (#5) the three prime ethyl ether/petroleum ether fractions. Of course, some pesticides, including several N-methylcarbamates, degrade on Florisil, adding another limita-

Figure 3. — Mills Procedure (PAM)

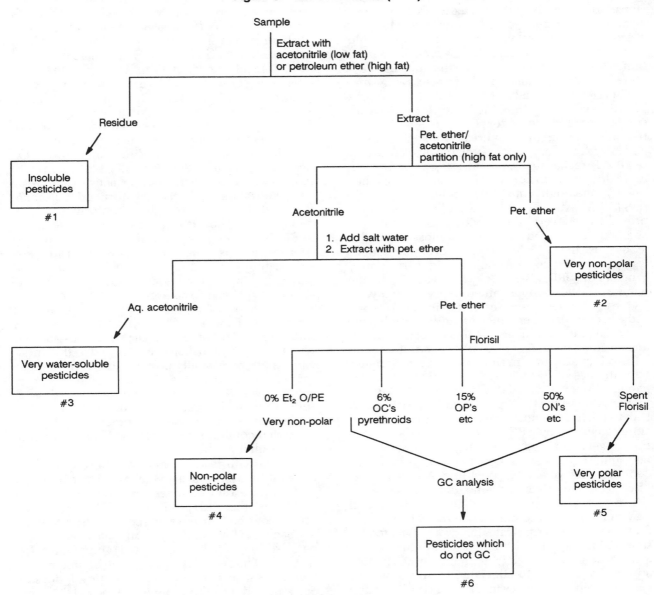

SOURCE: James Seiber, University of California, Davis, CA, 1988.

tion to the Mills procedure. Finally, success in this procedure depends on gas chromatography of the cleaned residues, so that non-volatile materials that do not elute or degrade upon GC (#6) as well as those showing poor response to the common selective detector will not be determined.

Thus, in essence, only pesticides within a range of polarity, volatility, and stability characteristics will survive the Mills determination. In fact, that number is about 200 (in fatty foods) or 274 (in nonfatty foods) for pesticides, transformation products, metabolites, etc. (5). Some pesticides are not recovered at all, or only partially, because of failure in one or more of the steps described above. Limitations exist in all multiresidue analytical methods, so that several pesticides simply "fall through the cracks" in Federal/State regulatory monitoring programs (1). How can the Mills method be expanded?

One approach is to alter or eliminate the limiting steps. For example, loss in the discarded aqueous acetonitrile phase (#3) could be minimized by using a stronger solvent (ethyl acetate or methylene chloride) than petroleum ether in the preceding partition. The tradeoff here could be the appearance of more interfering material in the final extract, which might raise detection limits. Alternately, this entire partition could be eliminated and the acetonitrile concentrated directly for Florisil cleanup. The tradeoffs here might be increased detection limits and lower recovery of some volatile pesticides (v.p. > 10-3 Torr) because concentrating acetonitrile is more difficult than concentrating petroleum ether. Finally, one might substitute a solid phase extraction (SPE) cartridge for the liquid/liquid partition, providing recovery of a slightly broader range of compounds and reduced volatility losses—the latter because the SPE elution solvent volume is much less than that used in liquid/liquid partitioning. Whether the SPE raises or lowers the detection limit would need to be determined experimentally.

One could thus critique each step in the Mills procedure, optimize to enhance breadth of applicability while maintaining acceptable detection limits, and in some cases (such as SPE substitution) perhaps achieve savings in time. Our own experience with the use of SPEs to isolate metabolites of organophosphorus pesticides from urine (13) would tend to support the time-savings notion, particularly because several samples (up to 10) may be extracted simultaneously by SPE. Manufacturers are offering gadgets built upon the SPE concept that facilitate simultaneous extraction and elution as well as concentration of eluate, providing overall savings of considerable time and amounts of solvents.

The Florisil cleanup can be attacked in several ways; miniaturized columns are already in wide use for relatively clean substrates (many non-fatty foods), thus reducing solvent volumes, and elution and evaporation times. Deactivated silica gel can be substituted for Florisil to alleviate the breakdown of certain compound classes on Florisil. HPLC cleanup methods could be substituted, allowing for expansion of the range of polarities that could be accommodated, minimizing solvent volumes, and alleviating breakdown. HPLC also has the ability to be automated, which is difficult with gravity column chromatography. For example, gel permeation column cleanup has been automated and commercialized for use with fatty foods (PAM). Finally, the Florisil cleanup step could be eliminated entirely so that the extract normally entering this cleanup would go directly to GC determination. The tradeoff here is increased detection limits (because more "garbage" enters the GC), decreased GC column life (same reason), and increased chance for misidentification and misinterpretation (because the Florisil fractionation works to simplify chromatograms and help in result interpretation). However, the large time-saving provided by Florisil elimination, in such procedures as Luke (PAM Section 232.41, Figure 4), has led to reduced use of it for multiresidue screening. Note also that the Luke method still provides opportunities for loss of pesticides, but fewer than in the full Mills procedure. As might be expected, the Luke method is applicable to non-fatty foods and can not be used with electron-capture or flame ionization GC detection without prior cleanup. It should also be apparent that various hybrid techniques can be devised in which the extract prior to Florisil cleanup is injected on GC to screen for some chemicals or chemical classes (OPs are most successfully handled) and then subjected to Florisil before looking for other classes (OCs, for example) or for GC/MS confirmation.

As a matter of fact, there are many hybrids and variations of the PAM version of the Mills (and Mills-Onley-Gaither) and Luke procedures, most of which are not published. This is good in that innovations are continually possible, but it introduces some uncertainty in knowing what is the best procedure for a given analysis and in comparing results from one laboratory to another. An in-depth study of innovations already in practice might yield clues that could improve the PAM versions of the multiresidue methods.

For alternate pesticide multiresidue approaches, it might be useful to see what types of extraction and fractionation schemes are used for chemical pollutants other than pesticides. HPLC-based cleanup methods include the silica column used by Wehner et al. (12) for analyzing pesticides in air, which has also been applied to water (14) including fog water (3). The column has a long useful lifetime and maintains its resolution characteristics. It does require periodic calibration with standards to show where fraction cuts should be made, but this is a simple matter of injecting a mixed standard. The polarity range was successfully extended to include polar glycosides (11) and derivatized glyphosate in plant extracts (10) by adding a methyl-butyl ether (MTBE)-THF gradient after the hexane-MTBE gradient. On the negative side, HPLC cleanup requires sample concentration to a very small volume (< 0.5 ml) prior to injection on the HPLC, does not tolerate suspended particulate matter, and has a sample throughput of only 1 sample/hr/column. There

Figure 4.—Acetone Extraction Method (Luke)

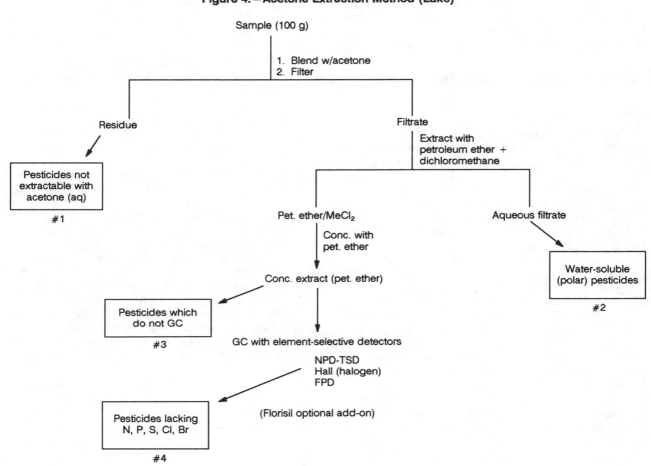

SOURCE: James Seiber, University of California, Davis, CA, 1988.

may be ways of increasing the throughput considerably (very short columns) but these remain to be proven. Also, the 1 sample/hr/column limitation is somewhat misleading because 24-hour operation might be possible if an autosampler were used.

A second HPLC cleanup approach used a cyano column with hexane to acetone gradient. This procedure was developed by Crowley et al. (3) for separating shale oil extracts, and it was used by our group (4) to separate mutagenic constituents of smoke particulate matter. It could probably be used for some pesticide residue analyses requiring fractionation. Other columns/mobile phases could be used as well.

It is somewhat interesting to note the diverging paths taken by pesticide residue chemists who have concentrated on column chromatography for cleanup and fractionation, and chemists involved with priority pollutant and drug analyses who have used acid-base partitioning against organic solvents for cleanup and fractionation. For priority pollutants in water, the total scheme uses purging with air or nitrogen to remove volatile pollutants (benzene, chlorinated solvents, etc.) and then acid-organic solvent extraction to separate acids (phenols) from base-neutral chemicals. This scheme would probably not be of general utility for pesticides in foods because (1) few pesticides are volatile or acidic, (2) some pesticides are not stable to acid conditions, and (3) the final base-neutral fraction (which would contain most common pesticides) might not be clean enough for low-level GC or HPLC analysis. The common drug schemes use a more complex acid-base partitioning system, which serves drug analyses well because so many of these agents are bases (alkaloids) or acids (barbiturates, salicylates, etc.). Thus, the cleanup technologies in these schemes are not applicable to the problem of multiresidue pesticide analyses in foodstuffs, where essentially neutral compounds need to be handled.

Other Stages of Pesticide Analyses

Once a residue-containing extract is provided, with or without cleanup, the steps of resolution, detection, measurement, and quantitation are performed, occasionally after derivatization. The gas chromatograph equipped with selective detection based upon the heteroatom (halogen, P,N,S) content of the pesticide analytes is the most common resolution-detection system employed.

Choices here include the following:
Column type —packed vs. capillary, phase choice
Detector type—Flame photometric (S,P)
      Thermionic (N,P)
      Hall electrolytic conductivity (C1, Br, N, S)
      Electron capture (halogens)

Voluminous literature exists on the applicability of each combination. Suffice it to say, the packed vs. capillary issue is still debated, with more converts to capillary following the introduction of reproducible splitters and megabore columns. These columns provide greater resolution and greater efficiency than packed columns, both of which generally lower detection limits and increase confidence in the results. They also minimize breakdown and irreversible adsorption of the more thermal-labile and polar pesticides, thus increasing breadth of applicability. They do not, however, have the capacity to accept very dirty extracts that might be chromatographable on packed columns. This represents another tradeoff, although in spite of it the technology is clearly leaning toward more capillary and less packed column use.

Regarding column phases, analysts already have a large selection (summarized in PAM Section 301), with the only new developments occurring in adapting conventional phases (or mimics) to fused-silica capillary columns.

Summarizing for columns, high load, bonded-phase megabore columns will suffice for virtually all GC systems and, through improvements in technology that are rapidly emerging, will extend the applicability of GC to even broader ranges of pesticide types. They will also minimize the need for derivatization (a time-consuming and error-prone procedure best avoided if possible) of some phenolic, carbamate, and polar metabolite chemical classes. More work in proving these points will pay rich dividends in improving conventional methods.

In GC detection, many improvements in virtually all detectors have occurred in the past 5 years, and these are being rapidly adopted by residue chemists. They include the following:

1. FPD detection limits have been improved almost tenfold. This is still the most reliable system for OP and S-containing pesticides.
2. Hall-type electrolytic conductivity detectors have improved dramatically and are now clearly the first choice for organohalogen compounds and near first choice for organonitrogen compounds.
3. The thermionic NP-TSD shows steady improvements and represents a viable choice for OP and ON analyses.
4. The pulsed-mode Ni63 EC is a vast improvement over earlier EC detectors and is still useful for some organohalogen compounds, particularly the more volatile ones resolved by capillary GC.

Newer detectors that may supplement the above improvements include the following:

1. Photoionization, particularly for aromatic compounds lacking heteroatans and for some poly-sulfur and polyhalogen compounds. There is now more than one supplier of this promising detector.
2. Mass selective (MS) detectors, for virtually all compounds.

The mass selective detector, or MS, is worth special note because of its universality, confirmatory power, rapidly improving detectability (particularly in the selective ion or SIM mode), and a healthy trend to lower priced, user-friendly systems of increasing ruggedness.

Many analysts have shied away from MS, including the mass selective detector (MSD) Ion-Trap version, and other GC/MS systems, feeling that it is more suited to dedicated analyses for a single analyte or small analyte clusters than for the range of analytes potentially present in a multiresidue sample of unknown origin. This is becoming a less valid objection because new MSs can be programmed to shift rapidly between pre-selected masses as the chromatogram develops, thus covering the broad range needed for many applications. Some industrial and contract labs have moved more to MS, to the point of replacing element-selective detectors. This is a very healthy trend and should be encouraged by increasing research funding in the area of tailoring multiresidue schemes to be compatible with the MS.

Aside from much improved versions of traditional pesticide analytical methods in the areas of capillary columns, improved selective detectors, and the

GC mass spectrometry-based systems, other conventional techniques and a few relatively new approaches are finding increasing applications in pesticide multiresidue methods. Chief of these is HPLC, which has become close to routine in handling analysis of some pesticides that are not amenable to GC, or for which HPLC provides an alternative to derivatization for GC. For example, some N-methylcarbamate insecticides (and their metabolites), for which derivatization and GC represented the only viable approach just a few years ago (8), are screened by HPLC using either direct UV/fluorescence detection, or detection following automated postcolumn derivatization. The multiresidue procedure of the California Department of Food and Agriculture (2) (figure 5), for example, integrates the use of SPE isolation with postcolumn derivatization HPLC, with detection limits for eight carbamates in the range of 0.2-0.5 ppm. Moye (6) provided other ex-

amples, including for glyphosate, phenoxy acids, and substituted ureas. Once again, technical improvements in HPLC columns and detectors have provided increased resolution, detectability, and reliability. Capillary column HPLC and supercritical fluid chromatography promise further advance: capillary columns in extending resolution and detectability further, and SFC in the ability to interface with the selective GC detectors (an area where HPLC is normally at a disadvantage relative to GLC). HPLC-MS is also improving, particularly with thermospray and other new interfacing systems, but is not yet competitive with GLC-MS in detectability and confirmatory power.

Still other instrumental advances may find future use in multiresidue analysis, including the following:

- *Headspace GC*—Volatile pesticides (methyl bromide, ethylene dibromide, phosphine)
- *GC-Fourier Transform Infrared*—Semivolatile-

Figure 5.—CDFA Multiresidue Screen

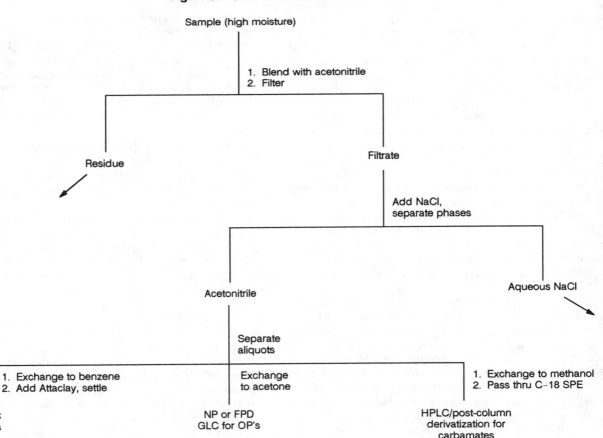

SOURCE: James Seiber, University of California, Davis, CA, 1988.

volatile pesticides; can be interfaced with GC-MS (GC-IR-MS)

- *Multidimensional GC*—More rapid screening for varieties of pesticides in single extracts.
- *Tandem mass spectrometry* (MS-MS)—Screening samples for classes of chemicals; confirmation.
- *High resolution mass spectrometry* (HRMS)—Screening samples for classes of chemicals; ultra-low level detection of specific chemicals; confirmation.
- *Immunoassay*—Screening samples for selected classes of chemicals, particularly those not amenable to low-level GC or HPLC analysis.

Finally, a few comments should be made on automation, and other time- and labor-saving approaches. Autoinjectors for GC and autosamplers for LC are commercially available in much improved versions over early devices introduced in the 1970s. Both can be considered routine and have extended sample throughput to 24-hour operations. A necessary adjunct to autoinjectors is a programmable integrating data system for data compilation, eliminating the need to have all peaks on-scale for quantitation. Another convenient adjunct is the use of internal standards (nonpesticide surrogates that chromatograph similarly to pesticides), bypassing the need for extensive standard curve preparation and reinjection of "out of range" samples.

Thus, microprocessor-controlled GLCs and HPLCs with autoinjectors and computer data systems are seen in increasing frequency in pesticide analytical laboratories and, combined with internal standards, can make large improvements in the time and costs of residue analysis. This trend will continue, as "smart" systems that identify (based on retention time) and quantitate suspected residues with less operator involvement are further refined and utilized. The data systems of GLC and HPLC instruments have the added advantage of providing records, which can help fulfill good laboratory practices requirements.

The use of SPE cartridges was mentioned previously as a sometimes more rapid and generally solvent-saving device in the extraction-cleanup phases of analysis. SPEs also provide an opportunity to conduct some sample preparation in the field. For example, we extracted water samples for pesticide residues by pumping water through C-18 SPEs immediately after the samples were taken in the field; very little extra time was added to that required for sampling and only the small SPEs needed to be transported to the lab for completion of analysis by GLC. This approach could perhaps be extended directly to milk, juices, and other fluid foodstuffs, and perhaps even to solid foods if a solvent extraction operation were set up close to the point of sampling.

Improved gadgetry for solvent concentration is gradually replacing the very clumsy, labor-intensive rotary evaporators and Kudera-Danish-Snyder column steam concentrators. For example, the N-Evap proved useful in simultaneously concentrating many samples of small solvent volumes when first introduced in the 1970s. A recently introduced programmable sand bath evaporator should also find use, particularly for concentrating aqueous samples. In fact, any move by technology toward smaller sample sizes and extract volumes should save time and decrease chances for in-house contamination because of the smaller glassware requirements.

Putting It All Together

Taking what appears to be the best of existing MR schemes, and extending to sample miniaturization and SPE cleanup-fractionation, leads to the hypothetical "method" in figure 6. The hypothetical method is broad-based in terms of handling pesticides over a range of volatilities and polarities, and it is quick because of lower volumes handled and the elimination of liquid/liquid extraction and solvent evaporation.

In this approach, all GCs are equipped with megabore capillary columns, autoinjectors, and data systems. LCs are equipped with short, small particle columns, autosamplers, and UV and fluorescence detectors with and without postcolumn derivatization. The GC/MS is programmed in the selective ion mode to search for ions diagnostic for individual pesticides. Quantitation is done vs. internal surrogate standards added to the first extract. Recoveries are calculated for the internal standards by occasional external standardization. Fluid samples, high fat, and low fat samples could potentially be accommodated with some modification of the first extraction step. All steps would need research and developmental optimization, using a variety of substrates and pesticide types. The point here is that most pesticide residue chemists could come up with a scheme that, conceptually, improves on existing methods by instituting newer technologies and miniaturization. Whether these conceptual schemes could extend multiresidue methodologies to new levels in the parameters in figure 1 is a question worth asking—and perhaps worth investing of public funds to answer.

Figure 6.— Hypothetical MR Scheme

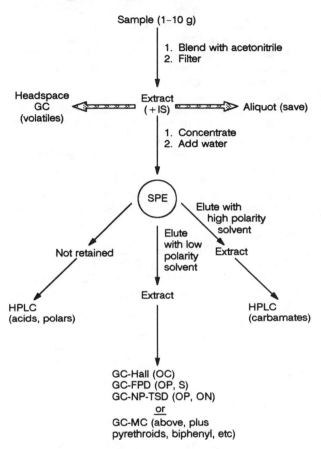

Sample (1–10 g)

1. Blend with acetonitrile
2. Filter

Headspace
GC
(volatiles) ⟸ Extract (+IS) ⟹ Aliquot (save)

1. Concentrate
2. Add water

SPE

Not retained

Elute with low polarity solvent

Elute with high polarity solvent

Extract

HPLC
(acids, polars)

Extract

HPLC
(carbamates)

GC-Hall (OC)
GC-FPD (OP, S)
GC-NP-TSD (OP, ON)
_or_
GC-MC (above, plus
pyrethroids, biphenyl, etc)

SOURCE: James Seiber, University of California, Davis, CA, 1988.

Conclusions

Can existing analytical methods be improved? The answer is certainly yes, and in fact they are continually undergoing improvement as new GC, HPLC, and MS systems are introduced and as new chemicals are included in the existing schemes.

How can they be improved? The following are offered as potential elements to improvement:

1. *Miniaturization*—Offers savings in time by processing smaller volumes, increases the possibility of automation, and might extend breadth (yet to be proved) through the use of commercial cleanup columns (HPLC or SPE cartridges).

2. *GC Technology*—Wide bore capillary columns interfaced with element-selective detectors will minimize the need for derivatization and pro-

vide more efficient resolution, thus lowering detection limits. When used with auto-injectors and integrating data systems, throughput and data quality will improve.

3. *HPLC Technology*—Will focus on those compounds that cannot be determined by GLC; critical need for selective HPLC detectors that go beyond UV, fluorescence, and electrochemical (SCF improvements will help here); if detectors were available, promises major improvement on breadth of MR technology. Even without super-selective detectors, HPLC will find specialty use in removing problem interferences and in postcolumn derivatization for specific classes of chemicals.

4. *MSD Technology*—This represents a real opportunity because this is an affordable, here-and-now technology that only needs a few well-designed studies to show applicability, particularly in the SIM mode with programmed ramping of ion masses through the chromatogram. MSD can be used as a detector (SIM mode) and also for confirmation (Scan mode).

Who Should Do It?

Industry has a responsibility for fitting new compounds into multiresidue schemes, but not for the development of the schemes themselves. Federal labs should take the lead, set the goals, and conduct the validation (with AOAC or other assistance). But they should not shoulder the burden of discovery and development alone.

A well-conceived, extramural funding program is needed, allowing for participation by academic institutions, research institutes, and state lead agencies. New funds in the range of $10 million would be needed, with half devoted to upgrading the equipment and scientific expertise in the residue labs of state agencies and the four regional Leader Laboratories of the USDA- CSRS - State Experiment Station's Minor Use Registration Program (IR-4), and half to competitive funding on a Request for Proposal (RFP) basis. Categories for the RFP would be the four mentioned above, in this section, and also a fifth dealing with extending multiresidue methods to new classes of pesticides (sulfonylureas, pyrethroids, etc.). Academic involvement is crucial, both to supply new ideas and also to stimulate involvement of graduate students and post-doctorals who will provide the invigoration needed for a longer-term, sustaining program of residue analytical excellence, which is needed over the long-haul.

References

1. Ambrus, A. and Thier, H.P., "Application of Multiresidue Procedures in Pesticides Residues Analysis," *Pure and Applied Chem.* 58:1035-1062, 1986.
2. California Department of Food and Agriculture, Multiresidue Pesticide Screens, California Department of Food and Agriculture, Sacramento, CA, 1988.
3. Crowley, R.T., Siggia, S. and Uden, P.C., "Class Separation and Characterization of Shale Oil by Liquid Chromatography and Capillary Column Gas Chromatography," *Anal. Chem.* 52:1224-1228, 1980.
3. Glotfelty, D.E., Seiber, J.N. and Liljedahl, L.A., "Pesticides in Fog," *Nature* 325:602-605, 1987.
4. Mast, T.J., Hsieh, D.P. and Seiber, J.N., "Mutagenicity and Chemical Characterization of Organic Constituents in Rice Straw Smoke Particulate Matter," *Environ. Sci. Technol.* 18:338-343, 1984.
5. McMahon, B.M. and Burke, J.A., "Expanding and Tracking the Capabilities of Pesticide Multiresidue Methodology Used in the Food and Drug Administrations Pesticide Monitoring Program," *J. Assoc. Offic. Anal. Chem.* 70:1072-1081, 1987.
6. Moye, H.A., "High Performance Liquid Chromatographic analysis of Pesticide Residues," *Analysis of Pesticide Residues*, H.A. Moye (ed.) (New York: Wiley-Interscience, 1981), pp. 333-378.
7. Pesticide Analytical Manual, Department of Health and Human Services, Food and Drug Administration, Washington, DC, Sections 201.01, and 232.41.
8. Seiber, J.N., "Carbamate Insecticide Residue Analysis by Gas-Liquid Chromatography," *Analysis of Pesticide Residues*, H.A. Moye (ed.) (New York: Wiley-Interscience, 1981), pp. 333-378.
9. Seiber, J.N., "Analysis of Toxicants in Agricultural Environments," *Genetic Toxicology*, R.A. Fleck and A. Hollaender (eds.) (New York: Plenum, 1982), pp. 219-234.
10. Seiber, J.N., McChesney, M.M., Kon, R., et al., "Analysis of Glyphosate Residues in Kiwifruit and Asparagus Using HPLC of Derivatized Glyphosate As a Cleanup Step," *J. Agric. Food Chem.* 32:678-681, 1984.
11. Seiber, J.N., Brower, L.P., Lee, S.M., et al., "Cardenolide Connection Between Overwintering Monarch Butterflies from Mexico and Their Larval Food Plant," *J. Chem. Ecol.* 12:1157-1170, 1986.
12. Wehner, T., Woodrow, J.E., Kim, Y-H., et al., "Multiresidue Analysis of Trace Organic Pesticides in Air," *Identification and Analysis of Organic Pollutants in Air*, L.H. Keith (ed.) (Boston, MA: Butterworth, 1984), pp. 273-290.
13. Weisskopf, C. and Seiber, J.N., "New Approaches to the Analysis of Organophosphates in the Urine of Field Workers," Paper presented at the 194th National Meeting, American Chemical Society (AGRO 141), New Orleans, LA, Sept. 3, 1987.
14. Woodrow, J.E., Majewski, M.S., and Seiber, J.N., "Accumulative Sampling of Trace Pesticides and Other Organics in Surface Water Using XAD-4 Resin," *J. Environ. Sci. Health* 21:143-164, 1986.

Techniques for and the Role of Screening Pesticide Residue Analysis

Richard L. Ellis, Director, Chemistry Division, Food Safety and Inspection Service, U.S. Department of Agriculture, Washington, DC

Contents

	Page
Abstract	153
Background	153
Screening Method Concepts	154
Attributes of Screening Methods	155
Quality Assurance	156
Detection Systems for Screening Methods	156
Integrating Screening Methods into Multiresidue Regulatory Programs	159
Constraints on Use of Rapid Test Methods	160
References	160

Figure

	Page
1. Decision Tree for Regulatory Control Program	161

Abstract

Analytical testing for residues has progressed from relatively insensitive bioassays to highly technical procedures combining attributes of computer science, electronics, materials sciences, and biotechnology. Consumers, consumer action groups, the National Academy of Sciences, Congress, and others have highlighted public health concerns about the detrimental effects of pesticides residues in food, water, and other parts of our environment. Regulatory programs are designing improved statistical-based sampling programs to ensure a safe and wholesome food supply. These programs highlight the magnitude of testing required to accomplish that goal. Testing procedures, once the domain of relatively complex quantitative and confirmatory techniques run in well-equipped laboratories with trained personnel, are not adequate to meet analytical demands with available resources. Rapid test systems employing advanced technology are being produced that can make residue testing programs responsive to this need. Regulatory statutes require a preponderance of information to support enforcement responsibilities. Thus, integrating rapid test procedures with quantitative and confirmatory methods is needed. Rapid testing procedures may be used by personnel not experienced in analytical sciences. This requires strong quality-assurance and quality-control programs to ensure proper design and use of rapid test methods. Regulatory-agency policy development on roles for these screening methods as well as other technological developments for testing procedures will influence development and application for improved public health analytical testing programs now and in the future.

Background

Modern agricultural production uses commercially available pesticides to combat a variety of weeds, insects, fungi, and other agricultural pests. These pesticides contribute substantially to the high level of agricultural production we currently enjoy. As a result, consumers are exposed to pesticides, usually in minute quantities, in several food groups including meat, dairy products, fruits, vegetables, dried food goods, most processed foods and many other household staples. Some pesticides, however, are considered as either acutely or chronically toxic to humans and other segments of the environment, and they pose potentially serious health risks to non-target organisms and species. This presents a significant regulatory responsibility to public health-related agencies as well as to Congress.

The magnitude and complexity of the regulatory responsibility is well developed by the Congressional Research Service 1986 report and the National Academy of Sciences report, "Regulating Pesticides in Foods." Regardless of the number of pesticides registered for use on agricultural products, the number is small compared to the more than 8,000 food tolerances listed in the Food, Drug and Cosmetic Act, Section 408 and 409 (2). From data supplied by EPA, 53 of these pesticides have active ingredients identified as oncogenic or potentially oncogenic (2). This does not include some of the chlorinated hydrocarbons considered as oncogenic in animals or humans. Further, FDA has classified 81 compounds through its surveillance index as warranting residue monitoring because of their potential health hazard. Based on the GAO Domestic Food Report (3), 30 of these received little or no residue testing between 1979 and 1985, and several pesticides included in the two highest classes as potential health hazards are not covered by the five current FDA multiresidue methods, although these residues may be analyzed by other methods or other programs. Recognizing the universe of pesticides used on foods, there is agreement that more residue methods are needed for monitoring purposes. This becomes more important as higher levels of sampling are called for to improve confidence that regulatory agencies are providing greater assurance of a safe food and water supply to consumers.

Screening Method Concepts

Analytical methods play an important role in food production inspection systems to protect public health. A universal analysis scheme that can simultaneously quantify the presence of all compounds or classes of compounds of interest in foods, animal tissue, or fluid with acceptable accuracy and correctly identify the analyte or analytes would be a desirable, unified methods approach for regulatory control agencies. Yet at present, there are very few analytical procedures available to regulatory agencies that simultaneously quantitate and confirm the identity of such residues. Until universal methods are available, regulatory programs will have to employ methods with individual attributes of presumptive presence, quantitation, and positive identification. To accomplish this goal, methods with different attributes must perform in concert for a highly effective residue program regardless of individual regulatory mandates.

Terms such as confirmatory, reference, quantitative, semiquantitative, screening, rapid, and presumptive methods are well known. An alternative to the potential difficulty of categorizing methods, and the stigma associated with these descriptive terms, is to define the methods independent of in-

tended purpose, according to the attribute or qualities of method performance. Attributes and qualities of three levels of analytical methods are relevant to support regulatory programs. Though the focus will be on screening methods, a brief description of the method types is needed to understand their interrelationship.

Level I methods incorporate the ability to quantify the amount of specific analyte or class of analytes and positively identify their presence in a single analytical procedure. These are assays with the highest level of credibility and are unequivocal at the level of interest. They may be single procedures that determine both the concentration and identity of the analyte, or combinations of methods for determining and confirming a residue for definitive identification. These methods are most commonly identified as confirmatory methods.

Level II methods are those that are not unequivocal but are used to determine the concentration of an analyte at the level of interest and to provide some structural information. For example, these methods may employ structure, functional group, or immunochemical properties as the basis for the analytical scheme. These methods are often reliable enough to be used as reference methods. Level II methods provide a quite acceptable approach for residue testing.

They may be used to corroborate the presence of a compound or class of compounds. Thus, two Level II methods may provide information suitable for Level I attributes, providing they employ different chemical technologies. The majority of analytical methods now available and used by regulatory control agencies are Level II methods. These methods are usually the quantitative analytical methods used in laboratories for regulatory control programs.

Level III methods are those that generate imperfect, though useful, information. These testing procedures detect the presence or absence of a compound or class of compounds at some designated level of interest and often are based on non-instrumental techniques for analytical determination. Results on a given sample are not as reliable as Level I or II methods without corroborating information. Level III methods may, for example, provide reasonably good quantitative information but poor compound or class specificity or identity, or they may provide strong or unequivocal identification with very little quantitative information. Level III methods are not poorly described or sloppy methods; rather, they must have defined operating characteristics of reliable performance. Many microbiological assay procedures and immunoassay test systems may fall into this category. They are used because of convenience and potential suitability to non-laboratory environments, analytical speed, sample efficiency through batch analysis, portability to non-laboratory environments, sensitivity, and the ability to detect classes of compounds. The hallmark of Level III-type methods is that action based on individual positive results require substantiation using Level I or II methods as required by the uncertainty of an individual result. However, epidemiological information may provide substantive data, reducing the uncertainty of individual results. These are typically screening or rapid test methods and may offer several advantages to a regulatory control program.

The reliability of Level III methods should be measured in part by their performance characteristics as well as their ability to handle relatively large numbers of samples within a given timeframe. Two key characteristics requiring definition include their percent of false positives (reporting a positive response when no analyte is present) and percent of false negatives (reporting a negative response when the analyte is present) when measured against a validated quantitative assay in a statistically designed protocol to derive the test method operating characteristics. When the operating characteristics are defined for false negative and false positive results, the operating range of the screening method may be established. Individual programs may select those false negative and false positive values to suit their particular program needs. The percent of false negatives must be quite low at the levels of interest (less than 5 percent), while slightly more flexibility may be acceptable for false positives for screening tests. A minimum level of residue detection can be described based on a balance between these two parameters.

Attributes of Screening Methods

Methods suitable for regulatory purposes must be reliable. To ensure analytical reliability, performance characteristics of a method must be determined by multilaboratory evaluation. In most cases, minimum standards should be set, designed to fit the needs of specific program requirements. By consensus with public health standard-setting organizations or agencies, the principal attributes of analytical methods are specificity, precision, systematic error, and sensitivity. Other attributes relevant to screening methods will be described as well.

Specificity is the ability of a method to respond only to the substance being measured. A residue control method must provide for unambiguous identification of the compound being measured. One set of measurements of specificity is the percent of false positives and false negatives. This characteristic is often a function of the measuring principle used and the analyte functionality—key factors for rapid test methods. Methods should be able to qualitatively differentiate the analyte from analogues or metabolic products of the compound(s) of interest under the experimental conditions employed.

Precision is a measure of the variability of results when the method is applied to separate portions of a homogeneous sample. Precision is usually expressed as standard deviation. This term is sometimes used to describe other method characteristics such as limit of detection, limit of decision (4), and limit of reliable measurement (5). Another useful term is the relative standard deviation because it is relatively constant over a considerable concentration range (an order of magnitude, for example), ideally covering the level of interest.

Systematic error is analytical method bias, the difference of the measured value from the true, assigned, or accepted value (mean 8 value). It is commonly expressed as the percent recovery of added analyte to a sample blank. At relatively high concentrations, recoveries are expected to approach 100 percent. At lower concentrations and particularly with methods involving a number of steps, recoveries may be lower. Regardless of what average recoveries are observed, low variability is a desirable feature. Commercial rapid test systems should be designed so that parallel curves for standard solutions of the analyte and sample extracts of analyte added to a sample are routinely achieved.

Accuracy refers to the closeness of agreement between the true value and the mean result. The accuracy requirements of different types of methods will vary with the use being made of the results. For screening methods, characteristics of false positive results and false negatives define a methods operating range.

The sensitivity of a method is a measure of the ability to discriminate between small differences in analyte concentration. A common practice is to define sensitivity as the slope of the calibration curve with known standards at the level of interest.

Beyond these method characteristics are a number of collateral criteria particularly suitable for screening methods for regulatory control programs. Methods should be rugged or robust, cost-effective, relatively uncomplicated, portable and capable of handling a set of samples simultaneously in a time-effective manner. Ruggedness of a method refers to its capability to be relatively unaffected by small deviations from the established values in the use of reagents, quantities of reagents used, time factors for extractions, and reaction or temperature. This does not, however, provide latitude for carelessness or haphazard techniques. Cost-effectiveness refers to use of relatively common reagents, efficient use of resources, and using instrumentation commonly used for trace environmental analyses. A method of being relatively uncomplicated refers to use of simple, straightforward mechanical or operational procedures throughout the method. Portability is the characteristic of the method that enables it to be transferred from one location to another without loss of established performance characteristics. The capability to analyze a set of samples simultaneously reduces the analytical time requirements of sample analysis. This is particularly important for screening methods in which large numbers of samples are to be analyzed in short or fixed timeframes.

The importance of establishing the attributes and performance criteria cannot be overemphasized. It provides the necessary information to allow regulatory control officials to develop and manage programs responsive to their public health responsibilities. Performance criteria for analytical methods also provide a basis for good management decisions in future planning, evaluation, and product disposition.

Quality Assurance

Regulatory control agencies responsible for monitoring foods are routinely made aware that any analytical discrepancy may require the inevitable defense of our analytical programs. A principal objective becomes one of assuring we have a well planned and executed quality-assurance program. Quality assurance is an important part of all regulatory control programs. With screening methods, or any rapid test system, established policies and procedures are needed to ensure that these methods are being properly conducted and the testor is evaluating the test response in the appropriate manner. The implications of poor performance of rapid test methods would be difficult for regulatory control agencies to deal with.

Quality assurance begins with the method development process. Activities include experimental optimization of each procedural step or manipulation to determine the critical control steps—those having a substantial impact on method performance. Other activities include identifying when an analytical method may be stopped without adversely affecting the results; determining the ruggedness or process variability that may be employed in any particular method step without reducing the method's performance; and determining the sample requirements necessary to ensure reliable, interference-free results. Instrument parameters should be optimized and a mechanism to test instrument performance established if instruments are required. Mass transfers in the procedure should be minimized. Lastly, the method must be written in thorough, concise, unambiguous language. These factors will facilitate method transfer and training for end-users of a method into a regulatory program. The focus on quality assurance cannot be overemphasized. In the long-term, it is less expensive to do it right the first time. It ensures credibility to a regulatory program and esprit de corps among analysts.

Detection Systems for Screening Methods

Two important reasons for using screening methods are 1) their capability to analyze a relatively large number of samples in a given unit of time, and 2) their robust nature. This latter characteristic allows latitude for using screening methods in non-laboratory surroundings. In these instances, methods will often be used by individuals not necessarily experienced in analytical chemistry techniques. This places a constraint on certain types of methodology. It limits use of certain types of equipment, instruments, and reagents. Further, methods need simple, unambiguous test instructions that will enable a testor to correctly prepare the test material, conduct the analysis, and interpret and report the test findings. Process controls defining critical steps in the test procedure are very relevant to the success of such a testing program.

Thin layer chromatographic procedures satisfy a significant number of desired attributes for screening methods. The capability to analyze a set of samples in a given timeframe is usually higher than other common chromatographic systems. There is a wide variety of adsorbents, chromatographic solvents, and reagents facilitating residue detection. In addition, residue detection is a static process rather than a dynamic one; quality assurance is easier because control samples and reference standards can be analyzed simultaneously with the test samples. A comprehensive review on thin layer chromatographic systems and procedures has been published recently (6). It describes an extensive array of systems for pesticide analysis. One that has been reduced to practice for a regulatory program consists of thin layer chromatography for separation of 12 organophosphate pesticides using cholinesterase enzyme inhibition for residue identification (7). A recent project with Food Safety and Inspection Service (FSIS) for screening chlorinated hydrocarbon pesticides employing thin layer chromatography with a variety of detection systems for chlorine (including many in reference 6) was not successful because the sensitivity at the level of interest was not attainable (8). A further complication was the sample extraction procedure from animal fat being too complicated for use in a nonlaboratory situation. Detection systems focused on the chlorine atom because of the relatively high chlorine content in the compounds of interest. A successful application of thin layer chromatography for a rapid field test has been developed for sulfamethazine by FSIS. Although these are limited applications for regulatory programs, this technique offers promise for the future as new reagents improve sensitivity and thin layer chromatography systems provide new approaches for effective sample purification and analysis.

The detection limits of most color-producing or fluorescent-generating reagents provide sensitivity at low microgram per gram ($\mu g/g$, ppm) concentrations. Reagents using enzyme inhibition allow detection limits in some systems at low picogram per gram (pg/g, ppb) concentrations. For example, many herbicides employing photosynthesis inhibition as a mechanism of action have been detected at picogram (10-12g) levels using plant chloroplasts and a reduction-oxidation chemical indicator. In corn, potatoes, and carrots, detection limits without purification of the sample extract were less than 10 pg/g (ppb) (9). Classes of herbicides adaptable to this detection system include triazines, phenylureas, phenylcarbamates, 13 uracils, and acyl anilides. This suggests the possibility of broad-spectrum screening tests suitable to nonlaboratory use.

Immunobased assays are emerging as promising screening test methods. Test systems for a wide variety of organic residues in soil, water, food, plant, and animal tissues are being developed by a number of companies in the United States. These tests are being developed in rapid, very sensitive, easy to use, and usually highly specific formats. They show promise for rapid onsite testing as qualitative assays while some are now being designed for fast, quantitative laboratory tests. Their designed specificity, which is commonly very high, generally allows use of relatively crude samples as a test material and makes them attractive for use in non-laboratory environments. Generally, the cost of these assays is lower than traditional analytical laboratory methods. However, they are still dependent on sample preparation. Nevertheless, potential per-sample cost for such assays is less than $15.00, including administrative costs. Instrumental methods are usually $50.00 or more for similar analyses. The major constraint of these assay systems is their relatively high cost of development. It is estimated that they become practical economic investments by economy of scale, when 100,000 tests per year are run (10).

Within our current regulatory and statutory environment it is not reasonable to expect registrants of pesticides or other chemical entities used in food production to voluntarily provide screening methods. There is little interest in developing multi-residue methods, in particular, that may be capable of either identifying or quantitating residues in food products that may include a competitor's product. Where a residue control problem exists or is likely to exist, Federal agencies commonly take the initiative for developing these methods. Because of the costs involved, prudent decisionmaking on priorities is essential. It must be understood that in certain instances, other metabolism or metabolic research may be needed to provide a basis for developing an analytical system responsive to regulatory control needs.

Opportunities do exist to stimulate methods development in the private sector. Examples include the recent legislation allowing commercialization of Federal government supported patents, federally supported research contracts and grants, and advertisement for commercially available analytical technologies. Within the Food Safety and Inspection Service, the last two have been extensively explored with measurable success. It is likely other Federal agencies have similar and possibly other opportunities to stimulate private sector interest. A known long-standing or highly publicized residue problem often generates heightened interest.

The big advantage of rapid test systems is their simplicity allowing tests to be performed by testors that are not highly experienced in diagnostic or analytical procedures. A disadvantage on occasion is that they are designed specifically for only one compound and require separate test systems for a class of pesticides. In some instances, sufficient cross-reactivity to a class of pesticides will allow other compounds to be detected, usually at higher concentrations in a sample matrix. Thus, there is some tradeoff for development by laboratories and use in regulatory programs.

It is often possible to develop effective quantitative methods using the same technology. These assays require state-of-the-art instrumentation and being performed by analysts in fully equipped laboratories. Adoption of qualitative or quantitative immunochemical assays is likely to take time before confidence and recognized legal status for such methods is attained. It may require considerable experience and familiarization with the technology by regulatory agencies to use test systems containing unknown reagents ("black box" test systems) to develop procedures assuring themselves that public health protection is not compromised.

Experience and familiarization with rapid testing systems such as immunochemistry based "card tests" is best accomplished by hands-on experience with them and supplemented by appropriate training materials prepared by experts in theory and technology of the rapid test systems. This is comparable to the education analysts had to acquire when chromatography and associated instrumentation was introduced into regulatory programs. This basic understanding enables regulatory programs and analysts to properly diagnose and evaluate test results and serves as a foundation for developing quality assurance plans and subsequent training for regulatory control programs.

Occasionally, in the development and design of ready-to-use products such as these tests, reliability and consistent performance of the assay from lot-to-lot production can vary. Quality control for production will likely improve with gained experience. Nevertheless, users of these systems must employ good quality-control and quality-assurance protocols to ensure method performance. Developing criteria for manufacturers of such systems either by the industry itself or by regulatory agencies planning to use such methods would be a step in the right direction to facilitate their acceptance.

A concern facing regulatory agencies is that some of these assays are more sensitive than the traditional quantitative and confirmatory assays, so that these qualitative results cannot be confirmed. This may limit further regulatory action and force technology to develop new quantitative and confirmatory methods to match the sensitivity levels. Regulatory agencies need to confirm what they have the capability to detect, particularly at the level of interest. This level of interest is usually either an action level or tolerance established by EPA or FDA.

It is important to recognize that analytical programs designed to detect potential residue problems must have the capability to provide quantitative values and structure identity at or below the level of interest. For example, within the Contamination Response System in FSIS, an analytical result for a pesticide or environmental contaminant that is at or above 80 percent of the tolerance or action level will trigger a set of specified actions, including directed sampling programs if a significant residue issue emerges. Without having the needed quantitative and confirmatory assays to support results from a rapid test system, inappropriate regulatory actions may occur. For enforcement purposes, for residues above an established action level or established tolerance, confirmatory methods must be capable of unambiguously identifying the analyte of interest at these concentrations. In situations where a tolerance or action level is established with a zero residue limit, confirmatory and quantitative methods must work at sub parts per million (ppm, $\mu g/g$) to parts per billion (ppb, pg/g) concentrations based on the approved analytical method for the analyte.

Another limitation is the heavy reliance on using aqueous media for performing the test. For certain food types, this may be of little consequence, but for others it may be a measurable deterrent. For example, most chemical-based assays rely on use of organic solvents to release the analyte of interest from the test sample matrix. This requires developing solvent systems providing sufficient transfer from the organic extraction solvent to the test system while not denaturing or deactivating the immunochemical reagents. Progress is being made in this area. For example, Immunosystems has developed an assay for chlorinated triazines (Res-I-Mune[R]) (11) that allows low ng/g (ppb) detection using select aqueous organic solvent systems. This system is currently being evaluated by FSIS for meat products.

Today, immunochemical assays are available not only for chlorinated triazines but also for paraquat, chlordane (heptachlor, dieldrin, endrin, aldrin, and endosulfan are detected via cross-reactivity), 18 pentachlorophenol and polychlorinated biphenyls (PCBs) at levels of interest. FSIS has method-development contracts for developing immunochemical assays for heptachlor-related organochlorine pesticides; ivermectin; synthetic pyrethroids (permethrin, cypermethrin, and deltamethrin); and nitroimidazoles in meat and poultry tissue (12). These are expected to provide improved laboratory analytical capability for these analytes. Development of qualitative screening assays is possible.

A commercial pesticide detection system based on cholinesterase enzyme inhibition has been developed by EnzyTech, Inc. (13) The enzyme ticket system detects common insecticides that account for about 85 percent of all insecticides used in the United States at concentrations in the low ng/g (ppb) range. Shelf stability for the test system is estimated to be several years. The design of the system allows for a two-tier analytical scheme that will allow differentiation of organic sulfur containing organophosphate insecticides from their oxygen analogs. This advantage reduces some of the options of further analysis to quantify and confirm these analytes. Research is being done to enable analytes from an organic extract to be analyzed with the test system. Development of quantitative and confirmatory analysis using other analytical technologies may be needed to support these qualitative methods.

New column chromatography packing materials have simplified many sample purification analysis procedures. These solid phase extraction materials allow many solvent-to-solvent extraction and purification systems to be eliminated from traditional methods. Future applications may become the basis of rapid test systems requiring only solvent elution to isolate analytes of interest.

Integrating Screening Methods into Multiresidue Regulatory Programs

Applications of screening methods for pesticide-residue regulatory programs to some extent depend on residue violation rates. The first scenario covers instances when data indicate a low incidence of an above-tolerance residue for approved pesticide use. The second scenario applies to situations with a relatively higher percent of residue violation incidence for approved pesticide use. A third scenario would be for detecting and confirming pesticide residues from unapproved pesticide use. The first two may be influenced depending on whether or not agreements exist for residue avoidance programs between a regulating agency and a food producer. Where such agreements are available, one incentive to such programs would be to reduce sampling of such producers, assuming a history of good quality-control in their production systems.

Integrating rapid test methods into regulatory programs does not imply reducing emphasis on reporting quantitative values below tolerances or action levels. These quantitative values both below and above these levels of interest are important for analyzing trends and designing future residue control programs. However, integrating rapid test methods for regulatory control programs implies an intelligent design using rapid screening methods (commonly, Level III methods) with quantitative methods (analogous to Level II methods) and confirmatory methods (Level I methods) to optimize the limited resources available to regulatory control programs. With a low-level violation incidence from statistical-based random-sampling programs, screening methods are particularly attractive for field or in-plant use because they allow for methods with broad versatility to test large numbers of food products and related samples. Data indicate that with statistical-based random-sampling programs, the large majority of samples contain non-detectable and below level concentrations of residues (14). This provides programs with the opportunity to clear products with non-detectable residues or detectable below a tolerance, while retaining suspected positives for more definitive analytical procedures. This generally provides for more effective use of expensive laboratory facilities and resources as well as for reducing the significant costs involved in sample collection and shipping all samples to a designated laboratory. Data management systems have to be appropriate to the regulatory need in all cases.

For instances in which there is a known or high-residue violation incidence, quantitative immunochemical, enzyme-inhibition assays and thin layer chromatographic systems designed for rapid testing in laboratory environments become very attractive. In this scenario, where large numbers of samples are expected to give results in residue violations, the advantages to regulatory programs for reduced analytical costs for sample collection and shipping are diminished. The level of effort needed for field or in-plant personnel to use and follow-up on results from rapid tests could result in an increased workload for additional sample collection and shipping. Using another laboratory analytical method (another Level II method), in these situations provides an independent assay for the analyte of interest and is generally suitable for verifying initial results. This may require developing and validating new methods using improved analytical detectors, more sensitive color-forming reagents, fluorescent-generating reagents, or biochemical and color-forming reagent systems that match the sensitivity, specificity, and other screening method performance characteristics.

Another option is to allow well-defined sample-compositing schemes to be employed for laboratory analysis. This is particularly attractive when no known incidence of a residue problem exists. It is somewhat less attractive under the second scenario with known or high-residue violation rates because it calls for reanalysis of individual samples within the composite sample when an actionable finding is indicated by analysis of the composite sample.

In the third scenario (detecting residues of unapproved pesticides or pesticide use), residue screening tests are very attractive because detection of any amount of pesticide residue in specific products is a residue violation. It normally requires support by a confirmatory procedure. This assumes, as in all other cases, performance characteristics of methods are well defined. In this scenario, quantitation is not a specific requirement, although administrative level may be defined by an agency before initiating other regulatory action. Under any of these scenarios, epidemiological information should be incorporated to design effective subsequent laboratory-analysis programs. To facilitate design of an integrated residue control program, a decision-tree process may be a suitable objective. This will require some preliminary activities. The mission statement of the regulatory agency and the objectives of residue analysis must be clearly defined and adopted. Figure 1 is a suggested approach. Others may be developed based on specific needs or other regulatory and statutory considerations.

Constraints on Use of Rapid Test Methods

A perceived constraint in some programs with screening tests is that they are not specific and consume too large a portion of valuable resources to identify the residue of interest. A possible resolution to this would be to encourage development of more selective screening assays to improve the selection process of a multiresidue or single-residue analysis method. That is, develop a hierarchy of test methods based on current and emerging technology, focusing on the concept of simplicity in design and application, automation technologies, and commercially available systems and equipment with potential for broad application.

Rapid testing systems may be compromised by other constraints. A rate-limiting factor for application of rapid tests is, or may become, preparing an appropriate sample for analysis. Encouragement is warranted for research to develop improved sample preparation techniques amenable to rapid test systems in nonlaboratory and laboratory environments. For example, supercritical fluid technology may be a valuable research avenue for laboratory based analysis. An alternative could be to focus on physical or chemical properties of pesticide residues. A third possible approach would be research on pharmacokinetic or metabolism studies to correlate pesticide residues in food and tissue matricies to fluid extracts. Incentive is needed to encourage commercial organizations to develop rapid test procedures. It is primarily through the economy of scale and return on investment for manufacturers that tests will become available and provide regulatory agencies with sufficient potential low-cost onsite, laboratory onsite, and laboratory test procedures. Development of rapid tests for regulatory use can be fostered by offering contract funding to the relevant regulatory agencies. Recent examples of this method development process have shown promise, particularly with colleges and universities.

References

1. Taylor, S., *Pesticide Monitoring Program: Developing New Methods to Detect Pesticide Residues in Food*, Congressional Research Service, Apr. 24, 1987.
2. National Academy of Sciences, "Regulating Pesticides in Foods," Committee on Scientific and Regulatory Issues Underlying Pesticide Use Patterns and Agricultural Innovation, Board of Agriculture, Washington, DC; National Research Council, 1987.
3. U. S. Congress, Government Accounting Office, *Pesticides: Need to Enhance FDA's Ability to Protect the Public from Illegal Residues*, GAO/ RCED-87-7, 1986, 58 pp.
4. Official Journal of the European Communities, Commission Decision 87/410/EEC, July 1987.
5. U.S. Department of Agriculture, *New Zealand Journal of Science*, Food Safety and Inspection Service, Revised 1987.
6. Sherma, J., "Pesticides and Plant Growth Regulators," vol. 14, *Modern Analytical Techniques*, G. Zweig and J. Sherma (eds.), Academic Press, 1986.
7. Clear, M.H., Fowler, F.R., Solly, S.R.B., et al., *New Zealand Journal of Science* 20:221, 1977.
8. U.S. Department of Agriculture, FSIS, Contract 53-A94-5-19, September 1985, personal communication, R. Ellis, Director, Chemistry Division, Science Program, Washington, DC.
9. Lawrence, J.F., *J. Assoc. of Anal. Chem.* 64:758-761, 1980.
10. McCausland, I., et al., *Emerging Technology For Testing Chemical Residues in Meat*, Report of Australian Meat and Livestock Research and

Figure 1.— Decision Tree for Regulatory Control Program

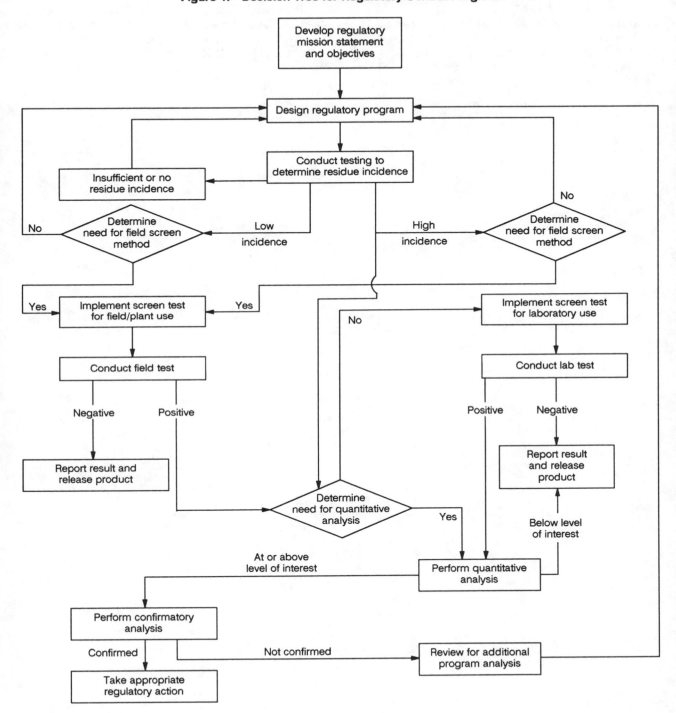

SOURCE: Richard Ellis, Food Safety and Inspection Service, U.S. Department of Agriculture, 1988.

Development Corporation, Sydney, NSW, Australia, October 1987.

11. ImmunoSystems, Inc., 8 Lincoln Street, P.O. Box AY, Biddeford, ME 04005.

12. R. Ellis, Director, Chemistry Division, Science Program, U.S. Department of Agriculture, FSIS, Washington, DC, personal communication.

13. EnzyTec, Inc., 8805 Long, Lenexa, KS 66215, *Product Bulletin, Pesticide Detetor Ticker.*

14. U.S. Department of Agriculture, Food Safety and Inspection Service, *Domestic Residue Data Book National Residue, 1985*, May 1987.

The Role of Robotic Automation in the Laboratory

Bruce E. Kropscott and Cynthia N. Peck, The Dow Chemical Company, Midland, MI, and
Harry G. Lento, Campbell Institute for Research and Technology, Camden, NJ

Contents

	Page
Abstract	163
Introduction	163
Robotics Definition	164
Advantages of Robotic Automation	164
Constraints of Robotic Automation	165
Key Elements to Implementation	166
Robotics Applications	166
Current Status of Automation in Pesticide Residue Testing	167
Constraints to the Use of Robotics for Multiresidue Testing	168
Future Prospects for Automation	168
Summary	169
References	169
Acknowledgment	169
Other Sources of Information	170

Abstract

Rapidly increasing numbers of samples for pesticide residue analysis have forced the analysts in analytical laboratories (governmental, industrial, and private) to look for ways to increase sample throughput. This trend has provided a need for the development of a variety of automated equipment for the analytical laboratory.

In support of the workshop on "Technologies to Detect Pesticide Residues in Food" sponsored by the Office of Technology Assessment (OTA), this paper will 1) provide an overview of laboratory automation, 2) assess the emerging robotic technology for the analytical laboratory, 3) review the current status of automation in pesticide residue analysis, and 4) identify research needed for expanded automation in the analytical laboratory.

Introduction

Scarcely an aspect of modern life has been unaffected by automation, yet defining automation is difficult without using automatic or automated in the definition. Consider Webster's definition: "the technique of making an apparatus (as a calculating machine), a process (as of manufacturing), or a system (as of bookkeeping) operate automatically" or the condition of being automated (1). Automation implies the integration of a self-governing system. Unlike mechanization, which is defined as simple replacement of human labor by machines, true automation must have the ability for feedback control and the ability to regulate. Four key elements of automation are 1) a source of power, 2) sensing mechanisms, 3) decision elements, and 4) control elements (2). For all practical purposes, laboratory automation is the use of devices that perform repetitive tasks. Reviews of large annual trade and equipment shows, such as the Pittsburgh Conference & Exposition on Analytical Chemistry and Applied Spectroscopy, provide an excellent overview of current automated equipment.

Laboratory automation can be divided into four basic categories:

1) Dedicated, single-task
2) Dedicated, multi-task
3) Computers
4) Robotics

The simplest type of automation is a dedicated, single-task instrument. These instruments may be commercially available or custom manufactured and perform just one independent function. Examples of single-task automated equipment include autoinjectors, electronic balances, timed shakers, centrifuges, switching valves, etc. Dedicated, single-task devices are well-established and widely used in most laboratories.

The next category of automation is the multi-task device. Instruments in this category perform multiple tasks such as diluting, mixing, filtering, solid phase extraction, chromatographic separations, etc.

Examples of dedicated multi-task automation include automated sample preparation devices that combine adding solvents, mixing, extracting, filtering, evaporating, etc. and multiple-step auto samplers that can heat or cool, add internal standards or derivating agents, serially dilute, etc. Most dedicated multi-tasking devices are highly specialized. For example, automated cleanup and extraction devices facilitate rapid processing of a highly selective number of repetitive, routine samples but remain subject to obsolescence and represent isolated, stand-alone equipment. The number of commercially available, multi-tasking devices is markedly less than its single-tasking counterpart. Additional multi-tasking devices include hyphenated technologies such as gas chromatography-mass spectrometry (GC/MS), liquid chromatography-mass spectrometry (LC/MS), and gas chromatography-infrared spectrometry (GC/IR), etc., which couple established, analytical technologies to enhance the automated detection and measurement of compounds.

Computers differ from the first two types of automation since they automate data handling and calculations instead of physical and mechanical manipulations. This category of automation includes hand-held calculators, integrators, personal computers for control and data handling, and networked laboratory information management systems (LIMS). Computers and associated microchip technology have developed into a modern "Industrial Revolution" that is extremely vast and important but beyond the scope of this paper.

Robotics evolved as hybrid systems incorporating technology from both mechanical and computer (microprocessor) automation. Robotics uses a computer-controlled, mechanical manipulator to incorporate both single- and multi-tasking automated devices into an integrated system. Since its commercial introduction and implementation in the early 1980s, laboratory robotics has provided reprogrammable, multi-tasking, computer-assisted automation in the laboratory for a variety of pesticide and non-pesticide applications. The cost of a laboratory robotics system typically ranges from $40,000 to $60,000. The return on investment depends upon the application but is typically 6 months to 3 years. Before discussing robotic automation, a working definition of a robot must be established.

Robotics Definition

A definition of a robot is in itself a formidable task, since there are so many misconceptions and preconceived ideas of what a robot is. A definition of a robot that has been adapted from the Robotic Industries Association's definition is as follows: A robot is a reprogrammable, multifunctional manipulator designed to move materials, parts, and specialized devices through a variety of computer-controlled motions for the performance of a variety of tasks (3). The key words are reprogrammable, multifunctional, and computer-controlled.

Misconceptions and preconceptions of robots are difficult to overcome. Most every equipment manufacturer wants products that are associated with the latest technology. An example of equipment that does not fit the definition is a "robotic" autosampler. The autosampler transports vials from a tray to an injector with precise timing, performs multiple injections, and varies the size or speed of injections. The autosampler is *not* a robot: it is an automated instrument that performs a single-task of repetitive, precision injections. In addition, most toys or mechanized trade-show mannequins do not fit this definition of a robot.

Several types of robots that do fit the definition include the following: 1) industrial, 2) research and development, and 3) laboratory robots. The first industrial robot in the United States was sold by Unimation to General Motors in 1961. Currently, industrial robots perform such tasks as welding, painting, parts assembly, and material handling. Research and development robots cover such areas as education, cybernetics, and space exploration. In 1982, another type of robot was introduced, a laboratory robot. Its major function has been automated sample preparation. The remainder of this paper will limit its scope to assessing the emerging technology of the laboratory robot, discussing its advantages, constraints, current applications, and future prospects.

Advantages of Robotic Automation

The advantages of robotics include many of the same advantages as conventional automation and are summarized in five categories:
1) cost-effectiveness
2) reproducibility
3) versatility
4) safety
5) automated documentation of procedures.

Robotics can be cost-effective. Like conventional automation, robotics provides a competitive advantage in that the robots can work extended hours and increase the use of existing equipment. Robots free personnel from performing repetitive tasks and devoting constant attention to minute details, thus allowing additional work or research to be performed. The robot is not subject to hunger, boredom, fatigue, or illness. Robots do not need promotions, pay raises, or medical benefits. However, robotics does not preclude the need for well-trained, competent analysts.

Reproducibility is a major attribute of a robotics system. Performing tasks with the exact timing and uniform sample handling, the robotics system separates the actual chemistries involved from variations in techniques, which may in turn lead to improved precision and accuracy in methodology. This is very useful in method validation, where conditions and parameters can be systematically varied to optimize new methodology during the validation process. Transfer of robotics technology could improve intra- and interlaboratory reproducibility.

Robotics is versatile automation and thus less subject to obsolescence. The reprogrammability of the robotics system allows method optimization or a complete change of application to meet changing needs in a laboratory. Robotics technology also bridges the gap between what is commercially available in dedicated automation and what is actually needed for a specific application (e.g., custom sample preparation, instrument interfacing, specialized autosamplers, etc.).

The use of robotics reduces human exposure to hazardous chemicals, extreme temperatures, and other undesirable conditions such as pinch points, defective glassware, and sharp objects.

Finally, the computer portion of the robotics system can provide automated documentation of the procedure. The entire program as well as sample weights, dilutions, timing, calibrations, etc., can be printed or transferred directly to a host computer, vastly reducing transcription errors. Computerized documentation thereby can establish an audit trail for the entire procedure.

Constraints of Robotic Automation

The present technology of laboratory robotics has several constraints, which are grouped into the following categories:
1) New technology
2) Mechanical and computer failures
3) Spatial and physical limitations
4) Safety
5) Associated technology lagging behind automation

Laboratory robotics is still an emerging technology. The world market for laboratory robotics in 1985 was estimated at 30,000 to 50,000 units (4), but this market has not been reached because there seems to be a general reluctance to change and a lack of wide acceptance of any new technology. As of December 1987, laboratory robotics systems numbered about 1,300, and only a limited number of personnel were trained in the operation and repair of robotics systems. To date, Zymark Corporation has more than 85 percent of the present laboratory robotics market. Other laboratory robotics companies include Lerkin, Fisher Scientific, and Hudson Robotics.

The majority of robotics systems have required significant cost and time to be fully programmed and functionally implemented. Newer robotics systems, such as the PyTechnology introduced by Zymark Corporation in 1986, have reduced start-up cost and time by providing systems that are pre-programmed and pre-positioned for basic laboratory operations.

Robots are hybrid systems that combine mechanical equipment with computers. This results in a combination of problems associated with machines (such as physical wear, mechanical failure, etc.) and with computers (electrical power, noise spikes, "glitches").

Spatial constraints also limit the robotics system because the robot is confined to its working envelope, typically less than a cubic meter. Exact positioning, spatial orientation and readily accessible work areas are necessary for the robot to interact with peripheral modules and support equipment. Modules and equipment are usually bolted on the table or placed in a rack to assure proper positioning. As a result, samples and solvents are limited in size (0.1 to 50 ml) and weight (less than 3 lbs.) to maximize the use of the working envelope.

A human has extensive systems of intricate sensors and feedback mechanisms that provide information about the environment (e.g., touch, pressure, temperature, hearing, sight). A human also possesses an extensive memory from which to recall and process that information. In comparison, a robot has a limited memory, limited feedback mechanisms, limited dexterity, and limited artificial intelligence. Thus safety, which was listed as one of the advantages of robotics, can become a liability when errors occur that require logical decisionmaking to recover from an unanticipated situation for which it was not designed or programmed.

Associated technologies (disposable supplies, glassware, ancillary equipment, etc.) are lagging behind the robotics technology. The associated technologies are not ready for a blind analyst with limited dexterity (4 to 5 degrees of freedom compared with more than 40 degrees of freedom in the human upper limb). A robotics system must be viewed as an **integrated system** consisting of the robotic arm, peripheral work-station modules (such as vortex mixers, centrifuges, evaporators, etc.) and supporting equipment (such as test tubes, pipet tips, extraction columns). Since robotics systems are integrated systems, they are only as good as the weakest component. Modules with moving parts such as shakers, centrifuges, and vortex mixers need to be manufactured for computer control and must be designed to return to an exact position to compensate for the blind analyst. Disposable items (such as pipet tips that are bowed, screw-capped bottles that will not seal, etc.) can produce spills, malfunctions in laboratory operations, or in the worst case, cause catastrophic failure in unattended operations. Although these types of laboratory supplies have been around for years, the specifications and quality control in their manufacture did not become an issue until they were used in conjunction with robotics systems. A failure is a failure whether it is caused by a $2 tip, a $7 centrifuge tube, or a $50,000 robotics system.

Key Elements to Implementation

At the Third International Symposium on Laboratory Robotics, Frank Zenie, president of Zymark Corporation, summarized the key elements to implementation of robotics. "Once adequate funds and people are available, the following four requirements are key to all successful automation projects: 1) motivated people, 2) proven chemistries, 3) disciplined planning, and 4) creative implementation" (5).

Robotics is an emerging technology and as such needs development from key, dedicated personnel. The technology is new enough that systems will fail from short-term problems (lack of time, lack of resources, lack of key people). There are many obstacles that can make a robotics system fail, but with motivated, dedicated people these problems can be overcome.

Automation without valid, proven chemistries is useless. If the application is not based on sound, reliable chemistry, robotics systems will only be automating the generation of meaningless numbers and useless results. On the other hand, robotics with its exact timing and uniform sample handling can be used as a research tool for separating the chemistries involved from the variability in the manual techniques.

Disciplined planning is another key element in successful implementation. Robotics systems have a great amount of versatility but actual applications are **well-defined** and **limited in scope.** The goal, tasks, and laboratory unit operations (LUOs) need to be well defined and focused to allow automation. Examples of well-defined applications versus open-ended applications are as follows:

Well-defined	*versus*	*Open-ended*
machine, tool and die; writing a calculations program; production of goods;		sculpting writing poetry basic research
analysis of organochlorines in corn using the Luke screening method	*versus*	determination of all pesticides in all food groups

Creative implementation is necessary since the robot can not emulate the human in task performance. "The analogy between the marvelously dextrous human hand and the robot hand is extremely crude, as is the analogy between human learning and robot programming" (6). The good news is that the robot does not have to emulate the human in task performance. The human hand has more than 50 distinctively different movements. That degree of dexterity is not necessary to pick up a test tube and move it to a balance, mixer, etc. In developing conventional laboratory methodology, humans incorporate unit operations that maximize their strengths and minimize their weaknesses. As a result, manual methods are validated with procedures, timing sequences, and specific laboratory tools that are most efficient and convenient for the human. If a manual application is to be performed by a robot, tasks must be modified, then optimized, and finally programmed for the robot's capabilities. Robotics systems can be used for automating method validation as well as for routine sample preparation. Methods can be developed and optimized by systematically varying parameters, eliminating the need for first developing manual methods that need to be modified for use with robotics.

Robotics Applications

Laboratory robots and workstations have automated a variety of laboratory unit operations (LUOs) including weighing, pipetting, diluting, filtering, centrifuging, evaporating, solvent dispensing, mixing, etc., which can be sequenced for specific applications. More than 100 applications have been developed in the pharmaceutical, chemical, biological, environmental, biotechnical, and food industries. More than 45 percent of those robotic applications are in the pharmaceutical industry. Currently more than 200 companies in the United States are using laboratory robotics. As of December 1987, the seven largest customers of laboratory robotics were The Dow Chemical Company, DuPont, Eastman Kodak, Eli Lilly, Merck, Monsanto, and Procter & Gamble, totalling almost 20 percent of the current robotics systems (7).

Current Status of Automation in Pesticide Residue Testing

The presence of several hundred registered pesticides has led to the development of multiresidue screening procedures. The FDA's pesticide analytical manual (PAM) describes screening procedures that are distinguished by both the type of food group and type of pesticide residue that are probably present. [8] All these methods have four basic, common operations: 1) obtaining a representative sample, 2) sample cleanup, 3) chromatographic analysis, and 4) data reduction and reporting.

Methodologies begin with procurement of a representative food material, preparation (peeling, grinding, homogenizing, etc.), and extraction with an organic solvent (acetonitrile, acetone, petroleum ether, etc.). The extraction step is usually a manual operation with large variations in sample and solvent sizes depending upon the food and levels of pesticides. This step is very labor-intensive, time-consuming and difficult to automate.

The sample cleanup isolates the pesticide from the rest of the matrix. This may be accomplished by techniques such as liquid/liquid partition, gel permeation chromatography, or solid phase extraction (SPE) columns (i.e., Florisil columns).

Sample cleanup is very labor-intensive and time-consuming. Developments in automating sample cleanup have been reported by several authors. For example, Stallings et al. applied automated gel chromatographic cleanup to the analysis of pesticides in fatty-food materials (9). Gretch and Rosen reported a cleanup procedure for multiresidue testing using automated solvent partitioning extractions interfaced with a column chromatography module for automated solvent partitioning extractions (10). Other automated gel permeation and chromatograph systems addressed the cleanup step by automating collection of eluent fractions, evaporation, and solvent substitution as well as injection into a gas chromatograph (11, 12). A review of papers from the *Advances in Laboratory Automation-*

Robotics indicated robotic automation of the cleanup step using solid-phase extraction (SPE) columns of a variety of pesticide and non-pesticide compounds from a variety of matrices (13, 14, 15).

The third step involves the actual chromatographic analysis. The three most common techniques are gas chromatography (GC), liquid chromatography (LC), and gas chromatography-mass spectrometry (GC/MS). Types of gas chromatography detectors used for pesticide residue analysis include electron capture, flame ionization, or Hall conductivity. High performance liquid chromatography (HPLC) with ultraviolet or fluorescence detection is also widely used for pesticides that are not readily analyzed by GC. Autosamplers coupled with chromatographic instrumentation facilitate the automation of the analysis step.

Finally, the data reduction and summary reporting step has been largely automated with the use of computers.

Due to the newness of automation technology and the timeframe required for method development, review, and publication, the literature does not reveal much in the way of published information on the specific application of robotics to multiresidue testing. It is very difficult to breakdown the percentage of work that is being done using automation versus manual preparation since there is so much variation from laboratory to laboratory in the type and amount of equipment, funding, and personnel. Private inquiries as to the status of automation by the authors of this paper indicated a considerable amount of research being done.

Automation of preparation, cleanup, and detection of pesticide residues in foods has typically focused on single, discrete operations. Specific tasks have been automated with single-task, dedicated equipment such as autoinjectors, which make repetitive, precision injections into chromatographic instruments. Reducing the variables in injection techniques allows more unattended operations and higher use of the analytical equipment. Automation in the final analysis step with the use of autosamplers and computerized data systems was a major accomplishment in increasing sample throughput in the analytical laboratory and has been incorporated in most of the laboratories, yet it did not address the labor-intensive extraction or cleanup. Dedicated, multi-task instruments have been developed for automated fraction collection, and solvent exchange can process several dozen pesticide residue samples sequentially. The $20,000 to $40,000 capital investment has prevented the incorporation of this equipment into some laboratories. Laboratories with large numbers of the same sample type and limited personnel resources may derive the most benefit from dedicated automation. On the other hand, a $50,000 robotic system may provide a better investment for these laboratories since the flexible, automated system may be used to process different types of samples as needed to meet the varying demands and optimize current methodology. As pesticide technology changes, the system can be upgraded to avoid obsolescence and reprogrammed to meet changing analytical needs.

At the Third International Symposium on Laboratory Robotics, Tillier et al. reported on their determination of deltamethrin (active ingredient in Decis insecticide) and its metabolite in milk and vegetables at the 50 ppb level (16). Their robotics system was used as a tool for optimization of various LUOs that are commonly used in screening techniques such as centrifugation, multiple solvent extraction, mixing, and solid phase extraction cleanup.

Applications using robotics for the automation of the Luke multiresidue screening procedure has been recently reported by Grady and Lento (17). Test results on several food matrices (tomatoes, corn, peas, and carrots) using several different organic, chlorinated pesticides gave similar results to those obtained by the manual assay. They predict continuing developments in the application of robotic techniques to other types of multiresidue screening tests, particularly in assays of fatty-type foods, organic phosphates, and methyl carbamates.

Constraints to the Use of Robotics for Multiresidue Testing

Regulatory and environmental samples are not readily automated because of some of the following factors:

1) Diverse type of samples and matrices
2) Widely varying classes and concentrations of pesticides
3) Large quantities of samples and reagents handled
4) Varying complexity and multiple sequences of extraction, cleanup, analysis
5) Lack of large series of similar samples
6) Need to show equivalency to official methodology

Samples requiring residue analysis have many variables (constraints 1-5), which interfere with the total automation process. In addition, many present day procedures were developed using equipment that is not suitable or compatible with other types of automation. The research cost for the development of new equipment to replace existing equipment is also a formidable problem.

The need to show equivalency to established methodology has placed a serious constraint on the practicality of automating current methods. Often it is cheaper for companies to stay with the manual techniques than to spend the time and effort on evaluating and implementing any new automation. Efforts need to be continued in the government and private industry to research and develop automated technology, particularly in the following areas:

1) robotics
2) laboratory information systems
3) automated cleanup apparatus
4) new, specific detectors
5) artificial intelligence/expert systems

Existing techniques and equipment need to be networked and integrated into working systems, not used solely as isolated workstations.

To test specifically for each of several hundred pesticides registered for use would be costly and extremely inefficient. Adoption of screening techniques (which could be automated) in conjunction with official methods (used for specific confirmation of over-tolerance samples) could allow for a rapid throughput of large numbers of samples without sacrificing regulatory methodology. The small number of suspect samples may be reanalyzed using the more lengthy, time-consuming, and specific methodology. A tolerance assessment system should be maintained with methodology that is shorter and instrumentation that is sensitive and specific. By narrowing the scope of the problem (i.e., from measuring for all types of pesticides in all types of foods to development of a series of screening techniques for specific classes of compounds in specific groups of foods), the possibility of automation then becomes more a reality.

Once a method is modified for the robotic system, subsequent method validation is not a constraint due to the exact timing, uniform sample handling, and reproducibility that is inherent in robotic systems. Transfer of robotic technology can easily be accomplished, making the multi-validation procedure required for official validation easier.

Future Prospects for Automation

Future prospects for robotic automation include improvements in the following areas:

1) robotics
2) computers
3) sensors
4) associated technologies

Although pre-programmed robotics technology is still not fully developed, advances in that technology could have the same positive impact that pre-programmed software packages had for the micro-computer systems, allowing an analyst to use the instrumentation without requiring an extensive knowledge of programming or theory of operation. Research and development is needed for improvements in existing electronics and mechanics of the robot. Expanded sample and solvent sizes (micro to macro-semi prep) are also needed for a variety of robotic applications.

Advances in computer technology will improve robotics, instrumentation, and data handling. The robots will need more memory, auxiliary control functions, graphics software, smaller physical size, and fewer hardware/software problems. Instrumentation must be able to communicate with computers as well as other dissimilar equipment without the need for extensive programming or additional interface modules. Computer technology must allow further integrated, networked automation in the laboratory.

Sensory technology such as sight, touch, hearing, temperature, and pressure need to be developed, miniaturized, and enhanced for the laboratory robot. Research and development of sensors will aid in the safety, performance, and feedback mechanisms of the new robotics systems.

One of the biggest opportunities for future improvement in robotics technology is with the associated technologies. Providing improved quality control and new designs in disposables (glassware, plasticware, etc.) can reduce the potential errors in unattended operations. Research and design of specific workstations (such as cappers, mixers, evaporation stations, etc.) that can be easily implemented with the existing robotics architecture will provide new application opportunities for the automated analyst.

"Laboratory automation is not based on a single technology, but rather on several technologies that can be focused on different parts of a lab operation. Some of those approaches are mature, others are evolving, and others are still experimental. Thus you should not attempt to implement a system in one grand stroke, but rather consider the options and plan a stepwise implementation" (8). If an advantage is to be gained using automation, all facets of the methodology must be examined. For example, while great strides have been made in automated analysis and data reduction, the sample preparation still involves much manual labor in many of the laboratories surveyed. Reviewing the prospects for future automation, several factors must be considered before choosing automated equipment such

as amount of funding, training, and availability of personnel; numbers and types of current and anticipated samples; and where the strategic advantage would be gained using a particular type of automation.

Summary

Robotics allows reprogrammable, multifunctional, computer-controlled automation for a variety of laboratory unit operations up to and including complete applications. Although robotics is an emerging technology, it has made great strides in laboratory automation by addressing the need to link isolated workstations with one another and has provided a means for an integrated, laboratory network with other automated systems. Robotics should continue to develop as a fundamental, integral tool for sample preparation, automation, and research and development in analytical laboratories.

Acknowledgment

The authors thank the following people and their companies for contributions to this paper in laboratory robotics: Albertha Paul, Zymark Corp.; William Kruka, Perkin-Elmer; Raymond Reilly, Hudson Robotics; Terry Hight, Radian; Ashok Shah, Fisher Scientific; and Frank McCullough, ABC Laboratories.

References

1. *Webster's Third New International Dictionary* (Springfield, MA: G&C Merriam Inc., 1981).
2. *New Encyclopaedia Britannica*, vol. 1 (Chicago, IL: Encyclopaedia Britannica Inc., 1987).
3. Conlan, Roberta (ed.), *Robotics: Understanding Computers* (Alexandria, VA: Time-Life Books, Inc., 1986).
4. Freifeld, K. "The One-Armed Chemist," *Forbes*, 135 (9) April 29, 1985.
5. Zenie, F., "Strategic Trends in Laboratory Automation-1985," Third International Symposium on Laboratory Robotics, Boston, October 1985.
6. Ullrich, R.A., *The Robotics Primer* (Englewood, NJ: Prentice-Hall, Inc., 1983).
7. Paul, A., personal communication 1/88, and Zymark Corporation—A Brief History, 12/4/87.
8. Pesticide Analytical Manual, vol. 1, 2nd ed. (Washington, DC: Food and Drug Administration, 1981).
9. Stallings, D.L., Tindle, R.C., and Johnson, J.L., *J. Assoc. Off. Anal. Chem.* 55:32-38, 1972.

10. Gretch, F.M., Rosen, J.D., "Automated Sample Cleanup for Pesticide Multiresidue Analysis III. Evaluation of Complete System for Screening Subtolerance Residues in Vegetables," *J. Assoc. Off. Anal. Chem.* 70 (1):109-111, 1987.

11. Johnson, J.J., Sturino, E.E., and Bourne, S. "An Automated Gas Chromatographic System for Pesticide Residue Analyses," EPA, 905/4-77-001.

12. Hopper, M.L., Griffitt, K.R., "Evaluation of an Automated Gel Permeation Clean-up and Evaporation Systems for Determining Pesticide Residues in Fatty Samples," *J. Assoc. Off. Anal. Chem.* 70(4): 1987.

13. *Advances in Laboratory Automation-Robotics 1984*, Zymark Corp., Hopkinton, MA, p. 61, 71, and 105, 1984.

14. *Advances in Laboratory Automation-Robotics 1985*, Zymark Corp., Hopkinton, MA, p. 111, 131, and 465, 1985.

15. *Advances in Laboratory Automation-Robotics 1986*, Zymark Corp., Hopkinton, MA, p. 37, 71, 291, 451, and 595, 1986.

16. Tillier C., Allegret, H., and Devaux, P. "Applications of Robotics in Residue Analysis," *Advances in Laboratory Automation-Robotics 1986*, Zymark Corp., Hopkinton, MA, pp. 291-311, 1986.

17. Grady, M. and Lento, H., "Application of Robotics to Multiresidue Testing in Foods," Pittsburgh Conference and Exposition on Analytical Chemistry and Applied Spectroscopy, New Orleans, February, 1988.

18. Liscouski, J., "Issues and Directions in Laboratory Automation," *Anal. Chem.* 60(2), 95-99, 1988.

Other Sources of Information

Osborne, David M., *Robots-An Introduction to Basic Concepts and Applications*, Midwest Sci-Tech Publisher, Inc. (Detroit, MI: 1983).

Krasnoff, Barbara, *Robots: Reel to Real* (New York: Arco Publishing, Inc., 1982).

Reichardt, Jasia, *Robots: Fact, Fiction, and Prediction* (New York: Viking Press, 1978).

Joseph, Michael, *The Timetable of Technology* (London: Marshall Editions Limited, 1982).

Potential of Immunoassays in Monitoring Pesticide Residues in Foods

Ralph O. Mumma, Department of Entomology, Pesticide Research Laboratory, The Pennsylvania State University, University Park, PA

and

Kenneth W. Hunter, Jr., Biotronic Systems Corporation and Westinghouse Bio-Analytic Systems Company, Rockville, MD

Contents

	Page
Abstract	171
Introduction	171
Immunoassays for Agrochemical Analysis	172
Preparation of Anti-Chemical Antibodies	172
Hybridomas and Monoclonal Antibodies	174
Principles of Chemical Immunoassays	174
Practical Applications of Chemical Immunoassays	176
Real-Time, On-Line Agrochemical Monitoring	178
Comparison of Immunoassays With Conventional Methods of Pesticide Residue Analysis	178
Conventional Methods Versus Immunoassay Methods	178
Advantages and Disadvantages of Immunoassays	179
Constraints, Opportunities, and Recommendations	179
Regulatory Agencies	179
Legislative Actions	180
References	180

Figures

Figure	Page
1. Antibody Affinity and Specificity	173
2. Monoclonal Antibody Preparation	174
3. Applying Reagents to 96-well Plate	175
4. Competitive Inhibition Enzyme Immunoassay	176
5. Standard Curve: Parathion Immunoassay	177
6. Computer, Printer, and Spectrophotometer	177
7. Generalized Biosensor	178

Abstract

The principles of immunoassays are presented, and selected applications of these assays for analysis of pesticide residues are cited; the advantages and disadvantages of immunoassays are compared with conventional analytical methods. The constraints and opportunities of immunoassays are discussed in light of regulatory and legislative influences.

Introduction

Analysis of agricultural commodities for agrochemical residues is usually time-consuming and performed by highly skilled chemists utilizing expensive analytical equipment. Consequently, costs of analyses are high. Five commonly used multiresidue methods detect 203 different pesticide residues, but this is less than half of the pesticides that the Food and Drug Administration (FDA) claims may occur in foods. A number of the pesticides not detected in the multiresidue methods are classified as high health hazards and must be analyzed by single residue methods. Again, the cost of analysis is a major limiting factor in how many analyses can be performed. Regulatory agencies responsible for ensuring the safety of agricultural commodities, both grown at home and abroad, do not have limitless finances and can only analyze a fraction of the samples that should be analyzed. A small percentage of samples possess illegal levels of pesticides, but unfortunately, we have to analyze all the samples to determine the few bad ones. Not only are Federal and State regulatory agencies concerned about pesticide residues, but the general public is taking an ever-increasing interest and demanding greater assurances of the safety of food and water. United States' farmers also have raised questions about the importation of agricultural products from countries that fail to regulate pesticide usage, for the use of high levels of pesticides can certainly increase a farmer's yield per acre and provide a competitive edge in the marketplace.

There is a need for simple, rapid, cost-effective screening techniques for pesticide residues in raw and processed foods. Since most foods do not contain illegal residues, inexpensive semiquantitative techniques could screen large numbers of samples, and only those few samples found in violation could be further analyzed by more conventional means.

Immunoassays offer many of these advantages. They have been routinely used for many years in clinical and forensic laboratories for analysis of small molecules such as hormones and drugs. The procedures are becoming so simple that they are now being conducted in doctors' offices and even in private homes (e.g., pregnancy tests). Immunoassays should be equally applicable for the analysis of pesticide residues.

This article will briefly introduce the principles of immunoassays, present selected applications of these assays for analysis of pesticide residues, and compare the advantages and disadvantages of this technique to conventional analytical methods. We will also discuss our prejudiced views of the constraints and opportunities for adoption of these techniques and how the regulatory and legislative branches of government can and do influence evaluation and acceptance of immunoassays.

Immunoassays for Agrochemical Analysis

The use of antibodies to identify and quantify agricultural chemicals grew out of the clinical use of antibodies in infectious disease diagnostics and therapeutic drug monitoring. The immunologic principles behind the technology have been known for some time, so the relatively late onset of antibody-based analysis of agrochemicals was probably due to a failure to recognize its potential outside the medical arena. Even after the publication of the first chemical immunoassays in the scientific literature, no commercially available or regulatory agency-approved chemical detection system based on anti-chemical antibodies was seen until recently.

Preparation of Anti-Chemical Antibodies

Antibodies are produced and secreted by plasma cells, the end-stage differentiated cell of the B-lymphocyte series. Plasma cells can be thought of as antibody-producing factories. The immunological rule of "one cell, one antibody," means that only one kind of antibody is made and secreted by one plasma cell (27). The antibody molecule evolved as one of an animal's major lines of defense against foreign substances such as pathogenic microbes. Antibodies are proteins whose primary amino acid sequence dictates a tertiary or three dimensional structure that bears a site into which a distinct chemical structure can bind (26). Some of the structures that can induce and interact with antibodies include sugars on the capsules of bacteria, viral glycoproteins, or glycoopids on tumor cells, but nearly any chemical structure, if presented to the immune system in the proper configuration, can induce and bind with a particular antibody. The analytical capabilities of antibodies have been appreciated for a long time (2, 17). Indeed, to measure the amount of a particular substance, one can inject the substance into an animal, isolate the antibodies to the substance, and in one of many modifications of immunoassay, detect and quantify the substance. Such is also the case with antibodies to small organic chemicals, but another tenet of immunology must first be considered before these chemicals can induce antibodies. The small size of nearly all agrochemicals forestalls their ability to induce the production of anti-chemical antibodies. Nevertheless, by attaching the small chemical to a larger immunogenic carrier molecule such as a foreign protein, the immune system of an animal can be coerced into producing an anti-chemical antibody. A chemical structure too small to induce an antibody by itself, that when conjugated to a larger carrier molecule induces a specific antibody, is termed a hapten (17).

When injected into an animal, a chemical hapten-carrier complex induces an array of different antibodies. There are antibodies to the carrier molecule in abundance, antibodies that bind to the hapten-carrier combination, and antibodies that bind only to hapten. It is only those antibodies that recognize the haptenic structure alone that are of value for the development of immunoassays. However, the antibody response to a particular hapten is extremely heterogeneous. Again, another tenet of immunology is based on the clonal selection theory (5). This theory states that foreign substances, such as the haptens, do not instruct the immune system to manufacture an antibody with structural complementarity to the hapten. Rather, there pre-exists in a mammalian immune system a B lymphocyte that is programmed to produce and secrete, upon stimulation by the proper chemical structure, an antibody with binding affinity to that structure. In essence the hapten selects from a pre-existing repertoire of B lymphocytes. In a typical immune response to a hapten, even with the limited size of a typical haptenic molecule, dozens or even hundreds of B lymphocytes with surface receptors capable of interacting even weakly with the hapten are stimulated to undergo proliferation and subsequent differentiation into end-stage, antibody-secreting plasma cells. Each of these clones of plasma cells secretes an antibody that recognizes in some way the haptenic structure. The family of antibodies that accumulate in the plasma of an animal following immunization with hapten-carrier are termed polyclonal in that they issue from many clones of plasma cells. The serum of such an immunized animal can be used as a source of anti-chemical antibody, and this antibody can be manipulated in ways to be discussed later for the quantification of the chemical.

The property of antibody binding to a chemical can be described by two closely related terms. The first is affinity, a term used to describe the strength of the interaction between chemical and antibody. Affinity is determined by the sum of all operant non-covalent chemical interactions (i.e., hydrogen bonds, van der Waals forces, hydrophobic and electrostatic interactions). A schematic representation of affinity is shown in figure 1. In this illustration, three antibodies are shown, all of which bind to the hypothetical chemical. The one on the left shows a perfect fit with the chemical and is thus a high affinity antibody. The middle antibody has one region of non-complementarity and is therefore of medium affinity, and the antibody on the right has only one complementarity region and is described as low affinity. The concept of affinity is important because, for most immunoassays, the higher the affinity of

Figure 1.—Antibody Affinity and Specificity

ANTIBODY AFFINITY

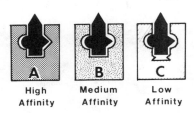

High Affinity | Medium Affinity | Low Affinity

ANTIBODY SPECIFICITY

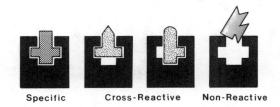

Specific | Cross-Reactive | Non-Reactive

SOURCE: Ralph Mumma, Pennsylvania State University and Ken Hunter, Westinghouse Bio-Analytic Systems, Co., 1988.

the antibody for the target chemical, the greater the sensitivity of the immunoassay.

The specificity of antibody-chemical interactions is illustrated in figure 2. Specificity and affinity are closely related terms, but they can be differentiated for illustration. Here we have one antibody and four chemical structures. On the left is a very specific interaction between antibody and chemical, and on the far right there is no interaction at all. The two chemicals in the center show a degree of cross-reactivity with the antibody due to a degree of structural homology with the chemical on the left. Specificity is of considerable importance because an immunoassay, as any analytical method, must be able to distinguish between related chemicals.

As mentioned earlier, the serum of an immunized animal can serve as a useful source of anti-chemical antibodies for the development of chemical immunoassays. However, there can be drawbacks to the use of serum polyclonal antibodies. First, the population of antibodies in serum is dynamic with respect

Figure 2.—Monoclonal Antibody Preparation

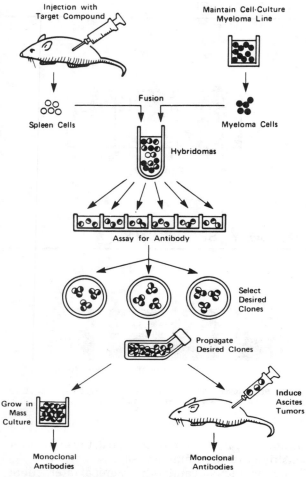

SOURCE: Ralph Mumma, Pennsylvania State University and Ken Hunter, Westinghouse Bio-Analytic Systems, Co., 1988.

Hybridomas and Monoclonal Antibodies

In 1975, two British scientists, George Kohler and Cisar Milstein, discovered that somatic hybrids between B lymphocytes and myeloma cells could produce antibody of "predefined" specificity (16). That is, the donor animal could be immunized with a target substance and immortal clones of these hybrids that secrete one particular antibody (monoclonal) with binding affinity for the target substance could be isolated. The hybrid tumors are known as hybridomas, and the monoclonal antibodies secreted by these cells have certain advantages. A generalized schematic of the hybridoma production procedure is shown in figure 2. Briefly, the spleen from an appropriately immunized mouse is removed and dissociated into a single cell suspension. These cells, some of which produce antibody to the target substance, can be maintained in nutrient medium (tissue culture) outside the mouse, but only for a few days. Although some specific antibody can be identified in the culture medium, it is too little to be of practical value. However, these short-lived cells can be physically fused in the presence of an agent such as polyethylene glycol (10) to myeloma cells, tumors of B lymphocyte origin that can live indefinitely in tissue culture (28). The resulting hybrids are heterokaryons, bearing the combined genetic information or genotype of both parental cells. Of paramount importance, the hybrids express two critical phenotypic characteristics, one derived from each parental cell; they secrete the antibody of the parental B lymphocyte, and they have unlimited growth potential, a trait of the parental myeloma. An elegant biochemical selection system is used to isolate the hybridomas (18), which are subsequently cloned to insure homogeneity. The cloned hybridomas can be grown in mass culture where the secreted antibody accumulates in the culture medium, or they can be adapted as ascites tumors in the peritoneal cavities of mice where very high levels of antibody accumulate in the ascites fluid. In either case, the product of the cloned hybridomas is a monoclonal antibody, a homogeneous reagent. The hybridomas can be cryopreserved and stored indefinitely in liquid nitrogen, and the monoclonal antibody is stable indefinitely under a variety of storage conditions. Therefore, the hybridoma technology can produce an unlimited, stable, and homogeneous supply of monoclonal antibodies.

Principles of Chemical Immunoassays

An enormous variety of immunoassay configurations have been developed, and a thorough review is beyond the scope of the present paper. However,

to concentration and quality. Secondly, the presence of an array of qualitatively different antibodies may in some cases obscure the analytical capability of the serum. Finally, the serum often bears unwanted antibodies that bind to the carrier molecule or the spacer unit between carrier and hapten; these antibodies, whether of natural origin or induced, may confound the analytical application. The unwanted antibodies often can be moved by purification steps (e.g., affinity, chromatography). Notwithstanding these problems occasionally encountered with polyclonal antibodies, many excellent immunoassays have been developed using these biological reagents. However, a recent technological advance now allows a single form of anti-chemical antibody to be produced in unlimited quantities.

as all immunoassays obey the same laws of mass action and thermodynamics, some general statements can be made. Immunoassays for small molecules such as pesticides must operate by competitive inhibition or displacement in which the binding of the free pesticide molecule to the antibody competes or displaces a tracer molecule. By way of example we will briefly discuss enzyme immunoassay, the most widely used method that employs an enzyme as the tracer and generates a color reaction as the read-out. Other tracers include radioisotopes, fluorescent molecules, magnetic particles, electron spin labels, etc.

The enzyme immunoassay, a modification of the original enzyme-linked immunosorbent assay of Engvall and Perlmann (7), is conveniently performed in a 96-well plastic microtiter plate (see figure 3), but it can be done with tubes or test strips. Prior to the first step in the enzyme immunoassay, the surface of the microtiter wells is coated with an optimal concentration of target chemical-protein conjugate (figure 4). Another popular configuration uses surface immobilized antibody, but the basic principle of both assays is the same. The conjugate adsorbs to the plastic surface by hydrophobic interactions, and following an incubation to assure maximum binding, the nonadsorbed conjugate is removed by washing with buffer containing a mild nonionic detergent. The first addition to the coated plate is a mixture of anti-chemical antibody and a known concentration of target chemical. If no target chemical was added to the antibody, most of the antibody would bind to the target chemical-protein conjugate adsorbed to the solid surface of the plate. The higher the concentration of target chemical added with the antibody, the lower the number of antibodies that bind to the solid phase due to the competitive inhibition of their binding sites through interaction with free target chemical in the fluid phase. After an incubation period, the reactants are washed away, leaving only the antibodies bound to the target chemical-protein conjugate on the plastic.

The second step of the procedure involves the addition of a tracer to detect the surface-bound antibodies from step one. In the case of the enzyme immunoassay, the tracer is a second antibody to which an enzyme is attached. This second antibody-enzyme conjugate binds to the surface adsorbed anti-chemical antibodies, and following an incubation, unbound second antibody is removed by washing. The third step in the enzyme immunoassay involves the addition of a solution of colorless enzyme substrate, which is converted by the enzyme into

Figure 3.—Applying Reagents to 96 Well-Plate

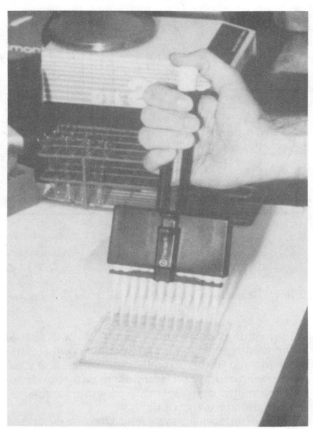

SOURCE: Ralph Mumma, Pennsylvania State University and Ken Hunter, Westinghouse Bio-Analytic Systems, Co., 1988.

a colored reaction product, the concentration of which is a direct measure of the concentration of antibody-enzyme tracer bound to the anti-chemical antibody on the plastic surface.

Because the color reaction is directly proportional to the number of anti-chemical antibodies bound to the plate, it is inversely proportional to the concentration of free target chemical. The higher the concentration of target chemical, the lower the color reaction. By running a series of known concentrations of target chemical, one can create a standard curve such as that shown in figure 5. A plot of optical density (color) versus target chemical concentration yields a curve with a linear portion often extending over several orders of magnitude. The enzyme immunoassay becomes an analytical tool when unknown samples are run at the same time and their optical density values compared with the standard curve. The apparatus for analyzing the

Figure 4.—Competitive Inhibition Enzyme Immunoassay

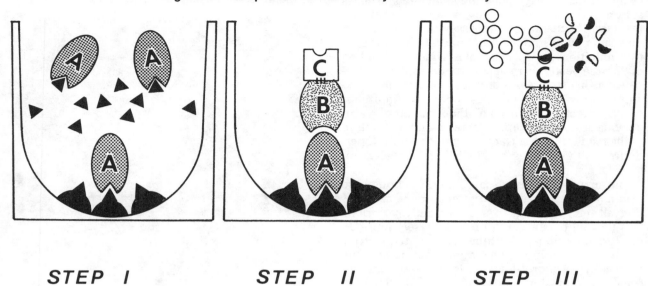

STEP I   STEP II   STEP III

SOURCE: Ralph Mumma, Pennsylvania State University and Ken Hunter, Westinghouse Bio-Analytic Systems, Co., 1988.

color reaction consists of a commercially available automated spectrophotometer that can evaluate the color in each of the 96 wells in less than one minute, a microcomputer interfaced with the spectrophotometer, and a software program for analyzing the data (see figure 6).

Enzyme immunoassays such as the one described earlier require 2 to 4 hours to perform, and most of this time is devoted to incubation. This assay format is highly quantitative, but other formats such as tube and test-strip enzyme immunoassays can be performed in minutes, and the results can be quantitative or semiquantitative. The criteria of sensitivity, specificity, accuracy, precision, and ruggedness, all critical to any treatment of conventional analysis, must also be addressed in chemical immunoassay. The enzyme immunoassay and similar assays that use a standard curve for comparison and determination of values in unknown samples are very amenable to statistical treatment. Although there is variation between particular chemical immunoassays due to the nature of the target chemical and the idiosyncratic properties of each antichemical antibody, chemical immunoassays can generally be as sensitive as conventional analysis techniques. Specificity is an inherent property of the antibody and is defined as the spectrum of cross-reactivities with related chemicals. It is not unusual, however, to see discriminatory capability at the single atom level, or even stereochemical selectivity

(4). Accuracy and precision are more related to the performance of the immunoassay than the properties of the antibodies, and for such assays as the enzyme immunoassay, these criteria are comparable to most conventional analysis methods. The variation between assays and between laboratories running the same immunoassay is also comparable. Immunoassays have component parts just as conventional assays, and these components must be standardized. For antibodies, this means that large batches of purified reagents must be prepared, stored in a way that preserves their integrity, and tested in standardized assays to ensure their quality.

Practical Applications of Chemical Immunoassays

Ercegovich (1976) was one of the first persons to recognize the potential of immunoassays to pesticide residue analysis. His students and colleagues (one of the authors, ROM) pioneered work in developing immunoassays for the organic phosphate insecticide, parathion (1, 9, 30). Similarly, Bruce Hammock's laboratory was actively developing immunoassays for pesticides (32), and Ken Hunter and colleagues (13, 14) developed antibodies to paraoxon and other organic phosphates recognized as war gasses. Subsequently, antibodies have been developed and reported for more than 30 pesticides, and a number of papers have appeared reviewing this

Figure 5.—Standard Curve: Parathion Immunoassay

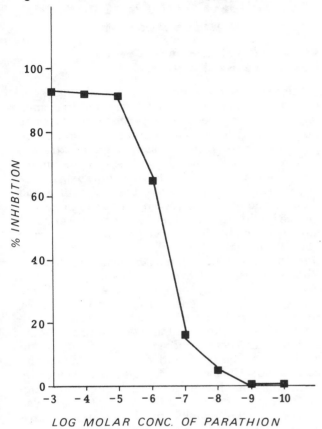

LOG MOLAR CONC. OF PARATHION

SOURCE: Ralph Mumma, Pennsylvania State University and Ken Hunter, Westinghouse Bio-Analytic Systems, Co., 1988.

Figure 6.—Computer, Printer, and Spectrophotometer

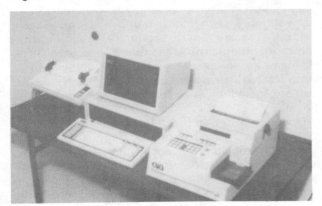

SOURCE: Ralph Mumma, Pennsylvania State University and Ken Hunter, Westinghouse Bio-Analytic Systems, Co., 1988.

progress (11, 12, 21). Industrial companies, some with commercial interest in mind, have developed many more immunoassays for pesticides, plant growth regulators, antibiotics, and other xenobiotics, but these data have not and may never be published.

Antibodies have been developed for various classes of pesticides, e.g., organic phosphates, carbamates, triazines, halogenated hydrocarbons, chlorophenoxy herbicides, pyrethroids, chitinase inhibitors, and biorational insecticides (21). Immunoassays also exist for a number of fungicides that cannot be grouped easily into a chemical class, such as Benomyl, Iprodione, maleic hydrazide, Metalaxyl, and Triadimefon. Interestingly, the antibodies for the pyrethroid S-bioallethrin exhibited chiral specificity (32), which cannot be achieved by any approved conventional method. An important potential use is with the biorational insecticides, such as the exotoxins from Bacillus thuringiensis, which can be quantified using immunological techniques. In the future, many biological agents derived through molecular biological techniques may be targeted for pest management practices, and immunoassays may be the only practical method to quantify these organisms or agents. Two environmentally sensitive chemicals, dioxin and pentachlorophenol, can also be analyzed in this manner, and an EPA-approved immunoassay for the latter compound is expected shortly.

Most of the early developmental work of immunoassays has been performed in academic institutions and with polyclonal antibodies. Unfortunately, very few examples of practical applications are documented in the literature. An exception is that of the contribution of W.H. Newsome from the Food Research Division, Bureau of Chemical Safety, Health and Welfare, Canada. Newsome has developed immunoassays for several fungicides and comparatively evaluated these with conventional methods (22, 23, 25, 24, 33). Van Emon et al. (31, 1987) have also compared immunoassays and conventional techniques in worker exposure studies with the herbicide paraquat. The authors of this article feel that many more application experiments need to be performed before we can thoroughly understand the influence of the matrix on immunoassay results.

The detectional limits of currently developed immunoassays for pesticides usually range from 0.1 to 1,000 parts per billion. Pesticide tolerance limits on many raw agricultural commodities are in the order of parts per million, and thus, immunoassays are sensitive enough to immediately make a contribution. With aqueous products such as water, fruit juices, and milk, immunoassays can be directly performed without any cleanup steps (3, 11).

Real-Time, On-Line Agrochemical Monitoring

Almost all of modern analytical chemistry deals with discrete measurements. Unfortunately, chemicals often present dynamic problems, concentrations waxing and waning over time (e.g., groundwater contamination with pesticides). Even the immunoassay cannot provide real-time (instantaneous), on-line (continuous) monitoring of these chemicals. However, a revolution in sensor technology is upon us that may provide both capabilities and may do so utilizing the same biological molecules generated for immunoassay.

The interface of biologic molecules like antibodies with microelectronic sensor systems to create hybrid devices known as biosensors promises to provide analytical capabilities beyond those now available. A biosensor is defined as a microelectronic device of one kind or another that utilizes a biologic molecule as the sensing or signal-transducing element. The structural requirements of a biosensor are shown in figure 7, and they include the following: a means of introducing the sample matrix to the sensor surface; an antibody or other biological molecule with binding affinity for a particular analyte in the matrix; a transduction mechanism whereby the binding event generates an electrical signal; appropriate amplification, processing, and storage of the generated signal data; and a means of outputting the information in a usable format.

A review of the many potential biosensors and the principles upon which they are based is beyond the scope of this report, and the reader is referred to recent reviews (6, 19, 20, 15, 29).

Figure 7.—Generalized Biosensor

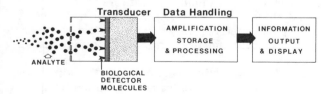

SOURCE: Ralph Mumma, Pennsylvania State University and Ken Hunter, Westinghouse Bio-Analytic Systems, Co., 1988.

Comparison of Immunoassays With Conventional Methods of Pesticide Residue Analysis

Conventional Methods Versus Immunoassay Methods

Before we compare conventional analytical methods to immunological assays, we must first summarize the steps used in both procedures. In a tradiional analysis the raw agricultural commodity or processed food is first subsampled and extracted or homogenized with an organic solvent to remove the pesticide residue from the insoluble debris. The organic extract is concentrated to small volume, and then an aliquot is analyzed by gas or high performance liquid chromatography. Pesticides are usually identified by the relative time it takes them to come through the chromatographic column (retention time) and their response to selective detectors. Chemical specific detectors are usually used with gas chromatography, and these detectors indicate the presence of halogens, nitrogen, phosphorous or sulfur atoms, which may be components of the pesticide residue. Although these detectors are highly specific, many compounds contain these atoms, and analyses can be confounded by such interfering compounds. Ultraviolet detectors are often the preferred method of detection with high-pressure liquid chromatography, but these detectors are also sensitive to all ultraviolet-absorbing substances. Because of these interference problems, organic extracts of food and raw agricultural commodities usually have to be partially purified using organic-solvent partitioning steps and time-consuming column chromatography prior to analysis by gas or high pressure liquid chromatography. This partial purification is often referred to as a cleanup step. Conventional analytical techniques are time-consuming, require environmentally sensitive and ultrapure organic solvents, utilize expensive chromatographic equipment, and require highly trained technicians. This results in expensive analyses for pesticide residues even for the most simple compounds.

However, when all procedures are followed, conventional analytical techniques are reliable, repeatable, and sensitive. Gas chromatography using atom-specific detectors usually can detect residues at the 1 to 100 picogram (10^{-9} grams), level but only a small amount of sample (1 to 5 microliters) can be analyzed in this manner. With high pressure liquid chromatography, a much larger aliquot of sample can be analyzed (25 to 50 microliters), but ultraviolet detectors usually require at least 1,000 picograms of residue. Gas chromatography separations require the chemicals to be volatile enough for separation as a heated gas, but unfortunately, many pesticides and their degradation products are not volatile and cannot be identified by this method. This is particularly true of the more polar, water-soluble pesticides and their metabolites. Also many pesticides do not absorb strongly in the ultraviolet and cannot directly be quantified with high sensitivity by this technique.

Immunological assays for pesticides may also involve many of these basic procedural steps. For the purpose of this presentation, we may think of an antibody as a very selective detector that is particularly useful for polar and water-soluble materials. In fact, immunological techniques are superior to conventional techniques in the direct analysis of pesticides in water. As for conventional methods of analysis, immunoassays require that processed food and raw agricultural commodities be extracted prior to analysis. However, the cleanup steps may be much abbreviated with the immunological technique. Also with liquid products, such as fruit juices, milk and soups, immunological analysis can be performed directly (3, 35). A potential drawback to immunoassays is that they are compound-specific and therefore most useful for single residue analysis. In contrast, conventional multiresidue procedures can detect and quantify many pesticide residues simultaneously. However, an antibody's great specificity does not always have to be an issue since antibodies can be selected that detect several chemicals of related structure, and different compound-specific antibodies can be combined in one analysis. Alternately a number of aliquots of food extract can each be analyzed with antibodies selective for a specific compound or for classes of compounds.

Immunoassays can be as reliable and repeatable as conventional methods of analysis, but usually the more highly quantitative immunoassays require more time to run than less quantitative immunoassays. Other immunoassay configurations can be quicker and simpler (1 to 10 minutes), but they are usually semiquantitative. However, if the emphasis is only on pesticide levels in food that exceed a certain concentration requiring regulatory action, the immunoassays are superior screening techniques. Immunoassays are also readily automated, while conventional analytical procedures are not.

Advantages and Disadvantages of Immunoassays

From an application standpoint, most immunoassays for pesticide residue analysis are simple and rapid, and in some cases, they may be used without any cleanup step. They are particularly useful for polar or water-soluble pesticides and their degradation products, and often immunoassays can easily be developed for compounds that are difficult to analyze by conventional methods. Since regulatory laboratories do not routinely analyze for pesticides not included on their multiresidue procedures list, immunoassay has the potential of filling this important void.

On the negative side, we should cite that the more rapid versions of immunoassay are usually not as sensitive and probably not as reproducible as conventional analytical techniques. Immunoassays may not be useful in a broad multiresidue procedure, even though several antibodies can be combined in one analysis. Other disadvantages include the lack of extensive commercialization, the lack of personnel with immunoassay experience, and the lack of knowledge and practical applications to raw and processed food.

Constraints, Opportunities, and Recommendations

Regulatory Agencies

Regulatory agencies at both the Federal and State levels are too slow to adopt or encourage modern methods and immunoassay is no exception. They seem to be spending most of their time on validation testing rather than funding or conducting state-of-the-art analytical methods development. To cite some examples, use of capillary column gas chromatography is only now starting to be accepted—it has been a routine procedure in most academic laboratories for years. Solid phase extraction (SPE) or concentration is rapidly being utilized by industry and private laboratories but it is not being emphasized by regulatory agencies. SPE is particularly attractive, since it often eliminates the need for expensive and environmentally sensitive solvents; this alone should be reason to encourage their use.

Immunoassays for pesticides have been demonstrated for more than 10 years, and regulatory agencies should have been taking a lead role in the development of these new techniques. Since many agrochemical industries and private laboratories have utilized these techniques for several years, regulatory agencies should encourage these organizations to make their data public so we can get a better feeling for the capabilities of these new methods. The agrochemical industry would not be using immunoassays unless they felt they were useful and reliable for their desired goals. Why has not the EPA or FDA sought information on these analyses so they could make more knowledgeable decisions? Additionally, why do they expect all analytical methods to meet the same strict requirements when perhaps only a screening procedure would be sufficient? By making quantitative analyses so difficult and expensive, regulatory agencies are actually reducing our knowledge of environmental pollutants because present methods can analyze only a fraction of the samples that should be analyzed.

There is at least one bright light in this dim world. The State of California has contracted for the development and testing of a number of immunoassays for pesticides. It is a pleasure to see a State regulatory agency take the lead in developing and evaluating this potentially important tool for the future.

Legislative Actions

Both State and Federal legislatures have constrained the regulatory agencies because they have asked them to do too many things and have not provided the financial backing to perform these tasks. Legislatures could take the lead by encouraging development and applications of the new methods of analysis. They should require the regulatory agencies to set aside a reasonable fraction of their budget moneys for developing the methods of the future. They should support grants and contracts to companies willing to pursue developments of new methods like immunoassays. Many new technologies such as immunoassays, enzyme assays, biosensors, solid-phase extractions, and affinity scavenging are now emerging, and much work needs to be done to determine their capabilities. We do not envision these techniques as replacing conventional methods, but rather as supplements to these methods. Such legislative action would stimulate development of these areas, and the well-being of the general public would greatly benefit.

References

1. Al-Rubae, A.Y., "The Enzyme-Linked Immunosorbent Assay, A New Method for the Analysis of Pesticide Residues," Ph.D. thesis, The Pennsylvania State University, 1978.

2. Berson, S.A., Yalow, R.S., Bauman, A., et al., "Insulin-131I Metabolism in Human Subjects: Demonstration of Insulin-Binding Globulin in the Circulation of Insulin Treated Subjects," *J. Clin. Invest.* 35:170-190, 1956.

3. Brady, J.F., Fleeker, J.R., Wilson, R.A., et al., "Development of an Enzyme-Linked Immunoassay for Aldicarb," *Biological Monitoring Technology for Measurement of Applicator Exposure*, Ph.D. thesis, Series 3 (Washington, DC: Amer. Chem. Soc., 1988).

4. Brimfield, A.A., Lenz, D.E., Benschop, H.P., et al., "Structural and Stereochemical Specificity of Mouse Monoclonal Antibodies to the Organophosphorus Cholinesterase Inhibitor Soman," *Mol. Pharmacol.* 28:32-39, 1985.

5. Burnet, F.M., "A Modification of Jernes Theory of Antibody Production Using the Concept of Clonal Selection," *Austral. J. Sci.* 20:67-69, 1957.

6. DeYoung, H.G., "The Mating of Biology and Electronics," *High Technol.*, pp. 41-49, November 1983.

7. Engvall, E. and Perlmann, P., "Enzyme-Linked Immunosorbent Assay (ELISA). Quantitative Assay of Immunoglobulin," *G. Immunochemistry* 8:871-874, 1971.

8. Ercegovich, C.D., *In Pesticide Identification at the Residue Level*, Advances in Chemistry Series #104, R.F. Gould (ed.) (Washington, DC: American Chemical Society, 1976).

9. Ercegovich, C.D., Vallejo, R.P., Gettig, R.R., et al., "Development of a Radioimmunoassay for Parathion," *J. Agric. Food Chem.* 29:559-563, 1981.

10. Gefter, M.L., Margulies, D.H., and Scharff, M.D., "A Simple Method for Polyethylene Glycol-Promoted Hybridization of Mouse Myeloma Cells," *Somat. Cell Genet.* 3:231-236, 1977.

11. Hammock, B.D., Gee, S.J., Cheung, P.Y.K., et al., "Utility of Immunoassay in Pesticide Trace Analysis," *Pesticide Science and Biotechnology*, R. Greenhalgh and T.R. Roberts (eds.) (Oxford, G.B.: Blackwell Scientific Publications, 1987).

12. Hammock, B.D. and Mumma, R.O., "Potential of Immuno-Chemical Technology for Pesticide Analysis," *Pesticide Analytical Methodology*, Am. Chem. Soc. Symposium Series No. 136, pp. 321-352, J. Harvey, Jr., Zeig (eds.) (Washington, DC: Am. Chem. Soc., 1980).

13. Hunter, K.W. and Lenz, D.E., "Detection and Quantification of the Organophosphate Insecticide Paraoxon by Competitive Inhibition Enzyme Immunoassay," *Life Sci.* 30:355-361, 1982.

14. Hunter, K.W., Lenz, D.E., Brimfield, A.A., et al., "Quantification of the Organophosphorus Nerve

Agent Soman by Competitive Inhibition Enzyme Immunoassay Using Monoclonal Antibody," *FEBS Lett* 149:147-151, 1982.

15. Hunter, K.W., "Technological Advances in Bedside Monitoring," *Arch. Path. Lab. Med.* 111: 633-636, 1987.

16. Kohler, G. and Milstein, C., "Continuous Cultures of Fused Cells Secreting Antibody of Predefined Specificity," *Nature* 256:495-497, 1975.

17. Landsteiner, K., *The Specificity of Serological Reactions* (Cambridge, MA: Harvard University Press, 1945).

18. Littlefield, J.W., "Selection of Hybrids from Matings of Fibroblasts *in vitro* and Their Presumed Recombinants," *Science* 145:709-710, 1964.

19. Lowe, C.R., "Biosensors," *Trends in Biotechnol.*, March: 59-65, 1984.

20. Lowe, C.R., "An Introduction to the Concepts and Technology of Biosensors," *Biosensors* 1:3-16, 1986.

21. Mumma, R.O. and Brady, J.F., "Immunological Assay for Agrochemicals," *Pesticide Science and Biotechnology*, R. Greenhalgh and T.R. Roberts (eds.) (Oxford, G.B.: Blackwell Scientific Publications, 1987).

22. Newsome, W.H., "An Enzyme-Linked Immunosorbent Assay for Metalaxyl in Foods," *J. Agric. Food Chem.* 33:528-530, 1985.

23. Newsome, W.H., *Bull. Environ. Contam. Toxicol.* 36:9-14, 1986.

24. Newsome, W.H., "Determination of Iprodine in Foods by ELISA," *Pesticide Science and Biotechnology*, R. Greenhalgh and T.R. Roberts (eds.) (Oxford, G.B.: Blackwell Scientific Publications, 1987).

25. Newsome, W.H. and Shields, J.B., "A Radioimmunoassay for Benomyl and Methyl 2-Benzimidazolecarbamate on Food Crops," *J. Agric. Food Chem.* 29:220-222, 1981.

26. Nisonoff, A., Hopper, J.E., and Spring, S.B., *The Antibody Molecule* (New York: Academic Press, 1975).

27. Nossal, G.J.V. and Lederberg, J., "Antibody Production by Single Cells," *Nature* 181:1419-1420, 1958.

28. Potter, M., "Immunoglobulin Producing Tumors and Myeloma Proteins of Mice," *Physiol. Rev.* 52:631-719, 1972.

29. Thompson, M. and Krull, U.J., "Biosensors and Bioprobes," *Trends Anal. Chem.*, July, 173-179, 1984.

30. Vallejo, R.P., Bogus, E.R. and Mumma, R.O., "Effects of Hapten Structure and Bridging Groups on Antisera Specificity in Parathion Immunoassay Development," *J. Agric. Food Chem.* 30:572-580, 1982.

31. Van Emon, J., Hammock, B.D., and Seiber, J.N., *Anal. Chem.* 58:1866-1873, 1986.

32. Wing, K.D., Hammock, B.D., and Wustner, D.A., "Development of an S-bioallethrin Specific Antibody," *J. Agric. Food Chem.* 26:1320-1333, 1978.

33. Newsome, W.H. and Collins, P.G., "Enzyme-Linked Immunosorbant Assay of Benonyl and Thiabendozole in Some Foods," *J. Assoc. Off. Anal. Chem.* 70:1025-1027, 1987.

34. Van Emon, J., *Bull. Environ. Contam. Toxicol.* 39:489-497, 1987.

35. Ferguson, B., personal communication, 1987.

Federal Pesticide Monitoring Programs: Analytical Methods Development

Charles L. Trichilo and Richard D. Schmitt, U.S. Environmental Protection Agency, Office of Pesticide Programs, Hazard Evaluation Division, Residue Chemistry Branch, Washington, DC

Contents

	Page
Abstract	182
Background	183
Tolerances	183
Qualitative Data on Metabolism and Degradation	183
Metabolism in Plants	183
Metabolism in Animals	183
Quantitative Data on Magnitude of the Residue	184
Magnitude of the Residue	184
Processing Studies	184
Feeding Studies	185
Analytical Methods	185
Effect of Limited Tolerance Data on Analytical Methods	185
Importance of Analytical Standards	186
Summary of Key Inputs to Food Monitoring	186
Overview Of FDA, USDA, and EPA Needs	186
FDA	186
USDA	187
EPA	187
Analytical Methods Development Program	188
FDA	188
USDA	188
EPA	188
Sharing Information Among Agencies	189
Accessing Technology in the Private Sector	190
Dealing With Hazardous Pesticides	190
Areas For Improvement	190
Recommendations For Improving Methods Development Programs	190
Acknowledgments	190
References	190

Figures

Figure	Page
1. Residue Chemistry Data Requirements	184
2. Key Input to Food Monitoring	187

Abstract

This paper provides a brief overview of the needs of the U.S. Environmental Protection Agency (EPA), Food and Drug Administration (FDA) and United States Department of Agriculture (USDA) in the area of analytical methods for monitoring pesticide residues in food. The importance in developing effective methods for tolerance enforcement that are rapid, sensitive, and inexpensive is discussed. The congressional mandates and agency approaches related to food residue monitoring, tolerance enforcement, and methods development are also described.

The effects of (1) changes in agricultural use practices that increase the extent of pesticide residues in the food supply and (2) limited tolerance data on the methods development process are noted. The acquisition of adequate metabolism data is the single most important chemistry contribution to the methods development process. Without full knowledge of the chemical identity of significant metabolites that occur as residues in food, it is impossible to develop monitoring methods for all residues of concern. While the primary focus for tolerance enforcement is on analytical methods, of equal importance is the need for readily available analytical reference standards.

The contribution analytical methods have in providing monitoring feedback for tolerance enforcement and tolerance-setting, in addition to their role in reducing the uncertainty in risk assessment, is also noted. Finally, suggestions are made for improving analytical methods for monitoring pesticide residues in food.

Background

Prior to any discussion on analytical methods to improve the monitoring and enforcement of tolerances for pesticide residues in the food supply, a brief overview of tolerances and related terminology is needed. Since tolerances depend on the state of scientific and technical knowledge (including analytical methods) at the time they are established, any limits in the existing data used will impose a corresponding limit in the analytical method used. Without an understanding of the key data elements that lead to a tolerance, it will be difficult, if not impossible, to significantly improve the analytical methods or the method development process for better tolerance enforcement (1).

Tolerances

A tolerance is the legal maximum residue concentration of a pesticide chemical allowed in a food or feed. Tolerances minimize uncertainty about food safety with regard to those pesticide residues. If a pesticide is detected and residues exceed the tolerance or no tolerance is established, the crop may be considered adulterated and be seized by the Food and Drug Administration (FDA), the United States Department of Agriculture (USDA), or a State enforcement agency. EPA establishes tolerances for pesticides, while FDA, USDA, and the States carry out tolerance enforcement in foodstuffs. EPA also provides the analytical standards used in tolerance enforcement (2).

Tolerances are set under authority of the Federal Food, Drug, and Cosmetic Act (FFDCA). Section 408 of the FFDCA applies to residues on raw agricultural commodities (RACs) and Section 409 applies to processed food or feed. Section 409 includes the Delaney Clause, which specifically prohibits the use of cancer-causing agents as food or feed additives.

There are three types of residue chemistry data that are essential for establishing tolerances:

1. Qualitative Data on Metabolism and Degradation
2. Quantitative Data on Magnitude of the Residue
3. Analytical Methods

The purpose of these chemistry data is to answer two basic questions. First, what is the chemical residue? Second, how much residue is there? Analytical methods are essential in providing answers to these two fundamental exposure questions. The "what" and "how much" information is used by EPA toxicologists to determine whether the dietary exposure is acceptable. The first half of EPA's tolerance-setting job is completed when EPA has concluded what and how much residue is present and that this level of residue is safe. The other half of EPA's job is to be sure adequate enforcement methods are available to check that the residue levels in the food supply do not exceed the tolerances.

Qualitative Data on Metabolism and Degradation

In order to answer the "what is the residue" question, qualitative data are required to determine the identity of the pesticide residues resulting from the transformation in plants and animals. EPA refers to these transformation studies that include both pesticide degradation and metabolism as metabolism studies.

Metabolism in Plants

Plant metabolism data characterize the identity of the residue that occurs in crops intended for consumption as a food or animal feed. These data identify the pesticide residues that remain in agricultural crops as the result of environmental transformation processes (degradation and metabolism). The resulting residue at harvest may be different than the chemical applied, due to breakdown or metabolism of the applied pesticide.

Metabolism in Animals

Whenever use of a pesticide results in residues in a livestock feed, or when a pesticide is applied directly to livestock, animal metabolism studies are required. The resulting data identify the pesticide residues to look for in the edible tissues of livestock or milk and eggs that result from transformation processes in the animal. If feed items are not involved or if this exposure pathway is blocked by label restriction, these data are not required (see figure 1).

Figure 1.—Residue Chemistry Data Requirements

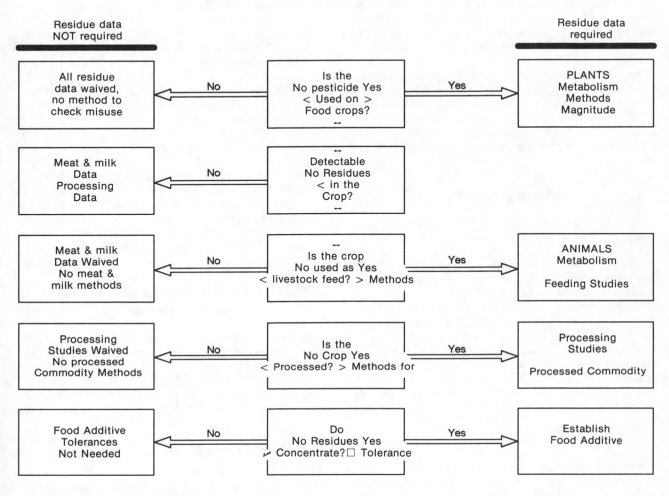

SOURCE: Charles Trichilo and Richard Schmitt, Environmental Protection Agency, 1988.

Quantitative Data on Magnitude of the Residue

Magnitude of the Residue

After the metabolism data have indicated what residue to look for in plants and animals (if applicable), methods are developed to measure these residues. Actual residue field trials are carried out to quantify the residues. These are the studies in which the pesticide is applied to crops at known application rates, in a manner similar to the use directions that will eventually appear on the label. The residue field trial studies result in residue data for the raw agricultural commodity (RAC) as it travels in interstate commerce.

Processing Studies

Processing studies are required to determine whether residues in raw commodities can concentrate or degrade on processing. If residues concentrate on processing, food or feed additive tolerances must be established. If residues do not concentrate on processing, the tolerance on the RAC applies to all processed food or feed derived from the RAC. It should be noted that the current EPA legal opinion on the Delaney Clause is that it applies to food and feed additive tolerances but not to RAC tolerances.

Feeding Studies

Livestock feeding studies are required whenever residues result in or on crops that are used as feed items. These studies provide data on the quantitative transfer of residues to meat, milk, poultry, and eggs. These studies are also required if a pesticide is applied directly to livestock.

Analytical Methods

Analytical methods serve two important purposes. The first is to generate residue data on which the dietary exposure assessment is based. The second is to enforce the tolerance after it is established. It should be noted that plant and animal metabolism data are the most critical data that precede the development of analytical methods. Without proper and complete metabolism studies to indicate which residues to look for, the development of analytical methods for all residues of concern may not be possible (3, 4).

Since risk assessment depends on exposure, analytical methods can have a significant impact on reducing the uncertainty in risk assessments by providing needed exposure data.

Analytical methods also serve an important role in providing feedback for tolerance enforcement and tolerance-setting procedures. Routine monitoring provides the obvious feedback on whether tolerances are being exceeded, or on whether tolerances have been set too high. However, sometimes the results of tolerance enforcement can lead to needed changes in the tolerance-setting process. For example, FDA monitoring uncovered over-tolerance residues of malathion in grain dust. Grain dust is now routinely collected at grain storage sites to prevent dust explosions and has become a disposal problem. Recently, the industry began pelleting this dust and using it as an animal feed. Due to the high concentration of pesticide residues in the dust, feeding of grain dust could lead to detectable residues in meat or milk. Furthermore, feeds formulated with grain dust as an ingredient are subject to seizure by FDA. As a direct result of the monitoring by FDA, EPA established a 135 ppm tolerance for malathion on grain dust (5). EPA also is revising its tolerance-setting procedures to routinely establish tolerances for grain dust to ensure that any potential residues in meat and milk are covered by tolerances and are safe.

Effect of Limited Tolerance Data on Analytical Methods

Any limits in the data that are used to establish tolerances will have a profound impact on the analytical methods. From EPA's perspective, there are two areas that can have a significant effect on the current state of the adequacy of analytical methods: 1) incomplete metabolism data, and 2) missing or impractical label restrictions that do not block exposure pathways.

Analytical methods can only be developed for those components of the residue that are identified in the metabolism studies. If metabolism studies do not fully identify the residues present, important components of the residue may remain undetected. Older chemicals whose metabolism studies fail to identify the significant residues present constitute the largest problem here. From EPA's experience in reviewing older chemicals as part of the re-registration process, it is not uncommon for 50 to 80 percent of the ^{14}C residues in radiolabeled metabolism studies to be unidentified. These limited data have an important effect on the ability to develop analytical methods. The development of analytical methods for chemicals with significant metabolism deficiencies will be delayed until the needed residue identification work is completed.

It should be noted that the complete set of residue data are not always required, particularly if the exposure pathways that lead to residues moving further into the food chain can be blocked by practical label restrictions. Determining what is practical is subject to much judgment and is further complicated by the dynamics of changing customary agricultural practices; this includes both economic and weather conditions that may affect the supply and demand of food or feed items.

In general, label restrictions are considered practical if three criteria are met: 1) the crop is under the direct control of the grower; 2) the economic value of the crop as a feed item is low; and 3) the U.S. customary practice is not to use the item as a feed. For example, label restrictions against feeding corn forage to prevent residues from moving into meat and milk commodities are not practical. Even though corn forage is under direct grower control, the high value of the feed item and the overwhelmingly common practice of feeding this commodity makes the restriction impractical.

What was practical at a certain period of time can change as use practices change. For example, until recently EPA considered the feeding directive, "Do not feed sugar beet tops" to be a practical restriction. Accordingly, data on metabolism, magnitude of the residue, and analytical methods were waived, since the feeding restriction was expected to prevent residues from moving into meat and milk. Therefore, analytical methods for determining residues in meat and milk were not available, since no pesticide residues were expected in these environmental media. In recent years, sugar beet tops have increased in economic value so much that California growers have changed their customary practice and now sell the beet tops for livestock feed. In this case, EPA was aware of the change and required data, including analytical methods, to cover any residues that could be expected in meat and milk.

However, EPA is not always aware of changes in use practices that result in residues moving further into the food chain than originally expected. The EPA Re-registration/Registration Standard process is one systematic scheme to identify such a problem area and call in the needed data. Again, however, until all chemicals are given a current review, the potential will exist for changes to occur in use patterns that result in more residue in the food supply with no corresponding analytical methods for enforcement.

It is important to note that no residue data are required for all nonfood uses. For nonfood uses, analytical methods are not required for detecting pesticide residues in food or feed crops, since residues are not expected in the food chain. Some older uses, previously considered as nonfood uses, may now actually be food uses that require residue data. Until these situations are identified, monitoring for food residues may not be possible because analytical methods are lacking. For these previously classified nonfood-use chemicals, analytical methods may not be available to FDA, USDA, and the States to check for accidental contamination or illegal use in food and feed.

Importance of Analytical Standards

Up to this point, the importance of analytical methods for monitoring pesticide residues in foods has been the primary emphasis of the Office of Technology Assessment workshop. Of equal importance, however, are the analytical standards that are used in the laboratory by those chemists conducting monitoring or enforcement activities. An analytical standard is a high purity reference standard used to calibrate the detector response of an analytical method. Chemists use a known analytical method together with a known analytical standard whose behavior and response is very predictable under laboratory conditions. Use of inappropriate standards

or standards of low purity will lead to erroneous methods results. If analytical standards are not of sufficient purity, enforcement becomes more time-consuming and difficult as predictable behavior cannot be obtained. If analytical standards are not available, enforcement becomes difficult, if not impossible.

When EPA is aware that analytical standards are not available, the agency can act under its authority under FIFRA 3(c)2(b) to require the pesticide registrant to submit additional quantities of the analytical standards. Failure of a registrant to provide or maintain analytical standards in the EPA repository can result in cancellation of the U.S. registration. EPA cooperates with FDA by providing analytical standards for those pesticides not having U.S. registrations that FDA needs to monitor imports. It should be noted that for pesticides used on imported foodstuffs that are not registered in the United States, there is no similar mechanism to obtain standards if the foreign registrant does not wish to cooperate.

Summary of Key Inputs to Food Monitoring

The importance of (1) changes in agricultural use practices that increase the extent of pesticide residues in the food supply, (2) limited tolerance data on residue identification (metabolism studies), and (3) the availability of analytical reference standards to food monitoring methods is depicted in figure 2. Without full knowledge of the chemical identity of significant metabolites that occur as residues in food, it is impossible to develop monitoring methods for all residues of concern. Similarly, the absence of analytical standards or the lack of knowledge about any increase in the extent of pesticide residue involvement of the food chain due to changes in agricultural use practice severely hampers the methods development process.

Overview of FDA, USDA, and EPA Needs

FDA

The Food and Drug Administration's (FDA) congressional mandate for enforcing tolerances is contained in the Federal Food, Drug and Cosmetic Act (FFDCA). The FDA is responsible for monitoring and enforcing tolerances for pesticide residues in all foods and feeds except meat and poultry. They need rapid, inexpensive methods for a wide variety of food matrices. FDA relies primarily on mul-

Figure 2.—Key Input to Food Monitoring

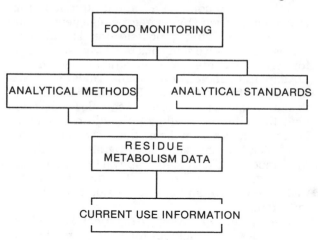

SOURCE: Charles Trichilo and Richard Schmitt, Environmental Protection Agency, 1988.

tiresidue methods that they have developed to handle the bulk of their monitoring efforts. The driving force for FDA to develop these methods is the great economic savings associated with methods capable of determining many pesticides at one time. The five multiresidue methods used by FDA detect approximately 60 percent of the pesticides with tolerances in food. FDA also uses single-chemical methods for monitoring pesticides of special concern when these pesticides are not detected by the multiresidue methods. The FDA also carries out market-basket surveys to determine the level of residues of many pesticides in ready-to-eat food. The FDA compiles the results of these quantitative analyses for pesticide residues in food. Data including incidence and levels of pesticide residues are available to EPA, the World Health Organization (WHO), and other interested parties (1). FDA also publishes their enforcement methods in the Pesticide Analytical Manual (PAM). Volume I (PAM I) (6) of this manual includes sampling procedures and a description of the multiresidue analytical methods. Volume II (PAM II) (8) of this manual includes methods for detecting individual pesticides.

USDA

The U.S. Department of Agriculture's (USDA) congressional mandate for enforcing meat and poultry tolerances is included in the Meat Inspection Act and the Poultry Inspection Act. The USDA enforces pesticide tolerances for meat and poultry. USDA is also responsible for enforcing drug resi-

due tolerances established by FDA. They also need rapid, inexpensive methods for meat and poultry products. (These include meat and poultry muscle, tissue, fat, liver, kidney, and processed meat products.) While USDA relies on multiresidue methods for chlorinated hydrocarbons (9), they also use individual methods for specific pesticides and animal drugs in their enforcement programs. These methods used by USDA are also developed by USDA. Recently, USDA has begun developing and utilizing rapid screening methods for specific compounds so that the more expensive laboratory methods will only be used on samples likely to be contaminated.

EPA

EPA's congressional mandates come from the FFDCA and the Federal Insecticide, Fungicide and Rodenticide Act (FIFRA). EPA sets tolerances under the FFDCA and registers pesticides under the FIFRA. EPA is responsible for establishing pesticide tolerances for all foods and feeds. Although EPA has no direct tolerance enforcement responsibility, the agency shares in the need for practical methods that are readily available. Practical methods need to be rapid, inexpensive, and reproducible, and they must involve equipment and reagents that are commercially available (10).

EPA does not normally develop analytical methods for tolerances. Rather, EPA requires the registrant of the pesticide chemical to develop methods necessary to enforce tolerances (11). EPA has provided written guidelines for the details on how this work should be carried out (12, 13, 14). EPA laboratories carry out method trials to assure that these written methods can actually be used to enforce tolerances.

To facilitate food monitoring and tolerance enforcement activities, EPA includes a methods availability statement in each Federal Register (FR) tolerance notice so that Federal and State enforcement agencies and other interested parties can more readily obtain copies of the methods. EPA also sends copies of methods for enforcing tolerances to FDA for publication in Volume II of the Pesticide Analytical Manual (7). In cases where no methodology exists for a pesticide of concern, EPA has taken the lead and developed methods such as was done to quantify dietary exposure to unsymmetrical dimethyl hydrazine (UDMH), a degradation product of daminozide (15). EPA's goal is to assure that a method suitable for enforcing tolerances is available before a pesticide tolerance is established as well as for all existing tolerances.

EPA accepts single chemical methods as being suitable for enforcement. In 1984, EPA regulations were revised to require data on whether existing FDA and USDA multiresidue methodology will detect and identify the pesticides (16).

To improve the quality of single chemical methods, EPA has encouraged more collaboration by method users, and it has encouraged petitioners to conduct an independent method check by a second laboratory prior to submitting the tolerance enforcement method to EPA. More recently, EPA (17, 18) has formally proposed independent laboratory confirmation for tolerance methods (19).

Analytical Methods Development Program

FDA

The FDA's primary method development efforts are in the area of multiresidue analytical methods (20). If multiresidue methods are impractical or impossible, single residue methods are developed to insure that residues can be determined. FDA uses information in the Surveillance Index to arrange in order of importance the methods development for pesticides used domestically. FDA has ranked pesticides according to the importance of generating monitoring data. This ranking scheme is called the Surveillance Index. The FDA Surveillance Index for pesticides was developed as a result of a recommendation of an FDA study group (21). The study group felt that selection of chemicals for monitoring should be based on potential health risk rather than analytical method availability.

FDA also uses a data base (22) on pesticide use in foreign countries to identify pesticides used outside the United States, for which methods must be developed. FDA has five major goals in the area of analytical methods development for pesticide residues:

Expansion of Existing Multiresidue Analytical Methods to Additional Pesticides and Alteration Products. Five multiresidue methods are regularly used by FDA, and each is undergoing study for expansion to additional chemicals. Multiresidue methods for groups of certain pesticides (e.g., triazine herbicides, chlorophenoxy herbicides, fumigants) are also available and used on occasion.

Extension of Methods to Different Food or Feed Commodities. This is a continuing activity dealing primarily with multiresidue methods. Modifications to existing methods are often required before the method can be used on additional commodities due to different physical or chemical composition or limits of detection.

Validation of Analytical Methods. It is the general practice to conduct a limited interlaboratory trial among a few FDA laboratories of a new method prior to introducing it for field use. The ultimate goal is collaborative study of a regularly used method for AOAC acceptance as an official method.

Adaptation of Newly Available Analytical Techniques for Integration into Existing Methods. Advances in instrumentation and sample preparation have the potential to allow for modification of existing methods so that the methods become cheaper and faster. FDA currently has programs on high performance liquid chromatography (HPLC), capillary column gas chromatography (GC), computer-assisted instrumentation, and a new residue extractor for fatty foods.

Development of "New" Analytical Methods or Techniques. This includes the development of immunoassay residue method capabilities (materials for use in FDA monitoring not now commercially available) being undertaken via contract.

In general, the methods development research could be divided into two broad types: 1) that which deals with the immediate program needs, and 2) that which is directed to future goals of greater scope to solve particular problems or to improve overall effectiveness or efficiency. Most of FDA's effort is forced into the first type.

USDA

Development of residue analytical methods by USDA comes under the purview of the Food Safety and Inspection Service (FSIS). The FSIS method development program is currently emphasizing the development of multiresidue screening methods, many of which are based on immunoassay techniques. Secondary emphasis is being placed on conventional chemical qualitative/confirmatory procedures. Methods are developed both in-house and under contract. USDA finds the meat and poultry methods developed by pesticide producers (PAM II methods) to be too long and expensive to be practical in a large-scale monitoring program. All methods used by USDA are subjected to collaborative studies prior to being used in FSIS laboratories. USDA does in-house collaborative studies and cooperates with the Association of Official Analytical Chemists (AOAC) in carrying out collaborative studies.

EPA

Since EPA has no direct responsibility for enforcing tolerances, methods development for residues in food is not generally carried out in EPA laboratories. Methods development at EPA is carried out primarily by the Office of Research and Development (ORD). ORD does not have a specific program to develop methods to detect pesticide residues in food; however, it supports such efforts by providing analytical reference standards and technical information through its Pesticides and Industrial Chemicals Repository (2). As noted previously, the availability of analytical standards are as important as analytical methods in tolerance enforcement. ORD does develop methods to meet specific congressional mandates under a number of laws:

Clean Air Act (CAA)
Clean Water Act (CWA)
Safe Drinking Water Act (SDWA)
Resource Conservation and Recovery Act (RCRA)
Comprehensive Environmental Response, Compensation and Liability Act (CERCLA, Superfund)
Toxic Substances Control Act (TSCA).

In some cases, these methods can be used as a starting point for detecting residues in food. The EPA organizations responsible for administering or implementing specific environmental laws request ORD to develop methods through research committees consisting of ORD and program office representatives. ORD laboratories are then directed to perform the requested work, which they perform internally or by contract, grant, or cooperative agreement. Most analytical method development activities are conducted by the Office of Acid Deposition, Environmental Monitoring and Quality Assurance (OADEMQA) in ORD.

As pesticides become of concern to the program offices, they are sometimes included in multiresidue methods. For example, six multiresidue methods have been developed by the Environmental Monitoring and Support Lab (EMSL) to detect approximately 120 pesticides and degradation products in ground water. Pesticide methods are also developed to monitor pesticide residues for specific projects requested by the Office of Pesticide Programs. In most cases, existing methods available from the literature, the FDA, or a pesticide manufacturer are modified for the matrix of interest.

The Office of Pesticide Programs has laboratories at Beltsville, MD, and Bay St. Louis, MS, that are primarily responsible for carrying out method validations to assure adequate methods are available to enforce tolerances. These laboratories have, on occasion, developed single chemical methods for pesticides or their metabolites when existing methodology was unavailable for important chemicals of concern, such as those chemicals involved in the EPA Special Review Process.

Sharing Information Among Agencies

Information on analytical methods is shared through implementation of Memorandums of Understanding (23) and periodic meetings. Currently EPA, FDA, and USDA meet quarterly to discuss specific problems associated with analytical methods. Past results from these meetings have included the following:

Protocols to be used by the pesticide registrants to determine whether pesticides would be detected by FDA multiresidue methodology (24).

User response sheets included in PAM II so that problem methods can be identified and better methodology required of registrants (25).

Identification and prioritization of problem methods so that better methodology can be developed.

Current projects under consideration at these meetings include the development of a protocol for determining the acceptability of a method and writing specific criteria on the acceptability of methods for enforcement purposes.

FDA and EPA cooperate on the Surveillance Index project. EPA provides FDA with pertinent exposure and toxicology information for those pesticides with tolerances so that FDA can rank the pesticides in order of priority for monitoring. Similarly, EPA representatives sit in on USDA's surveillance advisory team meeting to provide input on priority pesticides to be monitored in meat and poultry.

EPA has recently initiated procedures to make analytical methods submitted by pesticide tolerance petitioners more readily available to FDA, USDA, the States, and other interested parties. EPA now sends FDA and USDA copies of new chemical methods and method modifications for use on additional crops upon receipt of these methods. This provides the enforcement agencies an opportunity to comment on the suitability of these methods early in the tolerance-setting process and prior to approval of the tolerance. EPA also includes, in each published Federal Register notice for every tolerance, a specific statement on the availability of the analytical methodology. If the method has not yet been published in the PAM II, the FR notice includes the address of the EPA/FOI Office from which the method can be obtained.

Accessing Technology in the Private Sector

EPA requires registrants of pesticide chemicals to submit analytical methods as part of the data necessary to register a pesticide. These methods, developed by the agrochemical producers, are made available by publication in PAM II by FDA and released by EPA under the FOI Office. The publication of environmental matrix methods is done by the National Technical Information Service (NTIS). Since these methods must be made available to enforcement agencies and interested parties, EPA no longer accepts methods that are claimed to be Confidential Business Information (CBI).

Much residue data is generated by the food processing and distribution industry. EPA is currently working with the National Food Processors and the Grocery Manufacturers of America to make these residue data available for use by Federal agencies. EPA/FDA/USDA chemists are also meeting with technical committees of these organizations to suggest areas for monitoring pesticide residues and new methods development.

Dealing with Hazardous Pesticides

EPA evaluates potentially hazardous pesticides that appear to meet or exceed certain risk criteria through its Special Review process. Under the Special Review process, all available data on toxicity and exposure are reviewed. In addition, data essential to the determination of risk of a pesticide are required from the registrants when appropriate.

When necessary for Special Review decisions, EPA requests special monitoring programs from FDA and USDA to determine the level of residues in food. EPA also notifies the Grocery Manufacturers of America (GMA) and the National Food Processors of America (NFPA) so that residue data from the food industry can be made available. Increased cooperation in this area will improve the government's ability to deal with hazardous pesticides.

Areas for Improvement

Each agency should review its current regulations and guidelines with the goal of improving or modifying them if needed, so that analytical methodology needs can be better addressed. The EPA has issued regulation modifications involving multiresidue method protocols (27) and is considering second-lab validation of enforcement methods. Both

of these changes were initiated for the sole purpose of improving the capability of enforcement agencies to monitor for pesticide residues in food.

Recommendations for Improving Methods Development Programs

The major need among Federal and State agencies in the area of pesticide food monitoring is the development of quicker, more comprehensive multiresidue programs. The following are suggestions for improving methods development for food monitoring:

- Closer coordination between EPA, FDA, and USDA in methods research and prioritization. Agencies should identify lead organizations for each area of methods research and attempt to minimize overlap.
- Congress should consider providing incentives to industry, academia, and the States to develop methods for pesticide residues in food and to monitor for pesticides in food.
- The pesticide producers and the food production industry should increase their efforts at monitoring for pesticide residues in food and should share monitoring results with Federal agencies.

Acknowledgments

The authors express their appreciation to Paul Corneliussen for providing information of FDA's activities and to Bart Suhre for assisting with the section on USDA's activities. The authors also appreciate the diligence shown by Fannie Mosley in typing and retyping this manuscript particularly under the short timeframe.

References

1. Trichilo, C.L., "EPA Pesticide Contaminant Concern for Residues in Food and Feed," *Cereal Foods World* 32 (11):806, November 1987.
2. Analytical Standards are available from the U.S. EPA Environmental Research Center, Environmental Monitoring Systems Laboratory, Quality Assurance Division, Las Vegas, NV.
3. Kovacs, M.F., "Regulatory Aspects of Bound Residues," *(Chemistry) Residue Reviews* 97:1-17, 1986.
4. U.S. EPA, Pesticide Assessment Guidelines, Subdivision O, Residue Chemistry, Series 171-4 (a)(1)&(2), "Nature of the Residue: Plants," Addendum on Date Reporting (1987) Environmental

Protection Agency, Washington, DC. (Available from National Technical Information Service, 5285 Port Royal Rd., Springfield, VA 22161. Doc. No. PB 87-208641).

5. 21 CFR 56.270, April 15, 1987.

6. U.S. Department of Health and Human Services, Food and Drug Administration, FDA/EPA, *Pesticide Analytical Manual*, Volume I (Methods Which Detect Multiple Residues).

7. Read, et al., The FDA Pesticide Monitoring Program, JOACAC 591-595 (1987).

8. U.S. Department of Health and Human Services, Food and Drug Administration, *Pesticide Analytical Manual*, Volume II, Methods for Individual Residues.

9. *Official Methods of Analysis of the Association of Official Analytical Chemists*, S. Williams (ed.) 14th Ed., 1984, Section 29.037.

10. Trichilo, C.L., "The Challenge for Analytical Chemistry, Where Methods Came From," Food and Drug Law Institute Conference (Sept. 11, 1987) on "Pesticides in Foods Dealing with the Problem," page 2.

11. 40 CFR 158.125 (5)(4).

12. Pesticide Assessment Guidelines, Subdivision O, Residue Chemistry Series 171-4 (b), 1982, U.S. Environmental Protection Agency, Washington, DC. (Available from National Technical Information Service, 5285 Port Royal Rd., Springfield, VA 22161. Doc. No. PB 83-153981.)

13. U.S. EPA, Hazard Evaluation Division, Standard Evaluation Procedure, Analytical Methods, Draft of 1/19/88.

14. U.S. EPA, Data Reporting Guidelines - Addenda to the Pesticide Assessment Guidelines, Subdivision O, Addendum 2, Magnitude of the Residue: Crop Field Trials, Analytical Method(s), and Storage Stability Study; National Technical Information Service, PB 86-248192.

15. Wright, D., Jr., "New Method for the Determination of 1,1-Dimethylhydrazine Residues in Apples and Peaches," *J. Assoc. Off. Anal. Chem.* 70(4):718, 1987.

16. 40 CFR 158.125 (b)(15).

17. Trichilo, C.L., "Tolerance Setting Procedures for Residues in the Food Supply," National Agricultural Chemicals Spring Conference, 1987, page 9.

18. Kovacs, M.F., Jr. and Trichilo, C.L., "Regulatory Perspective of Pesticide Analytical Enforcement Methology in the United States," *J. Assoc. Off. Anal. Chem.* 70(6):940, 1987.

19. EPA Office of Pesticide Programs "Notice to Manufacturers, Formulators & Registrants of Pesticide Products" *Draft PR Notice 88-4*, Tolerance Method Trials—Independent Laboratory Confirmation April 1988.

20. McMahan, B.M. and Burke, J.A., "Expanding and Tracking the Capabilities of Pesticide Multiresidue Methodology Used in the Food and Drug Administrations's Pesticide Monitoring Programs," *J. Assoc. Off. Anal. Chem.* 70(6): 1072, 1987.

21. FDA Monitoring Programs for Pesticides and Industrial Chemical Residues in Food, Study Group on FDA Residue Programs, June, 1979, HEW Publication No. (FDA) 79-2116.

22. World Agrochemical Data Bank, an on-line service available only to subscribers to Battelle's World Pesticides Programme; Battelle Memorial Institute, Research Management & Economic Analysis Dept., Columbus, OH, 42301.

23. Memorandum of Understanding among the Food Safety and Inspection Service and Agricultural Marketing Service, U.S. Department of Agriculture and the Food and Drug Administration, U.S. Department of Health and Human Services, and the U.S. Environmental Protection Agency, October 5, 1984, 12 pages.

24. U.S. Department of Health and Human Services, Food and Drug Administration, Appendix II, *Pesticide Analytical Manual*, Volume I.

25. U.S. Department of Health and Human Services, Food and Drug Administration, Method Evaluation Form, November, 1985, Pesticide Analytical Manual, Volume II.

26. Methods are available from the Pesticide Analytical Manual, Volume II or Information Service Section, Program Management and Support Division (TS-757C), Office of Pesticide Programs, U.S. Environmental Protection Agency, 401 M Street, S.W., Washington, DC 20460.

27. Federal Register, Volume 51, No. 187, Friday, September 26, 1986.

Pesticide Analytical Methods Development at the State Level

William Cusick, California Department of Food and Agriculture, Division of Inspection Services, Chemistry Laboratory Services

and

James W. Wells, California Department of Food and Agriculture, Division of Pest Management, Pesticide Enforcement Branch

Contents

	Page
Abstract	192
Introduction	192
Pesticide Residue Monitoring Programs	192
U.S. Department of Health and Human Services, Food and Drug Administration	193
Florida Department of Agriculture and Consumer Services (FDACS)	193
Massachusetts Department of Public Health (MDPH)	194
Montana Department of Food and Agriculture (MDA)	194
California Department of Food and Agriculture (CDFA)	194
Analytical Methods Needed	196
Analytical Methods Developed at State Level	197
Impact of Local Regulatory Initiatives	199
Role of States in Analytical Methods Development	199
References	200

Abstract

The role of state regulatory agencies in the enforcement of pesticides residue tolerances and the development of new analytical technologies are determined by Federal policy and State legislative intent. State programs are focused to complement the regulatory activity of the various Federal agencies, but also to meet the state's sometimes more stringent regulatory requirements. This paper discusses the states' role in the national food protection program and highlights the differences between the state and Federal programs.

Introduction

The U.S. Department of Health and Human Services, Food and Drug Administration (USFDA) is the Federal agency responsible for monitoring pesticide residues in food. Over the years, a number of states have developed their own pesticide residue monitoring programs in response to specific needs identified by the states, perceived limitations in the Federal program, and perhaps most important, in response to the increased consumer concern regarding toxics in the food supply. The size and goals of these state programs vary, depending on the perceived need in the state and the funding available. This paper will examine the pesticide residue monitoring programs of several selected states in comparison with that of USFDA; discuss the kinds of analytical methods most needed, including a discussion of the applicability and potential for emerging analytical techniques; provide an overview of present analytical methods development in the states; discuss local regulatory initiatives that have placed special analytical requirements on the state laboratories; identify the present role of the state in analytical methods research and development; and make suggestions for what that role may be in the future.

Pesticide Residue Monitoring Programs

In order to present information that would be more representative of the national status of states' pesticide residue monitoring programs, examples are provided from several states with programs of different sizes and objectives. The states included are Florida, Montana, Massachusetts, and California.

U.S. Department of Health and Human Services, Food and Drug Administration

The U.S. Department of Health and Human Services, Food and Drug Administration (USFDA) analyzes approximately 10,000 samples of fresh fruits, nuts, and vegetables each year (7). Samples are taken of imported produce, as well as domestic produce destined for interstate shipment. The USFDA program consists of two major components: compliance monitoring and surveillance monitoring. In this paper we will deal with the surveillance monitoring component because it has the most applicability for comparisons with state monitoring programs. The objective of the surveillance monitoring component is primarily to enforce U.S. pesticide residue tolerances established by the U.S. Environmental Protection Agency (EPA). The tolerances are established by Federal regulation and published in Code of Federal Regulations 40 Part 180.

Sampling of imported produce is based on the regional import sampling plan, on headquarters-directed assignments, and on special emphasis surveys. In developing regional sampling plans, districts consider the dietary significance and production volume of the commodities, the compliance history of the country of origin, and pesticides used at origin identified through use of the Battelle World Agrochemical Data Bank. Because of resource limitations, USFDA headquarters places some restrictions on the commodities to be sampled based on the commodities' significance in dietary intake. For example, very few samples are taken of spices and herbs.

Headquarters-directed assignments are aimed at obtaining residue data for commodities or pesticides that have not sufficiently covered during previous years. Also included in these assignments are pesticides or commodities that, on a national level, are of increasing concern or interest. Examples of headquarters-directed assignments proposed for the 1988 Federal fiscal year include imported fresh cucumbers to be analyzed for organohalogen, organophosphorus, and carbamate residue; and imported fresh apples to be analyzed for organohalogen, organophosphorus, Ethylene Bisdithiocarbamates (EBDC), benomyl, thiophanate-methyl, Methyl 2-benzimidazdecarbamate (MBC) and daminozide residues.

Special emphasis surveys are based on selected high volume imports and on commodities treated with pesticides that are not allowed for food use in the United States. Each district is required to select and conduct a minimum of two of these surveys with priority given to country/commodity combinations not covered by previous monitoring in the district (3).

For domestic samples, USFDA districts prepare annual sampling plans based on local conditions such as pest problems, amount of production, past compliance history, or coverage. Headquarters specifies the minimum number of samples to be taken by each district and the resources to be expended on pesticide monitoring. In its annual guidance to the districts, the headquarter's office also specifics coverage of certain pesticides and commodities for each district. This special-survey element normally focuses on pesticides that are of potential health concern and that require analyses by single residue analytical methods, or it monitors the level of specific pesticides of importance to the EPA. For example, for several years a special survey was performed of EDB in grains and fruits. EPA needs information on the extent to which EDB residues were occurring because of carcinogenic concerns.

Other than specific surveys, districts are given considerable latitude in developing annual plans for domestic sampling. Most plans are designed to cover crops of local dietary importance, pesticides with high usage within the district, growers or commodities with past compliance problems, and commodity/pesticide combinations in which misuse is suspected.

Normally, samples are analyzed by one of five multi-residue techniques that detect from 24 to 123 pesticides. Single residues, or specific analyses, is performed during special surveys on specific pesticides, to confirm levels detected by multi-residue techniques, or when misuses of the pesticide is known or suspected (7).

Florida Department of Agriculture and Consumer Services (FDACS)

FDACS began monitoring raw agricultural commodities for pesticides residues in 1960. The Bureau of Chemical Residue Laboratory, under the Division of Chemistry, FDACS, is responsible for the analysis of pesticide residues in food and feed products produced or marketed in Florida. It is also responsible for the enforcement of Federal tolerances and guidelines adopted by the state. Each year the Bureau performs more than 10,000 determinations on approximately 4,000 food and feed samples. Each routine sample is analyzed by the chlorinated hydrocarbon and organophosphate multi-residue procedures. Samples of fresh fruits and vegetables are also analyzed by the carbamate screening procedure. Single residue analyses are performed on an "as needed" basis. Analyses of the majority of routine food samples are completed within 48 hours.

Since the late 1970s, the program has been set up to target the most probable problem areas in order to direct limited resources. Samples are taken of commodities throughout the channels of trade, including airports and docks. Samples may be of Florida-grown or imported produce, depending on the time of year. Florida's program is a combined crop-pesticide index. That is, in selecting samples for analysis, FDACS considers the propensity of the commodity to retain significant levels of pesticides, and the characteristics of the pesticides applied to the crop. According to W. George Fong, FDACS, the classification of crop groups from the standpoint of potential pesticide exposure of consumed plant parts is based on the book *Food and Feed Crops of the United States*, by J.R. Magness, et al. (2). Considerations of the characteristics of the pesticides applied to the crop include the following: acute oral toxicity, persistency in the crop, toxic metabolites formed, current EPA special review, systemic property of the pesticide, and human dietary exposure (2).

Massachusetts Department of Public Health (MDPH)

MDPH has been performing pesticide residue surveillance for about the past four years. Approximately 500 samples are taken each year that can be analyzed for about 30 different pesticides. Recently, MDPH has made a rather major change in its program direction. The department's program is tailored to identify and assess specific potential pesticide-related health risks. Potential risks are identified either through risk assessment analysis or through laboratory results. For example, if the laboratory detects significant levels of a chemical in food, risks assessments associated with that level will be initiated; conversely, if risk assessment demonstrates a concern for a particular chemical, the program will be directed toward analyzing commodities on which that pesticides may be used.

The objective of the program is to identify and assess the pesticide residues that may pose the greatest risk using information and criteria from the FDA surveillance index, data on file with the EPA and with other states (for example, from the FOODCON-

TAM program, a federally sponsored data-sharing program that collates pesticide residue analytical data from the laboratory. Emphasis is placed on the diets of those subgroups of the population determined to be most at risk from exposure. Samples are taken at the wholesale and retail level for both domestic and imported commodities (1).

Montana Department of Food and Agriculture (MDA)

MDA has been taking pesticide residue samples for about 13 years. An average of 250 samples are taken each year as part of agricultural pesticide misuse investigations. An additional 50 samples per year are specifically collected for residue monitoring (or tolerance enforcement) in food commodities. For misuse investigations, the pesticide analysis is normally limited to the specific suspect pesticide. For the monitoring program, any or all of the major pesticide groups are requested, e.g., carbamates, organophosphates, etc.

The majority of samples consist of agricultural commodities produced and marketed in the state that are known to have been treated with a specific pesticide. This normally occurs after a pest outbreak that has required extensive applications of the target pesticide. Samples are taken at the farmgate or retail level. The analytical laboratory is capable of analyzing for 70 to 100 different pesticides both through multiresidue and specific analyses. Analyses requested are dependent on the situation triggering the sampling.

California Department of Food and Agriculture (CDFA)

CDFA has had a pesticide residue program for more than 60 years. CDFA's pesticide residue monitoring program is organized into four major components: state routine, preharvest monitoring, focused monitoring, and processing foods monitoring. Altogether, the California program results in more than 43,000 determinations on approximately 13,000 samples each year. These samples are in addition to samples analyzed during misuse investigations, which account for an additional 4,000 samples per year. The state routine component is a commodity-based, tolerance-enforcement function consisting of approximately 6,500 samples of fresh fruits, nuts, and vegetables taken from throughout the channels of trade. Both domestic and imported commodities are included. Analysis for the majority of these samples is by multiresidue screens, capable of detecting approximately 100 pesticides. Analyses performed through multiresidue screens are normally completed within 4 to 6 hours from the time the sample is submitted to the laboratory. For this component, single method analyses are made on an "as needed" basis, with a turnabout time of generally less than 24 hours. The selection of 75 percent of the commodities sampled in this component is based on a statistical formula that takes into account the amount of consumption and historical residue data. Specialists are allowed to use their discretion in selecting the remaining 25 percent. Factors influencing discretionary sampling include knowledge of pest problems and pesticide usage within the production areas, data from the USFDA program, etc.

The preharvest monitoring component consists of approximately 2,500 samples taken from fields, prior to harvest. These samples are normally analyzed by the multiresidue screens. Specific analyses are requested on an "as needed" basis. Commodities to be sampled are determined by the amount of production in the county of origin, pest problems, pesticide usage within the production area, and by compliance history of the grower. Early detection and deterrence of pesticide misuse is one of the major goals of this program.

The focused monitoring component is a pesticide-based, rather than commodity-based, program. Each year, CDFA medical toxicologists identify pesticides of priority health concern. Commodities known to have been treated with those pesticides are sampled and analyzed for the specific pesticide. As with the Massachusetts program, emphasis is placed on the diet of those subgroups of the population determined to be most at risk.

The processing foods monitoring component consists of approximately 1,500 samples of raw commodities destined for processing. Samples are taken in the field, shortly before harvest or after harvest; at grading stations; and at processing plants prior to processing. These samples are analyzed by multiresidue screens. An important goal of this component is to provide information to the California Department of Health Services (CDHS) to assist them in designing their processed-foods-products pesticide monitoring program. The number of samples to be taken of each commodity is based on California production figures.

As can be determined from the previous discussion, there is quite a variety in the types of samples, types of pesticide analyses performed, and sizes of state programs. The objectives of state programs also vary dependent on resources and public concerns. However, similarities also occur. For example, the Massachusetts program, which is limited to 500 samples per year, has chosen to focus its sampling on specific pesticides as they relate to dietary risk. Though similar in size, this program is similar to California's focused monitoring program. The same theme can be seen in USFDA's headquarters-directed and specific emphasis assignments.

In Montana program, resource limitations have caused this state to restrict its monitoring solely to those situations in which the possibility of over-tolerances is the highest. The Florida program, though larger, has also directed its program in this way.

Most of the programs are, at least partially, developed to act as a deterrent to pesticide misuse. The California program, however, is the only one that routinely takes samples of commodities in the field prior to harvest, as well as in the channels of trade. The Massachusetts program appears to be based more on public health concerns than on deterrence.

All program have multiresidue screening capabilities. There is variation, though, in the number of pesticides that can be analyzed in this manner. Further discussion on analytical capabilities will follow.

All states contacted have the authority to adopt their own residue tolerance levels; however, all of them currently use those set by EPA. USFDA and some states also use "action levels" and "regulatory analytical limits" in determining whether or not to take enforcement action. The use of action levels and regulatory analytical limits is not uniform.

A recent decision by the U.S. Court of Appeals for the District of Columbia stated, in essence, that action levels set by USFDA were legislative rules rather than general statements of policy and, therefore, must be adopted according to the Administrative Procedures Act. The court found the Federal action levels to be invalid because they were not adopted according to this procedure. At best, action levels are useful as a guide and do not require or prevent USFDA from taking action (8).

The results of this 1987 decision have yet to be fully addressed. In Florida, where no tolerances or action levels exist for a pesticide in a particular commodity, a regulatory analytical limit is applied (9). Action levels are treated the same as tolerances. In cases in which no tolerance or action levels exists, Florida set its own regulatory analytical limited based on the lowest residue level the laboratory is able to reasonably detect, measure, and confirm with existing analytical methods (2). Historically,

California has acknowledged those Federal action levels as published in 40 CFR 180, but it has not acknowledged regulatory analytical limits set by Federal policy. California is currently re-examining whether or not action levels can continue to be used because of the Court of Appeals decision.

Analytical Methods Needed

In the past ten years, the need for and ability of pesticide residue laboratories to identify, quantitate, and confirm the presence of trace levels of pesticides in or on food crops has increased dramatically. California regulations require that the pesticide-residue analytical method submitted in support of a California registration for food-use pesticides not exceed 24 hours. The Florida enforcement program's mandate allows for food samples to be completed within 48 hours (2). The EPA currently has a *guideline* for analytical methods that emphasizes the desirability of a 24-hour method, but it is not mandatory.

Multiresidue screens currently being used by states are useful; however, they are not inclusive. Some pesticides do not lend themselves to a screening procedure because of their chemical constituents. Others, though they can be detected in water samples, require extensive preparation time for detection in the various crop matrices. When there is need for data on a non-screenable chemical, the slower single residue analytical method(s) submitted by the registrant or a PAM method must be employed.

There is a need for more multiresidue procedures that detect metabolites as well as the parent compound. For tolerances enforcement programs, time is of the essence, and analysis should be completed within a normal working day, making multiresidue screens ideally suited for this type of work. Many single residue methods also meet this criteria, although in some cases laboratories must modify submitted methods to achieve this time frame. Built-in quality-assurance features are needed, and methods should not require specific instrumentation that only a few state laboratories have or can afford (2).

Performance characteristics of the *ideal* analytical methods for pesticide residue in food crops would have the following minimum characteristics:

1. Methods would be validated on every crop type for which the pesticides is registered. As new registered food crop uses are approved, the analytical methods would be updated to reflect the new crop matrices. For example, an analytical method may be acceptable in selectivity and sensitivity for head lettuce, but when the same analysis is performed on green onions or parsley, the crop matrix interferences may reduce the analytical sensitivity to an unacceptable level.

2. All new analytical methods would be validated in a series of independent laboratories. This procedure would test the method to evaluate its reliability and reproducibility under various operating and management systems.

3. New methods or analytical regimes would have to include the ability to detect, identify, confirm, and quantify and and all metabolites included in the 40 CFR 180 tolerances. Ideally, this process should not exceed seven hours from the time the sample is received in the laboratory.

In addition to developing methods for new chemicals, review should be completed on the older chemicals, especially those with potential dietary impact. For example, the current approved methods for EDBC's are not product specific, and there are no known confirmational techniques. The only approved method is wet chemistry and involves CS_2 evolution and colorimetric quantification. Besides the obvious shortcomings of these types of methods, different tolerances exist for the various members of this family of chemicals on the same crop. There is no way, short of field investigation, to determine which tolerance applies and if an over-tolerance has occurred.

The needs of the pesticide regulatory programs for accurate data demand that the laboratories monitor their ability to provide accurate, timely, and reproducible analytical results. In order to assure these results, use of a well-managed quality-control or quality-assurance program is needed. In most states, such a program has been initiated. However, there is a need for development of new analytical quality-control methods with internal provisions. These internal checks could alert the analyst to developing problems and the need to effect timely corrective action. Such a system could greatly reduce the time currently being spent to investigate the causes of inaccurate analytical results, thereby reducing the analytical cost per sample.

Many of the newer pesticides being used on food crops are thermally liable and not easily analyzed by the high temperature GC systems. The other major analytical tool widely available for use is HPLC. The HPLC, however, lacks easy or reliable analytical confirmation. New methods that will provide quick, reliable, and cost-effective confirmation that will also be legally defensible are needed.

For pesticide residue enforcement, analytical methods that are specific for the parent chemical are needed. Currently, EPA does not require specific analytical methods for the parent compound. Metabolites included in the tolerances listed in 40 CFR 180 need to be identified. Currently, there are tolerances that state "and cholinesterase-inhibiting metabolites" or "and its metabolites" (40 CFR ed: 1980). Confusion exists regarding what parts of a commodity must be included in the analytical procedure. It is imperative that EPA of FDA take action to relieve this confusion. Suggestions would include publishing a single-source document such as that included in CODEX that provides this information or establishing a toll-free telephone number to an information officer to answer questions. This information center should be staffed around the clock to be of service to all states.

To facilitate detection of pesticide misuse, there is a need for development of residue analytical methods for various agricultural and environmental media, and for crops for which the pesticides in question are not necessarily registered. According to Laszlo Torma, Montana Department of Food and Agriculture, the methods in the PAM II are inadequate because they are not collaborated, and they are designed only for those commodities for which the chemical is registered. Companies and Federal laboratories with the assistance of state laboratories could set up and collaborate multiresidue methods for these compounds, and special consideration of a region could be acknowledged to meet these methods and regulations. For example, in Montana a relatively large number of the population consumes meat from wildlife on a regular basis; however, there is no official collaborative analytical method or established tolerance available for these foods. Another area that could be addressed is the pesticides that are not registered in the United States, but are registered in Canada. Frequently, these products enter Montana and other bordering states but when residue analyses are required, there is no method available (6).

Emerging techniques such as immunoassays and biosensors have potential for pesticide residue analysis. The initial impact of these new techniques is expected to be in the area of rapid screening of produce samples for a wide range of specific pesticides. Under this approach, the confirmation of the screening results would be via traditional GC, GC/MS, LC/MS, or other appropriate separation and confirmation systems. As the new techniques are proven to be accurate, dependable, and have internal quality-assurance checks, the classical confirmational steps could be reduced.

The major advantage of these new technologies would be their improved sensitivity and selectivity. CDFA is currently evaluating three ELISA techniques for use in the pesticide residue program. Two of the ELISAs are for the triazine class of compounds and one is for paraquat. The paraquat ELISA is of interest because it is potentially superior in sensitivity, selectivity, and reproducibility to the existing battery of available colorimetric methods.

Evaluation at CDFA indicates that the new technologies are rapid, reproducible, and inexpensive to use. These factors open the possibility of regulatory programs being able to perform more analyses per sample and to run more samples for selected pesticides. This would enhance the regulatory data base and provide statistically valid residue trends and dietary loads.

These new technologies appear to be "user friendly", and the amount of time and money to train staff to utilize these systems appears to be minimal. These procedures are "turn-key", and any laboratory could improve its capability without a massive infusion of funds.

At this time, however, most of these methods are qualitative, or at the most semiquantitative procedures. They do not promise, however, for being used as a preliminary screen (2). Research and field testing should be given high priority to make these tools available within the next few years.

Analytical Methods Developed at State Level

Analytical methods development at the state level varies with the objectives of the various state programs. Most state programs are primarily focused on enforcing Federal tolerances. To be effective, this type of enforcement requires rapid turnaround time. This often necessitates modifying existing analytical methods or developing a new analytical method. For example, CDFA laboratories have adapted a more rapid GC method for EBDC's in place of the Federal wet-chemistry method to be compatible with states' regulatory needs.

States that actively investigate pesticide misuse and pesticide illness incidents often must modify residue methods to meet their needs. For example, CDFA has modified analytical methods that were developed for food crop analyses to be applicable for different analytical uses, such as farmworker exposure monitoring or environmental drift and contamination of non-target areas.

Florida's laboratory has developed an HPLC-UV screening procedure for several families of herbicides, for example, triazines, uracils, phenylureas, etc., in water samples. When the sample preparation technique is worked out, these procedures can be used for vegetable and fruit samples as well (2).

In Massachusetts, EPA's decision not to ban the use of daminozide caused concern at the state level, and Massachusetts decided to take independent action. In order to perform the analytical testing of raw and processed apple products necessary to complete their risk assessment, this state's laboratory developed analytical methods to improve the sensitivity levels (1).

CDFA's resources for analytical methods development are devoted to modifying existing methods. Currently, the State of California may have the largest state-funded pesticide analysis program among states. CDFA's Chemistry Laboratory Services branch has a methods-development group staffed with one principal agricultural chemist (Ph.D.), two agricultural chemists III, which is the highest technical pay-grade in the state's system, and one experienced technical assistant. As part of the methods-development group, an in-house quality-control and quality-assurance program has recently been initiated and maintained by an agricultural chemist III and a technical assistant.

CDFA is involved in the evaluation of new analytical technologies such as the applications of super critical fluid chromatography in pesticide residue chemistry, ELISA, and tandem mass spectrometry through the methods-development group. Due to the geographical location and the past close working relationship with the University of California at Davis (UCD), CDFA is exploring the possibility of a state-funded collaborative effort for analytical methods-development research with UCD. This effort could include the following: (1) improvement, modification, and unique application of conventional analytical methods, for example, GLC, LC, and wet methods; (2) nonconventional analytical methods development, for example, ELISA, alternative detection of pesticides, novel separation science; (3) confirmation of analytical results through shared advanced instrumentation facilities, for example, HR MS, MSMS, Foumer Transfer Infrared Spectrometer (FTIR), and Nuclear Magnetic Spectrometer (NMR); and (4) training of appropriate personnel and technology transfer.

In the area of instrumentation review, California is currently looking for a better and more reliable confirmational technique for GC and HPLC systems. Currently, California is evaluating a GC/MS/LC for both GC and HPLC work. A GC Mass Selective Detector (MSD) will be purchased for evaluation along with further work with photodiode array detectors and supporting work stations. This type of work is very expensive for a state to fund and it is, therefore, limited in scope. The work conducted in California's laboratories is focused on addressing California's needs and may, therefore, not be of any utility to other regulatory or commercial pesticide residue laboratories.

In Florida, methods-development work has traditionally emphasized modification of existing techniques. To augment existing methods, this state is now extensively using Solid Phase Extraction (SPE). According to W. George Fong of FDACS, "SPE technique for sample preparation requires less sample and solvents and can be completed in much less time. It reduces the health hazards in the laboratory and generates less solvent waste. SPE also provides limited specificity" (2). FDACS has developed SPE techniques for carbamate analysis and adapted the techniques for most HPLC analyses. Some limited preliminary studies are also being done of SPE for gas-liquid chromatography. There are two chemist positions devoted to methods development and quality-assurance work in this state.

In Montana, methods-development is limited to determining the accuracy of a published method or adapting a published method for a given commodity to another commodity. Local needs further limit methods development primarily to areas of new herbicides (glyphosate, sulfonylurea herbicides, triazin, substituted ureas, etc.). This state has three chemists who expend approximately 70 percent of their times on residues analyses.

In Massachusetts, methods-development work has been on a case-by-case basis. This has involved pesticide-specific surveillance and compliance testing for chemicals that have been designated as public health priorities and have required state-level regulatory action. During 1987, activities include risk assessment and policy development for alachlor and 2,4-D, methods development and compliance testing for daminozide in apple products, and screening for heavy metals and organochlorine pesticides in bottled drinking water.

There is undoubtedly some duplication of analytical methods-development efforts by states and Federal government agencies when the objectives of the programs are similar, for example, monitoring for tolerances enforcement. In the past, little or no information was exchanged between state laboratories and Federal agencies regarding research or methods-development work being conducted. Currently, CDFA and USFDA Region IX are developing a memorandum of understanding (MOU) that will include a residue analytical section. Methods-development and quality-assurance procedures are being considered to be included in this MOU.

Impact of Local Regulatory Initiatives

State laws and regulations can place special analytical requirements on pesticide laboratories. Several examples from California illustrate this point. Historically, California law has provided that CDFA may seize a lot of produce if it is suspected of carrying excess pesticide residue. By statute, the lot may only be held for 24 hours unless laboratory analysis confirms the existence of the illegal residue. This has caused CDFA to modify or replace methods that take longer than 24 hours to complete. Proposition 65, passed by the California voters in 1986, provides that no person shall expose any individual to a chemical known to be a carcinogen or reproductive toxin without giving prior warning. While all of the ramifications of this law are yet to be understood, it is conceivable that the pesticide regulatory laboratories will have to modify or replace existing residue methodology to shorten turnaround time or to lower limits of detection for pesticides that are oncogenic or have adverse reproductive effects.

Recently, commercial laboratories in California have begun to conduct pesticide residue testing on produce for grocery stores. A bill has been introduced in the state legislature that would require such laboratories to be accredited by the state and to participate in a state-sanctioned quality-assurance program. Accreditation programs may place additional responsibilities on state laboratories to provide oversight, oversee and qualify control of uniform analytical methods.

Neither Florida nor Montana reported having legislation similar to Proposition 65, though Florida does have a regulation that suspends the use of aldicarb in an area where it has been found in well water in excess of 10 parts per billion. Massachusetts, with program emphasis on pesticides with potential chronic risks, may well have occasion to employ modified residue methods.

Role of States in Analytical Methods Development

Pesticides analytical methods-development at state laboratories has a different focus than that of academia, private industry, and Federal government agencies. Rather than the development of basic new analytical methods, state laboratories emphasize methods-application and subsequent methods-modification. This difference in emphasis has arisen from differences in the overall objectives of the various laboratories. Traditionally, academia has contributed in the aspects of basic, novel analytical methods-development, while industries have emphasized analytical methods for applications of a particular chemical. In general, state laboratories' needs for pesticide analytical methods are to monitor, regulate, and enforce the uses of pesticides within a given state, in accordance with federally-established standards. However, there are still differences in analytical needs between Federal and state laboratories.

The historical and current role of California in analytical methods research and development has largely been limited to modification of existing methods to meet our criteria of performance acceptance. There have been instances when new methods have been developed for residue analysis because existing approved methods were not specific, rapid, or sensitive enough to meet regulatory needs. For example, in 1985, contamination problems resulting from the misues of aldicarb on watermelons resulted in a recall of all California watermelons. In order to allow continued sales, California established a certification program that included sampling and analysis of melons, from all fields prior to shipment, for aldicarb and aldicarb sulfoxide. The original method was judged too time-consuming, as each of the four CDFA district laboratories was attempting to "clear" 20 fields per day, and each field required a minimum of five composite samples. With the single goal of certification in mind, an HPLC method was developed to provide the accuracy speed, and precision required (5).

In addition to ongoing methods modification, CDFA's methods-development group is addressing the use of new instrumentation technology in various residue applications. The pesticide registration laboratory works with pesticide registrants in order to resolve operational problems with their analytical methods. This activity is restricted to methods-modification, not conducting research, which is the responsibility of the pesticide registrant. Work conducted in CDFA's laboratories focuses on addressing California's needs and may, therefore, not be of any utility to other regulatory or commercial pesticide residue laboratories.

In the area of methods-development, Federal agencies should seek states' input to determine what the state's analytical needs are. Collaboration is necessary between state, Federal, and private laboratories. Additionally, states with smaller programs would benefit from a more vigorous training program provided by Federal agencies (6).

Massachusetts sees a need for FDA training programs for pesticide analytical laboratories. Training is necessary for comparability and accuracy of data, including analytical support and guidelines for data interpretation for a variety of analytical procedures and instrumentation. Also necessary, from this State's viewpoint, is the establishment of minimum criteria by which a laboratory would be considered a certified FDA laboratory. Such a program would include quality-control and quality-assurance, possibly including specified recovery rates and detection limits.

In order to provide uniform regulatory analytical results and assure consumer protection, consideration should be given to an EPA/FDA/NBS/state-managed laboratory accreditation program for all pesticide residue regulatory laboratories. As part of this program, EPA/FDA should conduct quarterly regional meetings with the state laboratories and a national meeting for all state chemistry managers. These meetings at the local and national level would provide state input into the national programs.

Many new pesticides are on the horizon which will require very different types of analytical methodology than are currently utilized in state programs. What role will states play in developing/modifying methods to analyze these pesticides? Will state laboratories be able to maintain the efficacy of their programs through modification of existing techniques? State programs have no role in *developing* analytical methods of support the registration of a pesticide. The responsibility to provide an acceptable analytical method at the time of product registration is clearly that of the registrant, whether that method is a modification of existing techniques or development of a completely new type of methodology. The role of states will continue to be working on published methods to improve their sensitivity, expanding the types of sample matrices, and optimizing registrants' methods for use in the state's analytical system.

The role of states in developing/testing new methods such as immunoassay, automation, and screening will be different depending on the size of the state's programs and the available funding. CDFA has defined its role in the development and testing of newer methods to include the identification of analytical needs, both short-term and long-range; and contractual support for development, or cooperation in product evaluation, such as with private immunoassay product suppliers. The use of automation and the development of expanded or new multiresidue pesticides screens are part of an ongoing process in California's program. CDFA is actively engaged in reviewing its analytical procedures for incorporation into an automated system, and expects to test a robotic system within the next 18 months. The expansion of current multiresidue pesticide screens and the development of new screens are priorities for CDFA's method development group.

The role of state pesticide residue monitoring is to supplement the broad Federal program, while focusing activities on crops produced within state boundaries. Cooperation is essential to minimize duplication of analytical methods-development. The Federal agencies responsible for food safety must provide the leadership in any cooperative effort. This leadership role must be open to address the real needs of the states and be sensitive to local conditions. The cooperative effort should include the development of a national set of methods-development goals that, in turn, could be monitored to ensure efficient use of resources. The technology sharing would reduce duplicative work and encourage state involvement in problem resolution.

Each state may have different analytical requirements and resources; however, there is common ground. On role that states could play would be in an advisory capacity to the Federal government. The establishment of a methods research and development advisory committee to the appropriate Federal agency should be encouraged. Such a committee would include representatives from the state's chemistry laboratory programs, along with representatives of consumers, production agriculture, academic institutions, pesticide registrants, and Federal programs. This advisory group could be composed of two subgroups: one to deal with policy issues, which would include the chemistry program administrators; and one to deal with scientific issues, which would include the principal chemists. This advisory group could be mandated to advise the Federal government on current problem areas, results of on-going state-sponsored projects, and recommend areas of research.

References

1. Chung, C., Weiss, L., Nassif, J., Ridley, N., Timperi, R., "Planning a State Program for the Surveillance of Pesticide Residues in Food," Presentation at the 1987 American Public Health Association Meeting, October 1987.

2. Fong, W. George, personal communication, 1988.
3. Food and Drug Administration, Compliance Program Guidance Manual, *Pesticides and Industrial Chemicals in Imported Foods*, (FY 88), 1988.
4. Gingery, G., personal communication, 1988.
5. Ting, K.C., Kho, P.K., "High Performance Liquid Chromatographic Methods for Determination of Aldicarb Sulfoxide in Watermelons," *Bulletin of Environmental Contamination and Toxicology* 37: 192-198; 1986.
6. Torma, L., personal communication, 1988.
7. United States General Accounting Office, *Pesticides, Need to Enhance FDA's Ability to Protect the Public from Illegal Residues*, October 1986.
8. Wessel, John R., personal communication to R.V. Peterson, 1988.

Pesticides Analytical Methods Development in the Private Sector

Lyle D. Johnson, Analytical Bio-Chemistry Laboratories, Inc., Columbia, MO

and

John E. Cowell, Monsanto Agricultural Company, Environmental Sciences Department, Life Sciences Research Center, Chesterfield, MO

Contents

	Page
Abstract	202
Introduction	202
Overview of the Private Sector	202
Pesticide Residue Analysis	204
Emerging Technologies	206
Multiresidue Technologies	207
Federal Interaction	208
Conclusions	209
References	209

Abstract

As a result of questions sparked by the ability to measure chemicals at increasingly minute levels, there has been an increased interest in the development of analytical methods for the detection of pesticide residues in foodstuffs. Among those in the private sector, most laboratories involved in pesticide method development have typically been university, industry, and contract laboratories. Food producers, food processors, and distributors also have an interest in analytical methods.

This discussion will focus on the objectives, the driving forces behind development, and the ramifications of these analytical methods. In addition, assessment of existing and emerging technologies will be performed from a private-sector viewpoint. Viewed constraints and opportunities will be addressed together with possible approaches to enhancing multiresidue method development. This multiresidue screening approach is necessary from an expedient and cost-effective perspective.

Introduction

Pesticides have evolved over the decades from persistent, long-term control, broad-spectrum efficacious chemicals toward short-term control, biodegradable chemicals used with integrated pest management practices. The resulting agencies have required the manufacturers to do extensive screening for toxicological and ecological concerns in the development of any new pesticide. Beyond requirements, each segment of the agricultural industry, whether it be grower, food producer, distributor, manufacturer of agricultural chemical, or regulating agency, has increased interest in the issue of pesticide residues in food.

A tremendous amount of expertise for analytical methods development exists in the private sector. The value of this actual experience in developing methods for the analysis of pesticide residues is often underestimated. The goal of this residue methodology development effort, whether the laboratory is a university, pesticide industry, food producer, food processor, or consulting contractor, is basically the same: to answer the question of how much residual pesticide is contained in the matrix of interest. The incentives and extent of participation of the different types of laboratories vary.

Overview of the Private Sector

The university laboratory may perform method development for the sake of knowledge and achievement, while the food producers and food processors are only concerned that the screening methods used, assure their products contain less pesticide residues than the corresponding tolerance (maximum allowable) levels. These tolerances, which are granted under the Federal Food, Drug and Cosmetic (FDC) Act, are established from supervised field trials at locations representative of each of the major crop-growing areas. The residue field trials are conducted by the pesticide registrant under the most extreme conditions of proposed use, such as the maximum application rate, the maximum number of applications, and the shortest interval from application to harvest. This measurement process ensures that the tolerance levels, established under the Federal Insecticide, Fungicide, and Rodenticide Act (FIFRA) and regulated by the Environmental Protection Agency (EPA), are not exceeded. The Food and Drug Administration (FDA) conducts a program of monitoring for pesticide residues primarily in raw, unprocessed food moving in the commercial channels of trade. Thus, the obvious interest on the part of the food producers is to ensure compliance.

Section 409 of the FDC Act, adopted in 1958, established the procedure for tolerances for processed foods and animal feed when pesticide residues on the raw agricultural commodity (RAC) concentrate in a processed fraction of the RAC. For instance, when raisins are processed from grapes, if a concentration of a residue occurs, then a food-additive tolerance is required for the pesticide in raisins. Conceivably, this concentration could make an undetectable residue in the RAC, detectable in the processed food. Some pesticides of toxicological concern concentrated in processed food would trigger the Delaney Clause. Food processors perform analyses to assure that their processed products contain undetectable residue levels or levels less than these food-additive tolerances.

Several contracting laboratories were surveyed (1, 2, 3, 4, 5) to determine their involvement in pesticide analyses and the level of methods development. Contract laboratories obtain analytical procedures from their clients, peer-review organizations, literature references, or when not available, develop a procedure from innovative research. In the cases of FIFRA registration projects, analytical methods are generally provided by the registrant. At best, research will be limited to adaptation of a method for additional sample matrices. Those laboratories concerned with minor-use pesticide registration, such as the regional IR-4 laboratories, respond in much the same way as a contracting laboratory. A method is provided by the company sponsor and used to acquire registration data (6). These IR-4 laboratories are usually affiliated with universities. These university laboratories have the analytical residue and method development experience and perform very cost-effective residue analyses. Other university laboratories have not shown a consistent interest in residue analysis except as an application for specific analytical techniques.

The contracting laboratory strives for a competitive edge by analytical method development for a purely monetary interest, while the industrial pesticide laboratory has the weight of economic and social responsibility to comply with the regulatory requirements for EPA registration. In addition to the development of residue field-trial data for estimation of the tolerance level, the pesticide registrant conducts reproduction and long-term animal feeding studies, using various species of test animals to establish the safety of the tolerance level. These toxicity studies determine the No Observable Effect Level (NOEL), the level at which the pesticide has no harmful effect on the most sensitive test animal. This NOEL is divided by a safety factor of up to 100 or more to set the Acceptable Daily Intake (ADI). The ADI represents the amount of pesticide residue that can be ingested by an average person every day for a lifetime without ill effect. Thus, the ADI usually is less than the sum of the normalized tolerances of the pesticide residue levels for all registered uses on crops.

The first step in the process of developing the crop residue and the environmental fate data base for a pesticide is the development of the analytical method. Subdivision O Residue Chemistry Guidelines (7), developed by the EPA, state that the pesticide registrants need to develop methods for residue analyses that serve two functions: 1) they must provide the residue data upon which judgments are made as to the identity and magnitude of residues from the proposed use, and 2) they must provide a means for enforcement of the tolerance. Sometimes, these two functions are best served by development of two separate methods. The initial role of developing analytical methodology justifiably belongs to the pesticide manufacturer. In addition to the production of the parent active ingredient of the pesticide, the manufacturer has had to synthesize the degradants or metabolites for identification purposes as well as for reference standards for the residue method development. The manufacturer is in the best position to develop data on the product chemistry, physical properties, and means of analysis of the pesticide.

As is inferred from the EPA guidance document, there are two driving forces in the development of analytical methodology. One is to develop an analytical method to provide data to quantitate the magnitude of residues from the proposed use to establish the residue tolerance. Toward this goal, there is a certain amount of pressure on the industrial chemist to develop methodology as quickly as possible, given that it takes approximately 5 to 7 years to perform the necessary toxicological, environmental fate, metabolism, and residue studies to fulfill regulatory requirements to ensure registration of a product to allow it to be sold. Thus, any time saved in this process or timeline can result in market entry advantage and greater profitability. During this rapid development, the optimal method speed and universality is not always addressed. The developing chemist is concerned mainly with quantitation of all required substances, with method sensitivity in that the method must be capable of detecting very low levels (i.e., an acceptable low level in food and feed matrices would be 10 to 50 ppb) and with method selectivity in that there are no interferences that would result in false-positive detections with use of the method. Thus, to achieve this high degree of sensitivity and selectivity in the most rapid fashion, the developer is compelled to use the most powerful state-of-the-art analytical techniques and instrumentation available. Additionally, the relatively large number of analyses needed to support a registration submission further serves as validation of this analytical methodology.

From a contract laboratory standpoint, the pressure to stay on schedule analytically with the various ecological, environmental fate, and residue chemistry studies is overwhelming. The registrant can be a very demanding sponsor as a result of the timeliness desired or imposed by the EPA. Methods are sent to laboratories for validation in both tested and untested matrices. Quite often, these methods have not undergone ruggedness testing to identify the critical steps of the procedure. Ruggedness testing through collaborative interlaboratory study determines the reliability of each step of the method by performance by several different analysts. Most laboratories have experienced, to the detriment of the analytical method, undesirable levels of method variability with different lots of reagents, absorbents, and column materials.

The other driving force is to develop a method that can be used to enforce the established tolerances. This methodology is usually different from the previous method because it has to be as simple as possible to minimize the cost of monitoring for pesticide residues. The EPA required enforcement method is expected to be rapid (less than 24 hours to completion), sufficiently sensitive in relation to the tolerance, interference-free, free of blanks or internal standards, and unencumbered by exotic equipment or reagents. The use of multi-detection methodology is extremely desirable. However, the method must measure the "total toxic residue", as determined in the metabolism studies [171-4(a), Nature of the Residue]. This total toxic residue includes the parent molecule and all metabolites of toxicological concern. Since most metabolites are not tested for toxicity, this means all metabolites isolated in sufficient quantities to be identified. This requirement greatly increases the level of difficulty in the development of multiresidue methodology and will be explained later in this discussion.

Pesticide Residue Analysis

Pesticide residue analyses can be classified into three groups for the purpose of examining applicability to multiresidue analysis:

1. compounds that do not degrade or metabolize quickly,
2. compounds that do degrade or metabolize quickly, and
3. compounds that degrade or metabolize at a rate that falls between these two groups; they are degraded to only a couple of additional compounds.

Compounds that are not degraded or metabolized either rapidly or significantly in the various environmental compartments (i.e., air, soil, water, plants, or animals) offer the best opportunity for multiresidue analysis. Only the parent molecule has to be isolated from the matrix for quantitation. Four general multiresidue methods for pesticide residues have been published by the Association of Official Analytical Chemists (AOAC) (8). These methods analyze for organochlorine, organophosphorus, fumigant, and carbamate pesticides. Examples of organochlorine pesticides that are addressed by the multiresidue method are as follows: dieldrin, heptachlor, DDT, lindane, methoxychlor, perthane, aldrin, endrin, and mirex. Organophosphorus pesticides that are addressed include the following: diazinon, ethion, malathion, methyl parathion, parathion, and fenchlorphos. Several fumigants are addressed: trichloroethylene, ethylene dibromide, chloroform, and carbon tetrachloride. And carbamate pesticides that are addressed are as follows: carbanolate, carbaryl, carbofuran, and propoxur. Most of these compounds are very stable, quite persistent, and tend to bioconcentrate in biological media or exhibit cholinesterase inhibition. Unfortunately, these descriptors coincide with what many feel to be environmentally obnoxious properties. From an environmental standpoint, one would prefer a pesticide that would degrade or metabolize quickly to naturally occurring compounds.

Compounds that are extensively degraded or rapidly metabolized in the various compartments (i.e., no parent molecule remaining) offer the least opportunity for multiresidue analysis. For these pesticides, the most prevalent method-development approach is to convert the multiple degradates or metabolites to a common chemophore for quantitation. An example of this is substituted aniline-based products such as diuron, neburon, and linuron, in which analysis is achieved by hydrolyzing metabolites to the common 3,4 dichloroaniline moiety. Thus, a multiresidue method using this approach could not address these three pesticides, since this procedure could not distinguish which one of the three produced the residue. Additionally, these types of conversion methods need specific optimization of each reaction (i.e., acid, base, or enzyme hydrolysis, oxidation, reduction, etc.). For instance, in the previous hydrolysis example, reaction conditions must be developed to maximize the yield of 3,4 dichloroaniline from diuron residues in a crop matrix to achieve the EPA minimum acceptable recovery of 70 percent. These conditions may be different for the reactions needed to obtain an acceptable recovery of 3,4 dichloroaniline from linuron residues in the same crop matrix not to mention in different crop matrices. Thus, pesticides that are extensively degraded or metabolized would probably not be suitable for multiresidue methods. As a general rule, the larger the number of metabolites, the more difficult the residue method development and the less likely the method would be able to measure many different pesticides.

Some compounds fall in between the two previously mentioned categories; they are somewhat degraded or metabolized to only a couple of additional compounds. These pesticides offer some hope for multiresidue analysis provided, that they are similar enough to other pesticides and they do not have common degradates or metabolites. For future convenience, metabolites will be referred to as degradates. These pesticides and degradates may not be amenable to direct detection because the degradates usually contain more polar functional groups, which require a modified analytical approach, than those used with the parent molecule. In these cases, the chemist uses chemical derivatization of the degradate(s) to convert them to a more measurable moiety. Derivatization reactions such as esterification, acetylation, acylation, silylation, and many others are used to improve the sensitivity, selectivity, or chromatographic behavior of the compound. Part of the difficulty in development of this type of method is in the isolation of the compo-

nents from as much of the matrix as possible. This goal is important in order to have the derivatization reaction more closely approach the optimized "neat reaction" with standard materials. The remaining matrix components could be considered to quench or in some cases compete with the derivatization reaction and thus lower recovery (yield). Thus, pesticides that require derivatization don't seem to fit as nicely with the concept of multiresidue methods due to the potential presence of competing reactants both from the matrix and other pesticide residues. This is not to say that with considerable developmental effort a multiresidue method could not be developed, but many parameters would have to be explored in such an endeavor.

Existing methods for detecting pesticide residues in foodstuffs can perhaps best be explained by breaking the method into two parts: 1) isolation from the food or crop matrix, and 2) the detection of the pesticide residue. Isolation of the residue is begun by solvent extraction of a solid food or by liquid partition extraction of a liquid food with a solvent for which the pesticide residue has a greater affinity. Thus, the residue is removed from the majority of the matrix components. However, numerous chemical compounds that are components of the matrix itself are co-extracted, and this is usually the most difficult part of the analytical method commonly known as the cleanup. These co-extracted compounds in fact possess properties similar to those of the pesticide residue and thus are more difficult to remove. Some of the usual cleanup techniques employed in analytical methods are the following: filtration, solvent-partitioning, absorption chromatography, ion exchange chromatography, solid-phase extraction, gel permeation, dialysis, and distillation. These techniques are all aimed at the removal of coextracted matrix materials from the sample extract. After the cleanup in many cases, chemical reactions have been used to convert residue components to a chemophore for enhancement of detectability, specificity, or improved separation from remaining components.

Two of the most common analytical instruments for the detection and quantitation of pesticide residues are the gas chromatograph (GC) and the high-pressure liquid chromatograph (HPLC). These instruments provide final separation of the pesticide residue from remaining components on a column of absorbent via several different mechanisms. The instruments also provide identification and a degree of confidence that the compounds eluting from the column at the same retention time as standard materials are indeed the pesticide residues. This is not always a certainty, however; it would be impossible to test every variety of every crop grown in every soil type and treated with every herbicide, insecticide, and fungicide for interferences in the residue method.

For each of these two types of instrumentation, there are numerous types of detectors. For instance, the gas chromatograph may be equipped with flame ionization, electron capture, alkali-bead flame, photoionization, flame photometric, Hall electrolytic conductivity detectors, or combinations thereof. These detectors operate under different principles and have the ability in some cases to detect only certain classes of chemicals. Residue chemists use this detector specificity to great advantage in method development and residue analyses.

High-pressure liquid chromatographs can have ultraviolet absorption, fluorescence, photoionization, photodiode array, or electrochemical detectors. Some researchers have developed specific reactions that are employed on-line after the column separation but prior to detection. This difficult type of in-situ derivatization, regardless of whether ultraviolet, visible absorption or fluorescent detection is used, is known as a post-column reaction detector. Symptomatically, this points out the great lengths the chemist is willing to go in order to achieve selective and sensitive analytical methods for the measurement of pesticide residues.

Emerging Technologies

Two of the emerging technologies for detecting pesticide residues in foodstuffs are the mass spectrometer and the immunoassay. The mass spectrometer, whether it is coupled with the gas or liquid chromatograph, can provide a positive identification of a pesticide residue component by virtue of its peculiar mass-fragmentation pattern. The specificity of the mass spectrometer is the real advantage, although for many compounds it also has great sensitivity. For difficult to detect compounds, there is always the option of derivatization, as with the other quantitation techniques. The mass spectrometer can also utilize several different ionization modes such as chemical ionization, electron impact, field desorption, or fast atom bombardment.

It is feasible to use the Luke-acetone extraction procedure (19) to isolate pesticide residues from the crop matrix, provide a gross cleanup with gel permeation chromatography (24, 25, 26) or florisil column absorption, and then proceed to GC-MS for detection. Coupling the resolving power of capillary chromatography with the specificity of GC-MS would allow screening a large number of compounds through its spectral library. Mass-fragmentation patterns matching particular compounds could be reanalyzed by selective ion monitoring (SIM) for confirmation and quantitation. By analogy, these techniques are now being used to analyze approximately 165 compounds in water and sediment for priority pollutants (26) Sensitivity of detection may in some cases be a severe disadvantage of this technique. As described in 40CFR180, crop tolerances in RACs vary widely by compound and crop type, which could result in some samples in violation being undetected due to the differences in tolerance levels of pesticides. For instance, one pesticide may have a tolerance of 50 ppm in corn grain, and another pesticide may have a tolerance of 0.05 ppm. An analysis screen set for the high-level tolerance would miss the low level and thus the sensitivity of the screen must by approached with knowledge of the tolerances. These tolerance levels could be easily identified by tabular presentation of compounds and RACs.

The use of mass spectrometry as a tool for analysis of pesticide use has been dramatically increasing, although instrument size and expense are a drawback. University and other small laboratories may not be able to justify the expense of dedicating a mass spectrometer for residue analysis. Contamination of the source with large amounts of chemicals from non-residue level use is an additional potential problem. Bench-top models with smaller price tags are being developed and could ultimately have significant impact for use as a multiresidue screening tool. One area for vigilance is that some classes of similar pesticides and degradants could conceivably yield the same fragment ions.

The other area of emerging method technology is the development of immunoassays for pesticide analysis. Immunoassays are generally applicable to pesticide chemistry, and these immunochemical techniques are highly specific, sensitive, rapid, cost-effective analytical methods (9,10). They owe their great sensitivity and specificity to biological systems that can produce the reagent antibodies that bind with high affinity to compounds of interest. Immunoassays are very sophisticated and require a certain proficiency to develop. Each intended use of the immunoassay has to be carefully considered prior to initiation of development efforts. Choice of the hapten, preparation of the conjugate, generation of the antibodies, and incorporation of the antibodies into an assay all have to be carefully and thoughtfully worked out prior to the very important demonstration of method viability by analysis of samples (11).

The most frequently mentioned concern with immunoassay results is the nagging possibility of unsuspected interactions with unknown components in the sample. This doubt is somewhat magnified because of the absence of color development in positive results, which is the opposite of the traditional color development in positive findings of derivatizational spectrophotometric methods. Thus, additionally colored solutions also create a concern (12). Since nearly all pesticide immunoassays are competitive binding experiments, any interferences that inhibit "complexation" of the antibody with the tracer yield incorrect positive findings.

Pesticide residues of regulatory concern in foods are often composed of mixtures of the parent and degradates (i.e., total toxic residue). In such cases, the extreme specificity of an immunoassay method may actually be a handicap. Knowledge of the ability of the antibodies to recognize the degradates is critical. In some cases, degradates could be substantially more sensitive than the parent. Therefore, a positive result above the tolerance level in a multiresidue screen may also be a false positive. In some literature studies, only 30 to 50 percent of the positive occurrences actually contained the analyte as confirmed by GC/MS(11). Thus, use of immunoassay for multiresidue screening has to have the potential for confirmation by other analytical techniques and should be evaluated to determine if the potential level of false positives is acceptable. In general, the immunoassay technique appears to offer excellent opportunity for use as a multiresidue method especially because of the low incidence of false-negative detections. Using this technique, the analyst can screen many more samples than previously possible with conventional techniques. However, more research directed toward field validation will be required to evaluate the immunoassay's reliability.

Multiresidue Technologies

The major advantage of a multiresidue method for the analysis of pesticides is that the method allows the analyst the opportunity to look for the presence of many pesticides at once. EPA could further encourage the development of these multiresidue methods by focusing on development of enforcement methods, not on the total toxic residue but on the identification and selection for analysis of the most significant analyte of a pesticide whether it be parent, metabolite, or degradate on a case-by-case basis. This would of course direct method development toward chemical classes or functionali-

ties, as with the existing multiresidue methods. The private sector, especially the food producers, food processors, and contracting laboratories, would benefit greatly from the ability to screen a raw agricultural commodity or processed food for multiple pesticides.

Companies who are processing food for distribution are conducting quality-control analyses. The National Food Producers Association (NFPA) uses PAM 212-2 (Luke) acetone extraction procedure. Four aliquots are taken to analyze for chlorinated hydrocarbons, organophosphates, carbamates, and substituted ureas. If they have special monitoring interests, they revert to specific methodology (13). Campbell Soup Company uses a similar ploy in using the 212-2 extraction procedure and expanding the florisil-elution parameters to include a large number of compounds. Analytical chromatographic conditions are also expanded to include the analytes of interest (14). The Dried Fruit Association in California operates under similar procedures (15). The NFPA also conducts research on the effects of pesticide residues in food processing (13).

Food processors generally conduct residue analyses (16,17) but they are not involved in methods development. They are contractually requiring pesticide-use history from growers to assure that pesticide label requirements were followed. Classical methods are then used for additional quality control (17).

The California League of Food Processors provides growers information on pesticides that may legally be used in California, that is, the tolerance, maximum-use rate, and the frequency of application for a particular crop. It also provides several forms dealing with pesticide treatment and crop history including guarantee forms, report forms, notices to growers, and refusal forms (18).

Quality assurance and litigation samples lead the analyst of a contract laboratory to the more general or screening procedures. In these cases, qualitative identification of the analyte can be as important as quantitation. The analyst will rely on methods from Federal regulating agencies such as EPA, FDA, and USDA, or from peer-review organizations, like AOAC or ASTM (19).

Actually, the regulating agencies are in the best position to coordinate multiresidue method development, especially EPA, since they are in possession of all the pesticide registrants' information on the physical properties, product chemistry, metabolism data, and means of residue analysis.

The pesticide registrants are required to submit an analytical method that is not designated as "company confidential'' for enforcement purposes. Additionally, EPA is requiring registrants to report the behavior of pesticides in the four FDA multiresidue protocols (20). However, some judgment is needed with respect to requiring the fit in these multiresidue methods for a parent molecule when the parent has been demonstrated in radio-labeled crop metabolism studies to rapidly and extensively metabolize. Whether expending a great amount of effort for multiresidue method development of pesticides with low toxicity (Category D or E) is worthwhile or not is also an issue to consider. Thus, the starting point for decisions on multiresidue development is in the hands of the regulating agencies.

Federal Interaction

Federal agencies should upgrade their technical approach to multiresidue technology. Industry seems to have the opinion that these techniques are antiquated, but in fact major gains can be made through modernizing the analytical step. Registrants are required to validate residue methodology used to develop the tolerance database by analysis of endogenous residues from the radio-labeled metabolism studies. This validation certainly identifies the solvent system needed for extraction in the enforcement method, as well as the potential selected analyte for multiresidue methodology. Standardization of chromatography materials with respect to size, surface area, moisture and absorptivity, for instance, would be beneficial to the analyst and help reduce inter-laboratory variability. Capillary and wide-bore capillary columns have become very practical in the laboratory since the advent of fused silica-bonded phase columns and they offer substantial increase in resolution from packed columns. Analytical detection systems in multiresidue methods are basically reduced to electron capture and thermionic specific for bas chromatography and UV-VIS and fluorescence detection for HPLC. Multiresidue technologies need to be expanded to include selective ion monitoring of mass spectrometry, especially for those pesticides or degradates that do not have a heteroatom to allow selective identification.

Perhaps the most visible item to be improved is presentation of the methodology in the Pesticide Analytical Manual Volume I (PAM-I). A wealth of information is harbored in its chapters if the analyst masters the system. Improvements could be made by using clear block-letter headings describing procedures instead of relying on the numerical codes. Methods should be presented in complete

form to allow a more concise flow of information, as in the style of the AOAC Manual (8). References to supplemental methods should be presented in the appendix to PAM-I while listing pesticide and cleanup procedures.

The most innovative step one could undertake would be the computer indexing of the PAM data base. Each pesticide entry file should have all the chromatographic conditions, approved methods, supplemental methods, and data on chemical structure. These data made available as public information in the form of a personal computer (PC) disk would give the analyst easy access to the analytical data. In those instances in which a class of compounds are to be analyzed, this would be a starting point in determining universal conditions and the development of multiresidue methods. The key to acceptance is ease of use (21).

An analyst could further narrow the scope of the multiresidue investigation by consulting an information center or database consisting of agronomic practices, crop registrations (22), pesticide fate, and toxicological significance. For example, Dr. Phil Kearney of the USDA-ARS developed a list of pesticides used on corn by consulting a half-dozen databases such as EPA information and state surveys (23).

Similar use patterns could be developed for vegetables, fruits, nuts, and other field crops based on regional use patterns. From these data, optimal selections of analytes would be made for the analyst. For example, the Arizona Department of Agriculture (ADA) requires certified applicators to register the compound being applied, the location of the field to be sprayed, and the registration form be filed with ADA. These data could also be compiled and made available to interested parties on a PC disk for easy access.

If the Federal government wanted to stimulate analytical method development, and particularly multiresidue methodology in the private sector, two things could be done to affect pesticide industrial development. The first would be to expedite the EPA review process. Currently, pesticide registrants are asked to internally review their petitions for registration package completeness. Still the EPA takes 12 to 18 months to respond to a submission. Expeditious review, whether by additional staffing or improvements in efficiency of the review process, could shorten the registration cycle.

The enforcement method seems to be the avenue that the agencies could use to encourage the pesticide industry to enhance multiresidue technology. Conditional registrations could be granted based on the submission of scientifically credible crop-residue studies with the proviso that the industry chemists attempt to fit the enforcement methods to the multiresidue scheme. Since it takes a while for a product to achieve widespread distribution and a "dent" in the marketplace, by this time the multiresidue enforcement method could be in place for screening purposes.

The pressure on the industrial chemist and the pesticide industry in general could be somewhat relieved by prolongation of the patent life to partially compensate for the 5 to 7 years spent in regulatory clearance studies. Since multiresidue method research is complex, time-consuming, and expensive, allowing industrial chemists greater freedom without delays in the pesticide registration could produce the desired results. Prompt evaluation of registration data would result in a longer market life, more profitability, and a propensity on the part of industry to provide resources toward developing methods for surveillance. In other words, if EPA reviews were expedited and patent-life prolonged, industry would not object to additional methodology requirements. Other options require the higher risk, and less advantageous, pouring of funds into long-term contracts or grants.

Governmental agencies should combine their resources to provide analytical pesticide residue training, similar to the Advanced Pesticide Residue Analysis workshop jointly sponsored by the US EPA National Enforcement Investigations Center and the New Jersey Department of Environmental Protection. The concept of this workshop could be enlarged to include analysts from the private sector. Recent demands in the analytical support of registration studies have resulted in qualified personnel being the limiting factor in laboratory expansion. Training sessions that reviewed the techniques of the PAM-I would be of value to the method development chemist as he researches for a sensitive and selective analytical scheme. Education of the researcher developing methods that coincide with EPA and FDA requirements would go a long way in attaining these goals.

Conclusions

The organization and direction of multiresidue methodology seem to rest with the EPA and FDA. The pesticide registration database complete with metabolic or degradate information is known by the EPA, and the pesticide monitoring techniques are known by the FDA. Incentives for development of these methods, whether in the form of appropriations, grants, or conditional registration, should be fostered by these agencies.

Industry should be requested to develop enforcement methods focused on analytes that are most likely to be present based on compound half-life calculations and the metabolic degradation pathway. FDA is facing an impossible task when asked to screen a crop for a few hundred compounds, as well as all their degradation products. It would be preferable to select one or two representative moieties as a biomarker to be incorporated into a multiresidue screen. If residues and the incidence of violation warrant further analyses, the total residue method should be used as supplied by the registrant.

The applicability of enzyme inhibition and immunoassays should be evaluated for pesticide residue analyses. Federal appropriations should be used to evaluate the number of classes of compounds that can be screened by these techniques. How broad are their applications with respect to sample matrix? Classical methods should be used simultaneously with the screening techniques to validate their accuracy. If these questions and conditions are satisfied, EPA could further promote promising techniques such as immunoassay, by acceptance as enforcement methodologies.

Multiresidue techniques are important and can be improved through a concerted effort. Revision of the PAM-I format, a PC disk database access, and upgraded analytical procedures including capillary chromatography and GC-MS-SIM would encourage this development.

Agency and private sector meetings or training sessions should be promoted to advance discussions for solutions to problems. Ultimately, the greatest step in solving the technical problems of pesticide residue analyses will be the enhancement of communication by all parties involved in the agricultural arena.

References

1. Pollack, Robert, Analytical Development Corporation, Colorado Springs, CO, personal communication, January 1988.
2. Craven, Don, Craven Laboratories, Austin, TX, personal communication, January 1988.
3. Ganz, Charles, ENCRS Laboratory, Winston-Salem, NC, personal communication, January 1988.
4. Hughes, Don, Hazleton Laboratories, Madison, WI, personal communication, January 1988.
5. Maliami, Nancy, Morse Laboratory, Sacramento, CA, personal communication, January 1988.
6. Spittler, Terry, Cornell University, Geneva, NY, personal communication, January 1988.
7. U.S. Environmental Protection Agency; Pesti-

cide Assessment Guidelines, Subdivision O: Residue Chemistry, October 1982; NTIS PB83-153981.

8. Association of Official Analytical Chemists, *Official Methods of Analysis*, S. Williams (ed.), AOAC (14th edition), 1984.

9. Hammock, Bruce, University of California, Davis, CA, personal communication, January 1988.

10. Hammock, B.D., Mumma, R.O., "Potential of Immunochemical Technology for Pesticide Analysis," In: *Pesticide Analytical Methodology*, J. Harvey, G. Zweig (eds.), ACS Symposium Series Number 136 (Washington, DC: American Chemical Society, 1979).

11. Wratten, S.J. and Feng, P.C.C., "Pesticide Analysis by Immunoassay," In: *Development and Applications of Immunoassays for Food Analysis* J.H. Rittenburg (ed.) (Elsevier, 1988).

12. Ferguson, Bruce, ImmunoSystems Inc., Biddeford, ME, personal communication, January 1988.

13. Elkins, Ed, National Food Processors Association, Washington, DC, personal communication, January 1988.

14. Lento, Harry, Campbell Soup Co., Camden, NJ, personal communication, January 1988.

15. Steffen, Ed, Dried Fruit Association, Fresno, CA, personal communication, January 1988.

16. Smalligan, Wayne, Gerber's Baby Food, Fremont, MI, personal communication, January 1988.

17. Vetro, Robert, Delmonte Foods, Walnut Creek, CA, personal communication, January 1988.

18. California League of Food Processors, Pesticide Lists and Program Forms, 1112 "I" Street, Suite 100, Sacramento, CA 95814.

19. U.S. Food and Drug Administration, FDA Pesticide Analytical Manual—Volumes I, June 1982; NTIS PB82-911899.

20. U.S. Environmental Protection Agency, Pesticide Assessment Guidelines, Subdivision O—Addendum: Residue Chemistry Data Requirements for Analytical Methods in 40 CFR Part 158.125—Multiresidue Protocols, May 1986; NTIS PB86-203734.

21. Williams, Michael, ABC Laboratories, Columbia, MO, personal communication, January 1988.

22. Crop Protection Chemicals Reference, Joint venture of Chemical and Pharmaceutical Press and John Wiley & Sons, (2nd Edition) 1986.

23. Kearney, P.C., USDA-ARS, Beltsville, MD, "Current Status of Herbicides in Groundwater," presented at the 28th Weed Society Meeting, February 1988.

24. Association of Official Analytical Chemists, "Organochlorine Pesticide Residues in Poultry Fat, Gel Permeation Chromatogaraphic Method, First Action," In: *Official Methods of Analysis*, S. Williams (ed), AOAC, (14th edition) Section 29.037-.043, 1984.

25. Hopper, M., "Automated Gel Permeation System for Rapid Separation of Industrial Chemicals and Organophosphate and Chlorinated Pesticides from Fats," *J. Agric. Food Chem.*, Nov/Dec: 1038-1041, 1982.

26. Method 3640, "Gel Permeation Cleanup," Test Methods for Evaluating Solid Waste, Physical/Chemical Methods, Laboratory Manual, SW-846-USEPA.

Pesticide Residue Monitoring in Canada

W. Harvey Newsome, Bureau of Chemical Safety, Foods Directorate, Health and Welfare Canada

and

Geraldine F. Graham, Bureau of Field Operations, Field Operations Directorate, Health and Welfare Canada

Contents

	Page
Abstract	211
Pesticide Residue Monitoring in Canada	212
Programs	212
Sampling Strategy for National Surveillance	213
Current Analytical Methodology	213
Research and Development	213
TLC-Enzyme Inhibition	214
Common Fragment	214
Immunochemical Methods	214
Robotics	215
Appendix 1	215
References	216

Figure

Figure	*Page*
1. Monitoring Programs	212

Table

Table	*Page*
1. Characteristics of Immunochemical Methods Developed at Health Protection Branch	215

Abstract

The Health Protection Branch of the Department of National Health and Welfare establishes maximum residue limits for pesticides in food in Canada, and it is responsible for ensuring that commodities offered for sale comply with these limits through surveillance and compliance programs. In addition, data are gathered on the levels of residue in a variety of foods to determine the dietary exposure of the population to these chemicals.

Approximately 3600 samples are analyzed annually through four programs designated as surveillance, compliance, data gathering, and total diet. The surveillance program is divided into regional and national components; the former generates data on residues and foods that are of local concern while the national component determines the state of compliance of selected foods in the marketplace across the country. The compliance program investigates and solves problems identified in the surveillance project. The data gathering program conducts analyses of a specialized nature in response to concerns arising from new toxicity data or gaps in the residue data base. The total diet study provides data on the actual dietary intake of pesticides from foods prepared as for consumption.

Methodology used for monitoring relies heavily upon a multiresidue procedure capable of determining 155 compounds. An additional 37 compounds are determined by specific methods. Current research is directed toward increasing the efficiency and scope of monitoring methods using immunochemical, degradation to a common fragment and robotic approaches. The characteristics and applicability of these methods are discussed.

Pesticide Residue Monitoring in Canada

Monitoring for pesticide residues in food is conducted at the federal level by the departments of Agriculture, Fisheries and Oceans, Canadian Grain Commission, National Health and Welfare, and in the provinces by the laboratories of the ministries of Agriculture and Food. The objectives of the various projects differ substantially—from providing assurances to farmers that pesticides used according to label directions will not result in residue problems and approving shipments for export to enforcing compliance with maximum residue limits (MRLs) established under the Food and Drugs Act. The Health Protection Branch of the Department of National Health and Welfare establishes the MRLs and is responsible for their enforcement through surveillance and compliance-type projects carried out in five regional laboratories situated across Canada. In addition, data are collected on the occurrence of residues in order to determine the dietary intake and to ensure that the lowest possible exposure consistent with effective pest control is attained.

Programs

Monitoring programs conducted by the Branch are divided into four categories: data gathering, total diet, surveillance, and compliance. A summary of these and an indication of the proportion of samples directed to each is given in figure 1.

The objectives of the Canadian program are very similar to those described for the United States (19) and the types of program also resemble each other closely, although the numbers of samples analyzed in Canada are smaller than those outlined for the United States (8). Thus, the total diet, data gathering, and regional surveillance projects in Canada are comparable to the total diet, selected survey, and district option in the United States. However, Canadian national surveillance and compliance projects do not have U.S. equivalents. Another major difference between the two countries' approach is that Canada does not have a separate program for imports but includes these items in most surveys in proportion to consumption.

Data gathering projects are designed to collect information on the occurrence of specific pesticides in the food supply, and they often involve biased sampling. Specific methodology, as compared to multiresidue methods, is often required, and projects are initiated as a result of new information on the probable occurrence of compounds or their

Figure 1.—Monitoring Programs

TOTAL SAMPLES-3585

National surveillance (1100)	Regional surveillance (525)	Compliance (525)	Data gathering (900)	Total diet (535)
1/1 dom./ import	4/1 dom./ import	1/2 dom./ import	national	224 composites

metabolites or in response to concerns arising from new toxicity data. Approximately 900 samples are analyzed annually in this program. The total diet program is similar to that conducted in the United States and, in its present form involves the preparation of 161 food items as consumed. One hundred and twelve composites of these items are then made, representing 99 percent of the Canadian diet. Samplings are conducted twice annually from different cities representing the five regions across Canada, such that all regions are covered in a two and a half year cycle. All composites are analyzed by the multiresidue method (9), and six additional compounds are determined by specific methods. The resulting data reflect actual pesticide intake that remains after trimming, washing, and cooking of foods.

The surveillance program consists of national and regional components. The national surveillance component is designed to determine the state of compliance of selected food commodities in the marketplace with respect to selected pesticides. Approximately 1,100 samples are analyzed annually, approximately one half of them by multiresidue methodology. A smaller number of samples (525) is analyzed in the regional surveillance project. Regional surveillance is planned separately by inspection and laboratory staff in each region and is designed to emphasize commodities and pesticides that are of local, rather than national, importance. This program uses information gathered on local pesticide usage, infestation problems, and crop conditions. Commodities are included where pesticide misuse is suspected.

Data obtained from surveillance projects are compiled each year, but are not published or stored in a computerized database. They are used internally to direct future surveillance and compliance projects and are available on request to other interested parties, including international agencies such as WHO/FAO.

The national surveillance component has only been in place in its present form since 1985. Eleven out of fourteen commodities tested have shown a state of compliance of at least 99 percent. The three exceptions are now included in the compliance project.

The compliance program is designed to investigate and solve residue problems identified by the national or regional surveillance components. This project is instrumental in preventing the sale of foods containing residues in excess of the MRL. Historically, a wide variety of pesticides have been found at violative levels. For example, in 1986/87, thirty-one different compounds were involved, with fungicides and organophosphates being the most numerous. Because the use of pesticides that are registered in other countries but not in Canada often results in residues that exceed our MRLs, residue problems have occurred more frequently with imported products than with domestic ones. Therefore, compliance efforts are concentrated on importers, who, under Canadian law, are responsible for ensuring the products they import comply with the Food and Drugs Act. Actions taken if violative residues occur range from refusal of entry to prosecution of importers who repeatedly import violative products.

Sampling Strategy for National Surveillance

The food supply is divided into 14 commodity classes such as vegetables, meat, dairy products, and fruit. These classes are ranked according to consumption, pesticide application, potential for residues, and data available from other agencies. Of these classes, fruit and vegetables represent approximately 35 percent of the Canadian diet and have the highest potential for residues. Thus, they are designated as constituting a minimum of two thirds of the surveillance samples. Thirty-five items from these commodity classes, representing 90 percent of the apparent consumption are selected for analysis once over a 10 year period. The highest consumption items representing 50 percent of the diet are analyzed twice over the 10 year period. For each pesticide-commodity combination, 100 samples are analyzed, so that a 4.8 percent violation rate would be detected with 95 percent confidence (2). These samples are procured in proportion to the geographic distribution of their origin, i.e., by province of production for domestic commodities and by country of origin for imports.

In Canada, 235 pesticides are registered for use on food. Those recommended in provincial spray calendars are considered to represent those in actual use and are ranked using such factors as volume of use, persistence, and toxicity. The selection of pesticides to be determined on imported foods is based upon the existence of a tolerance in the country of origin and weighted by the frequency of occurrence of previously detected residues. The FDA surveillance index (20) is also heavily relied upon to furnish a criterion for priority. Thus, a list of commodity-pesticide combinations is constructed. For those compounds that can be determined by multiresidue methods, pesticides can be included down to a low level of priority, while those requiring specific methods must be selected from the high priority portion of the list.

Current Analytical Methodology

As indicated previously, a multiresidue method (9) is used for surveillance wherever possible. This procedure, which is capable of determining 155 compounds in a variety of fatty and non-fatty foods, involves cleanup of an acetone extract by automated gel permeation chromatography followed by determination by capillary gas-liquid chromatography using at least two detectors—usually a Hall detector in the halogen mode and a thermionic nitrogen/phosphorous detector. HPLC with post-column derivatization as described by Krause (5) is used for methyl carbamate pesticides. An additional chromatographic cleanup on Florisil is required with some commodities.

Specific methods are used for an additional 37 compounds that cannot be determined by the multiresidue procedure. These compounds are examined as the need arises and, on average, each consumes the same resources as the multiresidue procedure. Often, members of this group of pesticides are insufficiently volatile for gas chromatography and do not contain chromophoric groups necessary for detection after HPLC. Examples are the ethylenebis(dithiocarbamates) fungicides and daminozide. Others such as maleic hydrazide, glyphosate, diquat, paraquat, and the organotin compounds cyhexatin and fentin require unique cleanup steps due to their polar nature. A complete list of these compounds is given in appendix 1.

Research and Development

In an effort to improve the efficiency of the monitoring process, as well as to identify new compounds such as metabolites and degradation products, research is conducted in the Health Protection Branch into the development of analytical methods. The private sector does not conduct method development as such but relies on methods published in the scientific literature or in manuals developed by Federal departments. The methods developed by the branch may classified as four types and will be discussed individually as: 1) TLC-enzyme inhibition, 2) degradation to a common fragment, 3) immunological, and 4) robotics.

TLC-Enzyme Inhibition

Two rapid screening techniques, qualitative in nature, have been studied in our laboratory to determine rapidly, and with as little sample purification as possible, whether a sample contained violative residues. Both rely on separation of the pesticides by thin-layer chromatography, followed by treatment of the developed plate with an enzyme or enzyme system and substrate. The first of these methods has been reviewed by Mendoza (10) and consists of detection of carbamate and organophosphate insecticides with an esterase preparation followed by a chromogenic substrate. Zones of inhibition indicated the presence of cholinesterase inhibitors, the identity of which could be indicated by the R_f. Several factors affected the sensitivity of the assay, including source of enzyme, substrate, and pretreatment of the plate with an oxidant to convert thiophosphates to their oxygen analogues. The disadvantage of the method, which prevented its routine use, was the presence of a number of naturally-occurring inhibitors in food extracts.

A more promising development is that of TLC-photosynthesis inhibition, which is applicable to those herbicides that inhibit photosynthesis such as phenylureas, phenyl carbamates, and triazines (6). After chromatographic separation, the plate is sprayed with a suspension of chloroplasts, followed by the redox indicator 2,6-dichloroindophenol and exposure to light. Photosynthetic inhibitors appear as blue spots of unreduced dye. The method requires little sample workup other than initial sample extraction and partitioning into dichloromethane, and it is relatively immune to interference. Detection limits are satisfactory for compliance purposes.

Common Fragment

This approach involves the conversion of pesticides with different properties, such as polarity and vapor pressure, to a common entity, permitting the determination of several compounds in a single analysis. The technique has been used for the detection of phenyl urea herbicides in a variety of sample types (4), and it provides information as to the total burden of a class of compounds in a food. This concept may also be used to determine alachlor,

diethatyl, and their 3,5-dichloroaniline-containing metabolites by hydrolysis to 3,5-dichloroaniline and determination of 3,5-dichloroaniline by GLC (15). Similarly, iprodione, vinclozolin, and procymidone are also determined by alkaline degradation to 3,5-dichloroaniline (18). The obvious disadvantage of this approach is that if excessive residues are encountered, individual determinations must be made to identify the offending compound.

Immunochemical Methods

The widespread successful use of immunoassay techniques (3) in clinical laboratories prompted us to evaluate its applicability to pesticide residues in foods. Both radioimmunoassay (RIA) and enzyme-linked immunosorbent assays (ELISA) have been developed for compounds ranging from the nonpolar polychlorinated biphenyls (11) to the water-soluble fungicide carbendazim (12, 15). Either immunochemical approach resulted in methods that correlated well with conventional chemical analyses for all compounds we have studied. The nonpolar PCBs posed the greatest problem, requiring sample purification as extensive as that required for gas chromatography if false-negative data were to be avoided. In contrast, carbendazim could be determined in crude ethyl acetate extracts without prior cleanup and was not subject to interferences. Similarly, methods for the fungicides metalaxyl (13), iprodione (16), and triadimefon (14) did not require any sample preparation other than initial extraction.

The specificity of immunochemical methods is generally sufficient for screening purposes but, as the data summary in table 1 indicates, varies greatly with the assay and is probably a reflection of the structure of the pesticide. For example, the selectivity of the assay for thiabendazole is very high, with low cross-reactivity for related compounds such as 2-benzimidazoleurea or carbendazim. In contrast, vinclozolin and procymidone react with antibody directed toward iprodione to a higher degree than does iprodione itself. Similarly, the herbicides metolachlor and diethatyl have considerable cross-reactivity with metalaxyl antiserum, further emphasizing the screening nature of the analysis.

The merit of ELISA compared with RIA lies in the relative safety and availability of reagents and in the simplicity of associated counting equipment. However, RIA is often more rapid, requiring fewer incubation steps and produces steeper inhibition curves, which result in greater sensitivity. A larger number of samples may be processed at one time with ELISA, resulting in low unit cost. Compared with conventional specific analyses, ELISA is ca-

Table 1.—Characteristics of Immunochemical Methods Developed at Health Protection Branch

Compound determined	Assay type	Quantitation limit (ppb)	Major Cross reactions	Sample
Aroclor 1260	RIA	2	Aroclor 1254	milk
Carbendazim	RIA	50	2-benzimidazole urea	cucumber
Metalaxyl	ELISA	100	metolachlor, diethatyl	tomato
Thiabendazole	ELISA	30	nil	potato
Carbendazim	ELISA	350	2-benzimidazole urea	apple
Iprodione	ELISA	100	vinclozolin, procymidone	tomato
Triadimefon	ELISA	500	triadimenol	apple

pable of producing four to five times the number of determinations per day.

Robotics

Robotics is being studied as a means of reducing the labor-intensive component of conventional multiresidue analyses. Two implementations of this technology are being evaluated—one that carries out the liquid-liquid partition step in the Luke et al. procedure (7), and another that prepares milk samples for the determination of a number of organochlorine compounds by gas-liquid chromatography.

The system used for partitioning (1) consists of a Cyberfluor Labotix robot arm, stirrer, and liquid handling apparatus under control of a microcomputer. Aliquots of sample extract are manually added to a flask where partitioning is carried out by a series of stirring actions with dichloromethane. After phase separation, the dichloromethane is recovered by the robot for concentration prior to cleanup. Recoveries of standards added to several commodities were comparable to those obtained with the manual partitioning procedure.

For milk analysis, the entire extraction and cleanup procedure was automated using a Zymark Corp. arm and custom-built series of workstations. This apparatus permits the weighing of sample, extraction with organic solvent, centrifugation, column chromatography, and collection and evaporation of three fractions prior to gas chromatographic analysis. Thirty-two compounds, in addition to PCBs are determined using an autosampler and data acquisition system. When evaluated against manual sample preparation, the robot was found capable of doubling the weekly output. The coefficient of variation at the 1 ppb level was 15 percent for the

automated system compared with 8 percent manually. Accuracy was equivalent for both systems.

Method development is now being conducted into the further application of immunochemical and robotic procedures, as well as such techniques as solid phase extraction for inclusion in the multiresidue method. In addition, new pesticides are continually being tested for inclusion into the existing multiresidue method. Since the analytical problems encountered in monitoring the food supply are common to both the United States and Canada, both countries benefit from new developments arising from research in North America or abroad. An excellent mechanism for communication and exchange of this technology is the Association of Official Analytical Chemists. This international organization of scientists from government, industry, and academia disseminates new findings at its annual meetings and through publication in a journal. In addition to being a forum for discussion of new approaches, methods are validated through a process of collaborative study in several laboratories.

Appendix 1

Pesticides Determined by Single Residue Methods: aldicarb, amitraz, *benomyl, bentazon, biphenyl, *chlorophenols, *daminozide, desmedipham, dichlone, diquat, *diuron, dodine, *EBDC, *ethylene dibromide, ethephon, ethylene thiourea, fluazifop-butyl, glyphosate, imazalil, iprodione metabolites, *maleic hydrazide, methiocarb, methomyl, *methyl bromide, napthalene acetic acid, naptalam, *organotin compounds, oxamyl, oxydemeton-methyl, *paraquat, o-phenyl phenol, pyrethrins, terbutylazine, thiabendazole, triallate, triforine, vinclozolin metabolites

Those compounds marked with * have been identified by GAO as needing single residue methods.

References

1. Calway, P., Internal Report, Ontario Region, Field Operations Directorate, Health and Welfare Canada, 1987.

2. Cochran, W.G., *Sampling Techniques*, 3rd Edition (New York: John Wiley and Sons, 1977).

3. Hammock, B.D., Mumma, R.O., *ACS Symposium Series*, No. 136, John Harvey, Jr. and Gunter Zweig (eds.), American Chemical Society 1980.

4. de Kok, A., Van Opstal, M., de Jong, T., Hoogcarspel, B., Geerdink, R.B., Frei, R.W., and Brinkman, Th.,U.A., *Intern. J. Environ. Anal. Chem.* 18: 101, 1984.

5. Krause, R.T., *J. Assoc. Off. Anal. Chem.* 68:726, 1985.

6. Lawrence, J.F., *J. Assoc. Off. Anal. Chem.* 63:758, 1980.

7. Luke, M.A., Froberg, J.E., and Masumoto, H.T., *J. Assoc. Off. Anal. Chem.* 58:1020, 1975.

8. McMahon, B.M. and Burke, J.A., *J. Assoc. Off. Anal. Chem.* 70:1072, 1987.

9. McLeod, H.A. and Graham, R.A. (eds.), Analytical Methods for Pesticide Residues in Foods (Ottawa, Canada: Canadian Government Publishing Centre, Supply and Services Canada, K1A 0S9, 1986).

10. Mendoza, C.E., *Residue Reviews* 43:105, 1972.

11. Newsome, W.H. and Shields, J.B., *Intern. J. Environ. Anal. Chem.* 10:295, 1981a.

12. Newsome, W.H. and Shields, J.B., *J. Agric. Food Chem.* 29:220, 1981b.

13. Newsome, W.H., *J. Agric. Food Chem.* 33:528, 1985.

14. Newsome, W.H., *Bull. Environ. Contam. Toxicol.* 36:9, 1986.

15. Newsome, W.H. and Collins, P.G., *J. Assoc. Off. Anal. Chem.* 70:1025, 1987.

16. Newsome, W.H., *Pest. Sci. Biotechnol.* (eds.) R. Greenhalgh and T.R. Roberts (Blackwell Scientific Publishers, p. 349, 1987).

17. Newsome, W.H., Collins, P., Lewis, D., *J. Assoc. Off. Anal. Chem.* 70:446, 1987.

18. Newsome, W.H. and Collins, P., *Intern. J. Environ. Anal. Chem.* 1988, In press.

19. Reed, D.V. and Lombardo, P., *J. Assoc. Off. Anal. Chem.* 70:591, 1987.

20. Reed, D.V., *J. Assoc. Off. Anal. Chem.* 68:122, 1985.

Pesticide Monitoring Program in Mexico

Silvia Canseco Gonzalez, Animal and Plan Health Office, Agriculture Department Mexico

The main objective of the Animal and Plant Health Law of the Mexican Republic is to protect animals and plants from pests and diseases. In addition, the law provides the Secretary of Agriculture and Water Resources the facilities to exercise control over the quality of biological and chemical products applied to animals and vegetables as well as to prevent agrarian activities from originating health risks and environmental contamination. This is carried out through the Plant and Animal Health General Direction, responsible for pesticide registration and control. This office takes care of setting tolerances and checking the quality of the formulations available for the growers.

The system to control these chemical compounds in Mexico involves separate aspects; the law requires the registration of import, manufacturing, development, and distribution firms. It may be considered that great advances have been made in the regulation of these firms in the past 18 months.

Equally, the registration of compounds sold in Mexico has kept a very acceptable level, as well as the registration of technicians who supervise the quality control in factories and who are responsible for usage recommendations in their own firms.

Pesticides, companies, and consultants are registered in the main offices in Mexico City; number registration of sales and distribution is done through the Agriculture Department officer in the Mexican states. In 1974, the construction of a network of laboratories was begun to bring about quality control of product formulas as well as to determine residue levels in affected crops. There are now 12 regional laboratories for pesticide analysis and one central reference laboratory for pesticide residues analysis of animal products. Five of these laboratories are able to conduct residue analysis as well, and the Vegetables Growers Union has built a laboratory for the same purpose.

Some colleges and universities in Mexico are making efforts to develop analytical methods, but the task is centered most often upon the pesticide industry and in the official laboratories. In both cases, it may be said that more important than the development of new methods is the implementation and verification of those methods developed by benchmarks or published in the literature.

Some efforts have been made with respect to pesticide residue analysis with the objective of modifying some methods to make them more economical, but no conclusive results have yet been reached.

This year, the program involves the analysis of 2,200 samples of vegetal origin, specifically of the following crops: chili peppers, green peppers, tomatoes, tomitillos, and strawberries. This is done using the FDA Pesticide Analytical Manual procedures already discussed and those modifications applicable to the country conditions.

The selection of the products to use against a pest problem should be made on the basis of the manual of Authorized Pesticides, which SAPAF edits and reviews each year and which lists those compounds that have complied with the requirements specified by the law. Also it includes information about pests, crops, and dosages that may be applied, safe intervals of application, and the residue limit that should be observed.

Let's use PAM procedures because the United States is the main consumer of our agriculture exports, thus we check both the domestic and foreign consumption.

However, during past years, economic factors have had the following negative effects on our work:
—lack of proper maintenance of the equipment
—no new equipment
—loss of training technicians and inability to contract replacement personnel.

This situation is aggravated by the problems of inflation and daily devaluation of the Mexican currency. This is reflected in the number of analyses that can be carried out, reducing it a considerable degree each year and thereby reducing the established capacity that the Secretaria de Agricultura y Proteci—opecuaria y Forestal (SAPAF) once had. During 1987, residue analyses were carried out on 970 samples of fresh agricultural produce. Since the tasks of analysis is very specialized and practiced by a small number of technicians, there is no interest in the reagent and solvent industry in Mexico in maintaining a quality product that satisfies the requirements of these analyses. For these reasons, the reagents and solvents are imported. In addition, much of the equipment and glassware is imported, so the prices for these materials have increased.

Considering that the main problem with pesticides is misuse, we are implementing the use of a prescription for selling pesticides. This means that in order to purchase a pesticide, the grower must present a paper written by a registered professional indicating the crop, the pest, product, and dosage.

As I mentioned before, residue analysis is carried out with the U.S. methodology whenever possible, but we don't eliminate the possibility of using those recommended methods from international agencies such as Codex Committee on Pesticide Residues.

We recognize the importance of fruit and vegetable trade between Mexico and the United States, and we are very concerned about it. To this end, we have instituted and analytical quality-control program between FDA and my office to assure that the pesticide residues in commodities involved in trade are below tolerance levels.

Nowadays the Agriculture Department has the tendency to implement pest control programs that are part of an integrated pest management program that that takes advantage of pests' natural enemies; and includes extending the use of old technologies such as biological control. Last year we had spectacular results on the soybean crop, reducing the use of pesticides by more than 50 percent.

Another technique is the use of sterile insects in the campaign against the Medfly and the cattle screwworm. Other pest control methods have been developed that originated from the EDB ban: hydrothermic treatment for the elimination of larvae in mangoes for export and the use of low temperatures as an agricultural sanitation treatment in citrus exportation.

The biological pesticides *Bacillus thuringiensis* is widely used for forestry pests in ecologically protected areas; we are conducting investigations on the use of fungi against soil pests.

Despite all these efforts, it is recognized that pesticide use will continue to be the extensively used means of pest control. Actions are being directed toward making adequate use of pesticides in which different government agencies, as well as the pesticide industry and professional organizations, participate by means of campaigns, qualification courses, refresher workshops, and symposia, all oriented toward keeping pesticides a useful tool without execessive risk.

Strong efforts are being made to get economic support from international agencies in order to let us continue this task.

Having the opportunity to participate in events such as this undertaking and others in which new technologies are expounded and revised, or at least having access to the information generated, can help Mexico maintain an acceptable level of technological development in this area. Visitation by specialists who might, upon observing conditions in the nation, be in a position to offer a more practical and acceptable assessment, would be equally useful. Nevertheless, the main problem is, and according to our perspective will continue to be, the lack of economic resources that permit us to incorporate innovations in day-to-day work.

It is necessary to identify sources of financing to continue the program and the technical assessment that allow research into other analytical possibilities.

Developing Pesticide Analytical Methods for Food: Considerations for Federal Policy Formulation

Sarah E. Taylor, Analyst in Life Sciences, Science Policy Research Division, Congressional Research Service

Contents

	Page
Abstract	219
Introduction	219
Federal Pesticide Residue Programs and Analytical Methods	220
Environmental Protection Agency	220
Federal Monitoring Program	220
Food and Drug Administration	221
U.S. Department of Agriculture/Food Safety and Inspection Service	221
Federal Pesticide Monitoring Program Evaluations	222
Analytical Technology and Program Design	224
Conclusion	226
Questions to Consider as a Research Strategy is Defined	226
References	227

Abstract

Technologies available to detect, identify and quantify pesticide residues in food have played a key role in defining the structure and effectiveness of Federal pesticide monitoring programs. Monitoring programs are used to assess public exposure to pesticides and as a basis for enforcing pesticide laws by detecting residue violations. Because of the volume of samples that must be analyzed and the dearth of information on the pesticide treatment history of food samples collected for analysis, Federal monitoring programs have been designed around the use of multiresidue methods. However, multiresidue methods are unable to detect all residues of interest, including a number of pesticides of high priority because of their widespread use and toxicity levels. This gap in detectable residues has served as a point of departure in recent policy debates concerning the appropriate direction of research in methods development.

This report examines Federal pesticide monitoring programs and how analytical technology has shaped them. It also considers program limitations that have been identified in recent policy studies, and raises questions about the role of analytical technology in addressing these needs. This report concludes that new analytical technology may offer an opportunity to address not only the gap in detectable residues, but to help achieve even more fundamental improvements in pesticide monitoring programs.

Introduction

Public health policymakers have long been concerned about the health implications of dietary exposure to pesticide residues. They have considered analytical methods capable of detecting and quantifying pesticide residues basic to any program designed to control such exposure. Even before a Federal pesticide monitoring program was developed under modern pesticide laws, this need for methods was recognized. For example, Dr. John Kerfoot Haywood, head of the Federal Insecticide and Agricultural Water Laboratory in 1905, was disturbed about possible health effects of pesticides and stated, "[i]t is essential that these [pesticide] compounds be analyzed by exact . . . uniform methods. . . ."(1).

During the past 3 years, several critical evaluations of Federal monitoring programs directed at pesticide residues in food have advised that improved analytical methods were needed to enhance the effectiveness of the programs. These recommendations have helped to focus public and congressional attention on analytical methods and have fueled the reevaluation of Federal policies currently underway inside the Federal agencies and by the Congress.

However, the interest of the public and of policymakers in analytical methods has been borne of a larger concern—that the government has been unable to supply to the public sufficient data to allay concerns about the safety of pesticide residues in the food supply. Some consumers have construed the gaps in residue data as indicative of a grave and unknown risk to public health (2). Some policymakers are desirous of more pesticide residue data because they believe it will more clearly show that the food supply is safe, and will help to restore public confidence in the effectiveness of the programs already in place (3).

This report examines Federal pesticide monitoring programs and the relationship between analytical technologies and the design and limitations of current monitoring programs. It considers recent recommendations regarding program needs to improve the analytical methods used in the programs. It also raises questions regarding how the goals and design of pesticide programs inthe future may influence the analytical methods policies developed and implemented today.

Federal Pesticide Residue Programs and Analytical Methods

Pesticide analytical methods are scientific techniques used to detect, identify, and quantify pesticide residues. The technology generally used for pesticide detection is gas-liquid chromatography (GLC) and high-pressure chromatography (HPLC) (4, 5). There are two general types of pesticide analytical methods in use today: multiresidue and single residue methods. Multiresidue methods are capable of detecting a number of pesticides having similar chemical and physical properties in a test of a single sample. Single residue methods are capable of identifying only one pesticide residue in a food sample. In general, multiresidue and single residue methods require comparable time and resources to conduct per sample. Therefore, multiresidue methods are considered more time and resource efficient than single residue methods (6). The advantages of multiresidue methods over single residue methods have helped to make them the basis of current pesticide monitoring programs. In addition, multiresidue methods capable of detecting large numbers of residues are useful in testing samples when reliable information about the pesticides used on the commodity is lacking.

The Federal pesticide program is actually a patchwork of programs administered by the Environmental Protection Agency (EPA), the Food and Drug Administration (FDA), and the U.S. Department of Agriculture (USDA). Analytical methods play a key role in the programs of each agency.

Environmental Protection Agency

The EPA has central authority for the regulation of pesticides under the Federal Insecticide, Fungicide and Rodenticide Act (FIFRA). Under the act, EPA is required to grant a license (registration) for pesticide chemical uses for which the applicant (registrant) has demonstrated, among other things, that "when used in accordance with widespread and commonly recognized practice it will not generally cause unreasonable adverse effects on the environment" (7). In determining whether a pesticide can be registered, among the factors EPA considers is whether residues that result from pesticide use pose a dietary hazard to humans or animals. For pesticides that will be used on a crop that will serve as human or animal food, EPA is required to grant a tolerance level for residues under the Federal Food, Drug and Cosmetic Act (FDCA). A tolerance level defines the maximum amount of pesticide residues that may remain in food (8).

A condition of registration for any pesticide for which a tolerance is granted is that the registrant supply to EPA a pesticide analytical method(s) capable of detecting and quantifying the active ingredient and the products of its degradation (9). An EPA laboratory tests the method (validation) to assess the validity and reliability of the method (10). The goal of the requirement is that the registrant supply to the agency the analytical means to enforce the pesticide tolerance. However, the requirement has been ineffective in achieving this goal largely because the methods supplied are often not practicable for regulatory purposes. Registrants generally fulfill the requirement for a method by supplying a single residue method. Because of the limitations of single residue methods when compared with multiresidue methods, as noted above, they are not feasible for routine use in monitoring programs, except in limited circumstances where some reliable information is available on the pesticide treatment history of the sample.

Federal Monitoring Program

Once a pesticide has been approved, the responsibility for monitoring residues in foods belongs to FDA and USDA. FDA is responsible for monitoring all domestic and imported foods for pesticide residues except for meat and poultry, which are monitored by USDA. FDA and USDA enforce the pesticide tolerances established by EPA. Foods containing illegal pesticide residues are considered "adulterated." FDA and USDA each have authority to inspect food to determine if it is adulterated and to prosecute those who are involved in interstate commerce of adulterated products.

FDA is also the Federal lead agency for the development of pesticide analytical methods for food products. Most of FDA's research focuses on the development and modification of multiresidue methods. FDA developed the surveillance index beginning in 1979 to classify pesticides according to potential health hazards based on toxicity, prevalence of use, and persistence in the environment. The index was designed to plan monitoring programs and has helped to prioritize research on methods for pesticides not detected by multiresidue methods.

USDA also conducts some research on analytical methods, but most of this work focuses on adapting multiresidue methods for special characteristics of meat and poultry samples (11).

Food and Drug Administration

FDA's pesticide monitoring program has been designed to accomplish FDA's legislative mandate under the FDCA within available resources to enforce EPA pesticide tolerances, and enforce the adulteration provisions of the Act (12). The two primary objectives of the pesticide monitoring program are 1) to enforce pesticide residue tolerances established by EPA, and to determine the incidence and level of pesticide residues in the food supply. FDA's monitoring program has two major components: general commodity monitoring and the total diet study. Only multiresidue methods are used for routine testing in these programs. Single residue methods are reserved for work targeted for a specific pesticide.

The general commodity monitoring program component involves sampling on an "as shipped" basis, raw agricultural commodities, processed foods, and animal feeds. The samples are analyzed for the purpose of enforcing tolerances established by EPA, and for determining the incidence and levels of residues (13). Although an express purpose of the FDA commodity sampling program is to determine the incidence and levels of residues in commodities, the program is incapable of providing data that can be used to estimate the general rate of residues that violate pesticide tolerances. This is because there is no statistically valid plan by which samples are collected. In fact, a sampling plan that would make such an estimate possible has not been

studied or compared with the plan in use. Some observers of the program have suggested that the sheer size, mobility, and decentralized nature of the U.S. food supply would make it impossible to collect a random sample of the food supply for pesticide analysis, even if the means were known (14).

FDA's sampling plan is made up of a set of guidelines to help officials in the district offices determine where to direct their inspection resources. Some guidelines provide commodity-specific quotas, e.g., "collect 12 egg shell samples," others are more general, "based on local usage, collect agricultural products for malathion analysis" (15). The plans specify that the sampling plan should remain flexible so that resources can be shifted to meet special needs that arise (16). Ultimately, the number of samples collected and analyzed for pesticide residues in a district is determined by available resources in that district. Pesticide monitoring must compete for resources in the districts with other significant public health functions, and sampling plans are sometimes derailed by emergency situations (e.g., a product tampering incident). In addition, even when resources are available, some guidelines are difficult to implement because of inadequate data. For example, the guideline noted above which directs testing pesticides based on local use patterns, is reliant on "detective work" done at the local level because little data is available on pesticide use patterns.

The total diet study (TDS) involves collecting a "market basket" of food samples several times per year in several geographic regions of the country, then analyzing the foods in a ready-to-eat form. The TDS is used to estimate dietary intake of selected pesticides by various U.S. age-sex groups (17). The design of the TDS provides a "snapshot" estimate of public exposure to those pesticides detected by the analytical methods used in the study. FDA relies on the TDS to make judgments about the public health risk presented by pesticide exposure through food.

U.S. Department of Agriculture/Food Safety and Inspection Service (FSIS)

Unlike the pesticide program of the Food and Drug Administration, the legislative mandate of USDA is not just one of enforcing pesticide tolerances in food (meat and poultry) or prosecuting those who engage in commerce of adulterated products. Instead, Congress has prescribed a system of ante-(18) and postmortem (19) inspection whereby meat and poultry products are affirmatively certified by USDA to be wholesome and in conformance with residue limits (20). The program is sometimes described as "continuous inspection." An explicit goal of both the meat and poultry antemortem inspection provisions is to prevent the entry of adulterated meat or poultry into commerce (21). USDA has implemented its inspection program by stationing Federal inspectors in meat and poultry slaughtering and processing facilities. USDA inspectors visually inspect animals and carcasses and collect tissue samples for analysis of chemical residues, including pesticide residues.

The USDA pesticide program is part of its National Residue Program, which also targets residues of animal drugs and environmental contaminants in meat and poultry. The program has been revamped in recent years to focus monitoring activities on pesticide residues according to hazard and estimated exposure (i.e., risk) (22). The program has three components: monitoring, surveillance, and exploratory projects. The focus of the monitoring program is to profile information on the occurrence of pesticide residue violations in specified animal populations on an annual national basis and to form the basis of enforcement actions (23). Samples are selected on a statistically random basis. Pesticides selected for analysis are based on an assessment of risk and the availability of an analytical method that is suitable for regulatory purposes (24). USDA tests for only those compounds that can be detected and quantified, and for which all metabolites can be identified by a practical analytical method. USDA has acknowledged that because of the large number of potential residues that may occur in the food chain, practical methods are not available for many compounds of interest. USDA has defined "practical methods" to be those that 1) require no more the 2 to 4 hours of analytical time per sample, 2) require no instrumentation not customarily available in laboratory devoted to trace drug or environmental analyses, 3) have a minimum proficiency level at or below the established residue limit (e.g., tolerance), 4) have aquality assurance plan, and 5) have undergone an interlaboratory validation study. Like FDA, USDA relies on multiresidue methods.

The surveillance program is designed to investigate and control the movement of potentially adulterated meat and poultry products. Samples are collected in a non-random, selective fashion directed at carcasses believed to be adulterated because of information obtained through investigation or through the monitoring program. The surveillance program is sometimes activated to follow the product of a particular supplier who was responsible for violations in the past. The program gives USDA the ability to trace problems to their source and take steps to prevent recurrence.

Exploratory projects can be likened to a research effort designed to examine a particular problem. Exploratory projects are sometimes used to evaluate new methods of monitoring or to study the occurrence of residues for which no acceptable limit (e.g., tolerance) has been established.

The design of the USDA program has enabled the agency to sample a statistically representative sample of the U.S. meat and poultry supply for pesticide analysis. This contrasts distinctly with FDA's commodity monitoring program, in which the actual sampling decisions are made on an ad hoc basis by inspectors in the field within the broad guidance of the pesticide sampling plans and within resource and information limitations. However, because the regulatory burdens placed on both agencies limit the resources that can be devoted to pesticide analysis, both agencies have opted to rely on multiresidue methods almost entirely. Therefore, those pesticide residues not detected by multiresidue methods generally escape without detection by any method. This contrast illustrates that in two agencies, with vastly differing legislative mandates, the capabilities of existing methods have been key determinants of the scope, limitations, and effectiveness of monitoring programs.

Federal Pesticide Monitoring Program Evaluations

Because analytical methods significantly influence the very nature of pesticide monitoring programs, improving methods has been viewed as a critical requisite of the programs in general. In the late 1970s, the Subcommittee on Oversight and Investigations of the House Committee on Interstate and Foreign Commerce, as well as the General Accounting Office, investigated the Federal pesticide monitoring program administered by FDA. Among the recommendations the subcommittee made was that FDA develop analytical methods to detect more pesticides, and to focus on methods that could be performed more quickly (25).

In FDA's own landmark study of ways to improve the pesticide program (26), FDA emphasized the importance of a "strong, continuously well-supported and closely coordinated analytical methods development program" (27) to the overall effectiveness of pesticide monitoring. The FDA study group highlighted the need for practical analytical methods, so that they could be used to handle the volume of samples necessary in a regulatory program. The group also suggested that research efforts focus on pesticides not detected by available methods, yet of concern because of toxicity and prevalence of use in agriculture (28).

The study group emphasized that for pesticides not detected by multiresidue methods" . . . research is needed on other kinds of surveillance analytical methodology to reduce the overall time and complexity of analyses."(29) Among the specific research projects suggested was the study of rapid bioassay screening tests that would indicate whether further residue analysis was needed by a more complex GLC method (30).

Although FDA reprogrammed resources to focus on these objectives, budgetary constraints and agency commitments to other public health needs curtailed the reprogramming possible (31).

Several recent studies of the Federal pesticide programs have stimulated interest in pesticide analytical methods. Among the most important of these was a 1986 study of the General Accounting Office (GAO) (32), which reported that there was a significant gap between the number of pesticides that could potentially be found in food and the number that could be detected practicably with the multiresidue methods being used in the pesticide monitoring program operated by the Food and Drug Administration (FDA) (33). FDA was found to rely on five multiresidue methods. The scope of coverage of each method ranges from 24 to 123 different residues. Together, the tests are capable of detecting 203 different pesticide residues.

GAO reported that the most serious limitation of the methods was that they could detect only 40.9 percent of the estimated 496 different pesticides that potentially could be found in food (34). Furthermore, the methods could detect approximately 64 percent of the estimated 316 pesticides for which EPA has established food tolerances and are either currently registered for use on food products or persist in the environment and appear in food despite cancellation or suspension of food uses (35). Although single residue methods maybe used to detect the estimated 59.1 percent of pesticides not detected by the multiresidue methods, as a practical matter, they are not used because the inefficiency of the methods cannot be absorbed in the program given resource constraints. GAO reported that pesticides not detected by the five multiresidue methods are not routinely monitored.

Although multiresidue methods detect a substantial number of pesticides of health concern, among those not monitored because of the limitations of existing methods are 33 of 81 of those pesticides identified in FDA's Surveillance Index (36) as being of high priority for routine monitoring (37).

Recognizing the relative cost-efficiency of multiresidue over single residue methods, GAO recommended that FDA expand the number of pesticides that can be detected by multiresidue methods and, until "comprehensive capability" exists to test for most pesticides, conduct more testing of pesticides not detected by multiresidue methods (38).

The manner in which limitations in analytical capability restrict the effectiveness of monitoring was highlighted in two recent studies of the USDA National Residue Program. In a 1985 study, the National Academy of Sciences (NAS) made broad recommendations that the National Residue Program be readjusted to direct inspection to reflect assessments of relative chemical risks and to emphasize residue prevention. NAS also advised, "[t]he analytical methods used must be appropriate to the task. . . .The testing program will require substantial support for research, including the development of more accurate, more sensitive, and less expensive tests as well as tests for new hazards"(39).

A 1987 GAO report pointed out that, as in the FDA program, a gap existed in the USDA program between the possible residues in food and the scope of practicable testing methods. GAO recommended that USDA systematically assess the status of methods for detecting harmful chemicals in food to provide a basis for deciding on the additional research needed to develop more effective methods (40). In addition, GAO echoed the advice of NAS that greater emphasis be given to new methods development including rapid, inexpensive screening tests to detect an array of hazardous compounds (41).

The issue of pesticide analytical methods was also the focus of a 1987 report of the Congressional Research Service (CRS) (42). That report considered whether new and relatively inexpensive rapid analytical methods based on such biological reagents as enzymes (e.g., enzyme bioassays) and antibodies (immunoassays) might have applications supplementary to those of the multiresidue methods used in the FDA monitoring program. The report concluded that enzyme bioassays may offer a relatively inexpensive screening method to use in identifying foods free of certain pesticides (negative results). CRS considered the potential applications of immunoassays to include uses as single residue methods, or chemical class-specific screening methods. Also, immunoassays were believed to hold promise as small-scale multiresidue methods. Some of the tests being designed were considered simple enough to be performed by relatively unskilled persons in the field. However, CRS noted that a policy decision to incorporate rapid test methods into the monitoring program, particularly as screening methods, would have implications for the cost and design of the monitoring program because screening is not a regular part of the current monitoring program (43).

The critical position of analytical methods in pesticide monitoring programs has been recognized repeatedly in evaluations of Federal programs. Each study that has recognized the limited scope of the existing, practical multiresidue methods, has recommended that more research dollars be devoted to expand the scope of practicable methods. Several studies have suggested the need for less expensive and more rapid methods to cover pesticides not detected by multiresidue methods. NAS and CRS have suggested that rapid screening tests may serve a valuable function in pesticide monitoring.

Analytical Technology and Program Design

In focusing on analytical methods as a technical issue bearing on the effectiveness of pesticide monitoring primarily in terms of how many pesticides can be detected, most policy analyses have treated methods as merely tools used to reach a predefined objective. This perspective obscures the fact that analytical technology serves to define program design and goals.

Analytical methods help to define program design and goals in several ways. First, the scope of pesticide coverage and limits of detection of analytical methods define what is and what is not detected in a pesticide monitoring program. Second, the complexity of the method influences who is able to do the testing and what kind of equipment and facilities are needed. Third, the level of confidence in the reliability and validity of the test results influences for what purposes they are suitable. Finally, the resources needed to run the test influence how many tests can be run within fixed resources. The cost of the method is influenced by a variety of factors including its complexity and whether it provides opportunities for economies of scale.

The development of gas chromatography (GC) during the late 1950s, has had a significant impact on the design and goals of Federal pesticide programs. GC technology is the foundation upon which modern GLC and HPLC multiresidue methods were developed. Before GC was available, analytical chemists had to use such relatively unsophisticated pesticide detection methods as colorimetry and paper chromatography, which provided limited quantitative information. The GC technology transformed analytical capabilities because it provided reliable quantitative measures of chemicals and pressed the limits of detection continually lower.

GC was first promoted as a useful method of detecting chemical subunits of fats, known as fatty acids. However, pesticide residue chemists soon adapted the technology for pesticide analysis, and eventually developed the broad scope multiresidue methods currently used in monitoring programs.

The timing of the GC discovery was significant. The period of the 1950s and early 1960s was a watershed period for both the analysis and regulation of chemicals in food (44). The 1954 Miller Amendments to the Food Drug and Cosmetic Act (FDCA) for the first time established in the law the concept of scientificially determined tolerances as a basis for restricting the sale of foods containing pesticide residues (45). The 1958 enactment of the Food Additive Amendments to the FDCA included the precedential Delaney clause (46), which reflected the view prevailing among scientists at the time, that for at least some health risks of chemicals, particularly carcinogenicity, no "safe" level of exposure could be defined. This view accentuated the role of chemical detection and fostered efforts to press the capabilities of analytical chemistry to ever lower limits of detection.

In 1962, as the Miller Amendments were being implemented and the potential of GC being explored, Rachel Carson's influential book *Silent Spring*, (47) was published. The book highlighted concerns about the health and environmental consequences of the organic pesticides (organochlorine and organophosphorus compounds) developed during World War II. The charges the book made about the accumulation and persistence of such pesticides as dichloro-diphenyl-trichloro-ethane (DDT) in the fat component of foods, including milk, gained the attention of regulators at FDA (48). As regulators made these organic pesticides a monitoring priority, they found GC to be particularly well-suited to detect these classes of chemicals.

The characteristics of GC worked to help shape the design of pesticide monitoring programs. For example, the methods had to be performed in the laboratory, by highly skilled residue chemists. These features meant that food samples collected had to be sent to equipped laboratories, and results were not available for several days. The complexity of the system caused the analysis of each sample to be relatively costly.

Although improved efficiency was gained through the development of GLC and HPLC multiresidue methods, these are still laboratory methods that must be operated by highly skilled staffs. The limited scope of multiresidue methods also has served to define goals of pesticide monitoring. Organic pesticides have remained a priority in the monitoring of food residues. However, because of the health and environmental dangers presented by the early organic pesticides, many have been phased out of use. Newer pesticides are of more diverse classes and have been designed to degrade more quickly into breakdown products to avoid environmental persistence and accumulation. The changes in pesticide formulation have increased the number and chemical class diversity of compounds to be analyzed in food, significantly increasing the scientific task of monitoring them. Many of these chemicals cannot be detected by the practical multiresidue methods being used in monitoring programs (49). Residue problems have gradually shifted outside the direct focus of multiresidue methods. The very methods that once provided the means by which regulators could rise to meet the challenge of monitoring pesticides in food now limit their ability to do so.

The limitations of the methods have, in turn, served to help shape the goals of monitoring programs. As noted above, because of resource constraints that prevent the use of single residue methods, both FDA and USDA have focused their monitoring efforts on those pesticides detected by multiresidue methods. USDA in particular has articulated as a premise of their monitoring programs that a pesticide will not be selected for monitoring in the National Residue Program unless a practical analytical method exists to detect it (50). Multiresidue methods have thus influenced both the design and the goal of the monitoring program. In this sense, the analytical technology of multiresidue methods has ascended beyond the role of a tool to accomplish a policy objective to one that helps define the policy objective.

Of course, analytical technology is not the only variable that influences the design of monitoring programs. The significant differences in the legislative mandates of FDA and USDA are largely responsible for the enforcement focus of FDA's commodity sampling program as distinguished from the certification focus of USDA's monitoring program,

as a component of the meat and poultry inspection system (although both programs serve enforcement purposes). In addition, the legislative mandate of an agency may also influence the technologies it adopts into its program by defining certain problems as within the jurisdiction of that agency. For instance, USDA has in recent years incorporated rapid screening tests for certain animal drugs, e.g., the "sulfa-on-site" test into the meat inspection program. These tests are helpful to USDA in achieving its mandate of not only enforcing drug residue limits, in which case they must be confirmed with a more sophisticated analytical method, but also in preventing the entry into commerce of food containing illegal residues by obtaining test results quickly. FDA may have a similar interest in on-site test results if the mandate of that agency were expanded to require FDA to prevent food containing illegal residues from entering into commerce.

While the studies discussed above (excepting the CRS report) have focused on a range of problems afflicting Federal pesticide monitoring programs, the recommendations regarding methods research have arisen from concern about the gap in pesticides potentially present in food and the coverage of multiresidue methods. Some studies have made vague reference to the costly nature of pesticide analyses (e.g., GAO Livestock Report; NAS Meat Inspection Report) and have implied a need for less expensive and more rapid test methods. However, the program studies have focused little attention on the possible relationship between other fundamental problems in pesticide monitoring programs and the currently used battery of analytical methods.

Some additional problems of Federal pesticide monitoring programs that have been recently documented include the following list.

1. The public is exposed to foods sampled and found to contain violative pesticide residues because the food passes into commerce while the samples are shipped to central laboratories, analyzed, and results reported (51, 52, 53).

2. Time delays and sample backlogs in FDA laboratories expand the time it takes to obtain analytical findings (54).

3. Because of limited program resources, a relatively small portion of the domestic food supply (no estimate available) and approximately 1 percent of imported food shipments are analyzed by FDA (55, 56).

Because most studies of Federal pesticide programs have not focused directly on the possible linkage between analytical methods and monitoring program design, the possible role of analytical methods in addressing the above problems has not been highlighted.

Conclusion

As the future of pesticide analytical methods development is charted, there is a danger in focusing only on strategies to fill the gap between potential residues in food and residues detectable by multiresidue methods. The so-called gap has been defined using current analytical technology as a reference point, rather than program needs generally. To focus on the gap alone propagates the limitations of the current program and the technology that has helped to define it to the arena of research objectives. Such a focus fails to consider the opportunities analytical technology may offer to improve pesticide programs in more fundamental, structural ways. Rather, it may inform judgments about the direction of future methods research to consider what the future of pesticide monitoring programs should be. The span between that goal and the status of current pesticide programs is a truer estimate of the "gap" that represents current program needs.

Examining the ability of current analytical technology to meet those needs within realistic estimates of program resources will help to suggest an appropriate research strategy.

Questions to Consider as a Research Strategy is Defined

As research priorities are established for pesticide analytical methods development, it may be useful to consider the following questions.

Studies of Federal pesticide monitoring programs not only have revealed a gap in detectable pesticides but also some structural problems that have been generated by a system that requires food samples to be sent to centralized laboratories for analysis. There, even a relatively small number of pesticide samples can add to and become enmeshed in laboratory backlog and delay. Can analytical methods be designed so that they can be performed in the field?

The studies also reveal a system in which many of even those relatively few foods that are sampled and found to be violative, are nevertheless consumed because there is no rapid way to identify foods containing illegal pesticide residues. Can analytical methods be developed to provide on-site results?

Reports show a system (FDA) in which resources run out after only spot-check sampling is done. Can inexpensive (e.g., screening) methods be developed so that more sampling and analysis can be performed assuming fixed resources? Can more expensive laboratory methods be reserved for confirming results of screening tests?

In addition to considering how methods development might address problems that have been identified inside existing monitoring programs, it also may be instructive to consider the assumptions of the existing Federal program.

Analytical methods have become a limiting factor in the enforcement of laws concerning pesticide residues in food. The premise of the pesticide registration system is that registrants will supply to regulators the analytical means to enforce a condition of registration, i.e., acceptable food residues. As discussed above, the current method requirement imposed on registrants has not fulfilled this objective. This fact spawns several policy questions regarding analytical methods development.

Would a requirement that the method submitted by a registrant be useful to regulators be workable? Would a required contribution by registrants to a Federal research fund for the development of practicable methods satisfy the need for such methods?

What resource commitment to analytical methods development would be necessary to keep pace with the advent of new pesticides?

Does the premise of the method development requirement for registrants expect more from technology than can feasibly be delivered?

Even if the scope of analytical methods were broad enough to detect all possible residues, how meaningful would it be if scaled-up affordable sampling with rapid analytical results were unavailable? From an ideal public health perspective, what should be the food sampling goal? What level of resources would be needed to achieve this goal, given current analytical technology? What would be the impact on cost if inexpensive screening tests could be used in the field to detect residues and laboratory methods reserved for confirmation? Can an ideal level of sampling be achieved assuming the use of screening tests and fixed Federal resources?

If industry (e.g., the fresh produce industry, the food processing industry) obtained private certification of the conformity of their products with pesticide requirements through the use of private analytical testing, what impact would it have on the goals for analytical methods development?

What are the regulatory implications of developing inexpensive, rapid, and simple pesticide analytical methods that may be used by members of the public?

Do the limitations of pesticide monitoring programs and methods suggest a need for enforcement policies that focus more attention on residue control than on residue detection?

References

1. Whitaker, A.H., "A History of Federal Pesticide Regulation in the United States to 1947," p. 49-50 (dissertation, Emory University, 1979). (Dr. Haywood was also head of the insecticide and fungicide section of the Association of Analytical Chemists.)

2. See, e.g., Montgomery, A. America's Pesticide-Permeated Food, Nutrition Action Health Letter, v. 14, June 1987. p. 5 ("Not all pesticides are unsafe. But some can cause cancer, birth defects, heritable genetic mutations, and nerve damage. Clearly, we need to spend more money and devote more resources to improving our testing procedures for detecting hazardous residues.")

3. Mr. Pasquale Lombardo, Division of Contaminants Chemistry, Food and Drug Administration, private interview, Wash., D.C., Jan. 26, 1988.

4. Both GLC and HPLC operate on a similar basic principle. A chemical mixture (food sample extract) is injected into the portal of specialized chromatographic equipment that contains a "separating column." The separating column permits pesticides to pass through it at different rates based on differences in their physical and chemical properties. As each chemical reaches the end of the column, each is in turn sensed by a detector, and a printer displays the chemical as a "peak" on a chromatographic print-out. Chemicals can be identified by comparing the time interval between sample injection and the appearance of a peak with the intervals of known standard chemicals. The amount of a chemical is determined by measuring the size of a peak.

5. The pesticide analytical methods in use in monitoring programs are detailed in U.S. Library of Congress, Congressional Research Service. "Pesticide monitoring Program: Developing New Methods to Detect Pesticide Residues in Food," by Sarah E. Taylor, Apr. 24, 1987.

6. The most costly part of pesticide analysis by GLC or HPLC, whether a single or mult-residue method, is in the perparation of the sample for injection into the chromatograph. Consequently, because multi- and single residues methods require similar sample preparation, and a multiresidue method provides methods information on many pesticides, multiresidue methods are considered more resource efficient that single residue methods. However, the cost of a multiresidue analysis costs up to $200 per sample of fruit, vegetable or grain, while fatty foods, including milk and fatty fish cost approximately $320 per sample analysis. Shroff, A. Regulatory Affairs Division, Food and Drug Administration, personal communication, Apr. 16, 1987.

7. 7 U.S.C. Sec. 135a(c)(5)(d). "Unreasonable adverse effects on the environment" is defined as, "any unreasonable risk to men or the environment, taking into account the economic, social, and environmental costs and benefits of the use of any pesticide." 7 U.S.C. Sec. 136(bb).

8. EPA has failed to company fully with the above described requirements of FIFRA. See, for example, General Accounting Office. Pesticides: EPA's Formidable Task to Assess and Regulate Their Risk. GAO/RCED-86-125. Washington, DC, 1986. p. 92-100. Registration processes are discusses in U.S. Library of Congress, Congressional Research Service, "Pesticide Regulation: Legislative Debate About FIFRA in 1986," by Aidala, J. May 11, 1987. p. 5. See also Conner, J.D. et. al. *Pesticide Regulation Handbook.* (Washington, DC, 1987.)

9. 40 C.F.F. 158.125.

10. The EPA validation should be distinguished from the formal validation required by the Association of Official Analytical Chemists (AOAC) for a method to gain official status (the "gold standard" for analytical methods). AOAC requires that at least six laboratories validate a method. The purpose of validation by AOAC criteria is to assure that the method is capable of performing as intended and that the results of an analysis are of acceptable accuracy and precision. See Hill, K.R. and P.E. Corneliussen, "Validation of Official Methods," *Analytical Methods for Pesticides and Plant Growth Regulators,* v. XV, Academic Press, New York, 1986. However, the AOAC validation method takes several years and is so resource-intensive, requiring the attention of the limited number of expert residue chemists in the U.S., that many EPA officials consider it an unworkable systems for their regulatory purposes. Dr. Francis Griffith, Residue Chemistry Branch, Environmental Protection Agency, personal communication, Feb. 23, 1988. (557-0826).

11. Discussed in U.S. Library of Congress, Congres-

sional Research Service. "Pesticide Monitoring Program, Developing New Methods to Detect Pesticide Residues in Food," by S.E. Taylor, Apr. 24, 1987.

12. See 21 U.S.C. sec. 342 (a)(2)(C), 374(c)-(d).

13. Reed, D., P. Lombardo, J. Wessel, L.A. Burke and B. McMahon. Division of Contaminants Chemistry. The FDA Pesticide Monitoring Program, *J. Assoc. Off. Anal. Chem.*, v. 70, no. 3, 1987. p. 59.

14. Duggan, R.E. and H.R. Cook, "National Food and Feed Monitoring Program," *Pesticides Monitoring Journal*, 5:37, June 1971.

15. Food and Drug Administration, Compliance Program Guidance Manual, Pesticides and Industrial Chemicals in Domestic Foods (FY88/89), Oct. 1, 1987.

16. Ibid.

17. CDP Associates. Assessment of FDA's Total Diet Study, Contract HHS-100-82-0076. 1982.

18. Poultry Products Inspection Act, 21 U.S.C. sec. 455(s); Meat Inspection Act, 21 U.S.C. sec. 603.

19. Poultry Products Inspection Act, 21 U.S.C. sec. 455(b); Meat Inspection, 21 U.S.C. sec. 604.

20. See Poultry Products Inspection Act, 21 U.S.C. sec. 455(b) (The Secretary, whenever processing operations are being conducted, shall cause to made by inpsectors, post mortem inspections of the carcass of *each* bird processes.") Federal Meat Inspection Act, 21 U.S.C. sec. 604 ("[A]ll such animals found to be not adulterated shall be marked, stamped, tagged or labeled as 'inspected and passed'. . . .").

21. Federal Meat Inspection Act, 21 U.S.C. sec. 603 ("For the purpose of preventing the use in commerce of meat and meat food products which are adulterated. . . .") Poultry Products Inspection Act, 21 U.S.C. sec. 455(a) ("For the purpose of preventing the entry into or flow or movement in commerce of, or the burdening of commerce by, and poultry product which is . . . adulterated.)

22. 1987 National Residue Plan, p. 3. A.3.

23. Food Safety and Inspection Service, United States Department of Agriculture. Compound Evaluation and Analytical Capability National Residue Program Plan 1987. Jan. 1987, p. 2.1.

24. 1987 National Residue Plan, p. 5.1.-5.2.

25. U.S. Congress. House. Committee on Interstate and Foreign Commerce, with separate views by the Subcommittee on Oversight and Investigations. Cancer-Causing Chemicals in Food. 95th Cong. 2d Sess. Washington, U.S. Govt. Print. Off., 1978. p. 37-38. Committee Print.

26. U.S. Dept. of Health and Human Services. Food and Drug Administration. Public Health Service. Study Group on FDA Residue Programs. FDA Monitoring Programs for Pesticide and Industrial Chemical Residues in Food. June 1979. p. 57 [1979 FDA Study Group Report.]

27. 1979 FDA Study Group Report, p. 58-59.

28. 1979 Study Group Report, p. 58-59. (FDA developed the surveillance index system as a response to this identified goal.)

29. 1979 FDA Study Group Report, p. 57.

30. Ibid.

31. See, e.g., U.S. Department of Health and Human Services, Food and Drug Administration. Public Health Service. Report on Proposals to Improve Control of Pesticide Residues in Imported Foods, Mar. 10, 1982. p. 9.

32. U.S. General Accounting Office, "Pesticides: Need to Enhance FDA's Ability to Protect the Public From Illegal Residues," Report to Congressional Requesters by the Comptroller General of the United States, GAO/RCED-87-7. Washington, DC, 1986. p. 31-33. [GAO Domestic Food Report].

33. While the GAO report focused on the FDA monitoring program, its conclusions regarding the adequacy of pesticide analytical methods also implicates the methods used in the monitoring program of the USDA because they are similar in nature to those of FDA's program.

34. FDA has disputed the relevance of comparing the scope of coverage of the five multiresidue methods to the reference point of 496 pesticides. FDA contends that the number includes pesticides that are not actually in use because registration is pending or has been cancelled, and it includes pesticides for which all food uses have been cancelled. They agency has implied that 230 may be a more appropriate reference point. Bowen, Otis R., Secretary of Health and Human Service. Letter to Charles Bowsher, Comptroller General of the United States, Mar. 20, 1987.

35. Domestic Food Report, p. 31-34.

36. The surveillance index is a system developed by FDA in 1979 to classify pesticides according to potential health hazard. The classification scheme was developed to help the agency put in priority its monitoring of residues not detected by multiresidue methods and to direct research efforts to develop new methods. Pesticide chemicals undergoing special review at EPA because of special health or environmental concerns have been given priority in being clas-

sified in the surveillance index. The index lists pesticides in Classes I, II, and III. with Class I being of highests priority based upon the toxicity, use pattern (poundage and crop), potential for food residues and persistence in the environment. See U.S. Dept. of Health and Human Services. Food and Drug Administration. FDA Monitoring programs for Pesticide and Industrial Chemical Residues in Food; Study Group on FDA Residue Programs, June 1979, p. 57.

37. GAO Domestic Food Report, p. 39.

38. Ibid., p.43.

39. Food and Nutrition Board, National Research Council, National Academy of Sciences. Meat and Pountry Inspection: The Scientific Basis of the Nation's Program, 1985. p. 55-56. In USDA's report responding to the recommendations of NAS, it largely attributed its limited methods to lack of adequate research funding. USDA suggested that it should be taking advantage of its potential as a significant purchaser of rapid test methods to stimulate developmental work in the private sector. U.S. Dept. of Agriculture, Food Safety and Inspection Service. FSIS Future Agenda: Response to the NAS Recommendations. June 1986, ch. II.

40. General Accounting Office. Imported Meat and Livestock; Chemical Residue Detection and the Issue of Labeling, GAO/RCED-87-142 Wash. D.C., Sept. 1987. p. 49-50. [GAO Livestock Report]

41. GAO Livestock Report, p. 38-39.

42. U.S. Library of Congress, Congressional Research Service. Pesticide Monitoring Program: Developing New Methods to Detect Pesticide Residues in Food, by Sarah E. Taylor, Apr. 24, 1987.

43. U.S. Library of Congress, Congressional Research Service. Pesticide Monitoring Program: Developing New Methods to Detect Pesticide Residues in Food, by Sarah E. Taylor, Apr. 24, 1987. p. 33-34.

44. U.S. Library of Congress, Congressional Research Service. Food Safety Policy: Selected Scientific and Regulatory Issues. IB83158 by S. E. Taylor and D.V. Porter (regularly updated) p. 2-5.

45. 21 U.S.C. Sec. 346a (amended by Act of July 22, 1954 ch. 559, 68 Stat. 511).

46. The so-called "Delaney," or "anti-cancer" clause was incorporated into the FDCA through the Food Additives Amendments of 1958, the Color Additive Amendments of 1960, and the Animal Drug Amendments of 1968. The essence of each clause provides that a substance shall not be deemed safe and shall not be deemed safe and shall not be approved if it is found to induce cancer when ingested by man or animal, or if it is found after tests that are appropriate for the evaluation of the safety of the substance to induce cancer in man or animal. The standard of safety embodied in the anti-cancer clause is sometimes termed as "zero-risk" or "zero-tolerance" standard. See, U.S. Library of Congress, Congressional Research Service. Food and Color Additives: "De Minimis" and "Delaney," by Sarah E. Taylor. Aug. 5, 1987. The Delaney Clause applies to pesticide residues in foods when residues concentrate during food processing to levels exceeding the tolerance approved on the food commodity. The implications of the Delaney Clause to perticide chemicals was considered in Board on Agriculture, National Research Council. Regulating Pesticides in Food: The Delaney Paradox. Wash., D.C., 1987.

47. Carson, R. Silent Spring. (Boston: Houghton Mifflin Co., 1962) (The book was first published as a series of articles appearing in The New Yorker.)

48. Carson, pp. 140, 169, 178.

49. Discussed in U.S. Library of Congress, Congressional Research Service. Pesticide Monitoring Program: Developing New Methods to Detect Pesticide Residues in Food, by Sarah Taylor, Apr. 24, 1987. p. 16.

50. 1987 National Residue Plan, p. 5.1-5.2.

51. GAO Domestic Food Report, p. 4.

52. General Accounting Office. Better Sampling and Enforcement Needed on Imported Food. GAO/RCED-86-219, Washington, DC, Sept. 1986. p. 4. [GAO Imported Food Report]

53. General Accounting Office. Problems in Preventing the Marketing of Raw Meat and Poultry Containing Potentially Harmful Residues. HRD-79-10, Washington, DC, Apr. 1979.

54. General Accounting Office. Laboratory Analyses of Product Samples Needs to be More Timely. GAO/HRD-86-102, Washington, DC, Sept. 1986.

55. GAO Domestic Food Report, p. 3.

56. Ibid.

Appendix C
Glossary of Terms

Glossary of Terms

absorption spectrum: a plot of the amount of light absorbed by a gas, liquid, or solid at particular wavelengths versus the wavelengths examined.

acetone: a solvent used to extract pesticides from foods.

acetonitrile: a solvent used to extract pesticides from foods.

adsorbent: a material that gathers a gas, liquid, or dissolved substance on a surface in a condensed layer.

adsorption chromatography: chromatography based on the interaction between a chemical dissolved in a solvent and an adsorptive surface, such as the surface of a diatomaceous earth particle.

affinity: The strength of the interaction between chemical and antibody. The higher the affinity of the antibody for the target chemical, the greater the sensitivity of the immunoassay.

alkali flame ionization detector (AFID): a detector that measures the presence of nitrogen and phosphorus within a molecule.

alumina: the natural or synthetic oxide of aluminum.

analytical columns: columns that are used to separate chemicals at the microgram level or below.

aromatics: chemical compounds containing one or more benzene rings.

atomic emission spectrometric detector: a detector that measures light emitted from atoms, ions or molecules following excitation by electrical energy, flame, or high temperatures; see flame photometric detector.

capillary column: long, open tubes ranging from 0.01 to 0.03 inch in internal diameter and from 30 to 500 feet in length; the inside wall of the tube is coated with a thin film of involatile liquid.

chemiluminescence detector: a detector that measures the emission of light produced by a chemical reaction.

cholinesterase: an enzyme that hydrolyzes choline esters.

chromatogram: the record obtained from a chromatographic analysis.

chromatography: the separation of mixtures into their constituents by preferential adsorption to, and elution from, a solid support.

compliance samples: commodities collected by FDA when a violation of pesticide residue tolerance levels is suspected or known.

derivatization, chemical: modification of a chemical, usually by the addition to or modification of, a functional group to enhance or permit detection of the compound.

detector, chromatographic: a device for measuring the amount of a chemical following chromatographic separation.

diatomaceous earth: a fine siliceous earth composed chiefly of the cell walls of diatoms (any of numerous microscopic, unicellular, marine, or freshwater algae having siliceous cell walls) used for adsorption chromatography.

distillation: the volatilization or evaporation and subsequent condensation of a liquid, as when water is boiled in a retort and the steam is condensed in a cool receiver.

electroactive functional groups: chemical groups of a molecule that can be oxidized or reduced electrochemically.

electrochemical detector: a detector that measures the flow of electrons that occurs with the oxidation or reduction of the chemical analyzed.

electron capture detector (ECD): a detector that measures amount and electron affinity of the chemical analyzed.

elute: to remove an absorbed material from an adsorbent by means of a solvent.

emulsion: an intimate mixture of liquids, one of which (the disperse phase) is distributed in large or small globules throughout the other (the continuous phase). The emulsifying agent, the third component, is present at the interface between the two liquids.

exploratory projects: a survey done by FSIS to determine if a pesticide not currently detected or a method not currently used should be included in a monitoring program.

fixed wavelength UV absorbance detector: a detector that can measure the absorbance of light by a chemical at one single wavelength.

flame photometric detector: a type of atomic emission spectrometric detector employing a flame as a source of excitation of the chemical.

Florisil: a diatomaceous earth adsorbent.

fluorometer: an instrument used to measure the intensity of fluorescence produced by a fluorophor.

fluorophor: a molecule or portion of a molecule that is capable of excitation by high-energy radiation and will subsequently emit low-energy radiation.

fouling (detector): contamination of a detector with material that decreases the sensitivity or stability of the detector response.

gas chromatography: chromatography in which the substance to be analyzed is vaporized and diffused along with a carrier gas through a liquid or solid adsorbent for differential adsorption.

gel chromatography: the separation of molecules on a column on the basis of size following their movement into and out of, or their total exclusion from, pores in the gel column.

Hall microelectrolytic conductivity detector (HECD): a detector that measures the presence of halogens (e.g., Cl, Br), sulfur or nitrogen in a molecule.

hapten: a chemical compound so small that it must be conjugated to a larger molecule before it can stimulate antibody production.

herbicide: a chemical for killing plants, especially weeds.

Hill reaction: the evolution of oxygen from a chloroplast in the presence of ferric ion following the introduction of light.

hybridoma: a cell type produced by the fusion of spleen cells and myeloma tumor cells which can produce monoclonal antibodies.

hydrocarbons: any of a class of compounds containing only carbon and hydrogen.

immiscible: incapable of being mixed.

immunoassay: the use of antibodies to identify and possibly quantify a substance.

integrators: computers used with gas and liquid chromatography in part to determine a chemical's retention time and quantity.

ion trap detector (ITD): a miniaturized mass spectrometer used in the detection of gas chromatography eluants.

ionic: pertaining to electrically charged atoms or groups or atoms.

liquid phase: the chemical that is bound to the inert supporting phase in a gas chromatographic column that separates the various components of a mixture placed on the column.

market basket: a selection of foods that represents the typical diet of a U.S. household.

mass selective detector (MSD): a miniaturized mass spectrometer used in the detection of gas chromatography eluants.

mass spectrometry (MS): an analytical technique in which a chemical is broken into fragments with positive or negative charge(s) and the mass and relative abundance of these fragments are analyzed to produce a mass spectrum.

matrix: the material in which the chemical to be analyzed is found, e.g., pesticides in food.

metabolite: a compound produced from another (known as a parent compound) as a result of physical and chemical processes acting on the original compound.

microgram: 10^{-6} grams.

mobile phase: the solvent that flows through a chromatographic column.

monoclonal antibodies: antibodies produced by a single strain of cloned cells (e.g., hydridomas) in culture.

multiresidue method (MRM): analytical method that can detect more than one pesticide during an analysis of a sample.

nanogram: 10^{-9} grams.

nanometers: 10^{-9} meters; used to describe wavelengths of light that are used to excite molecules and that measure the light absorbed by or emitted from an excited molecule.

neutral: having no electrical charge, positive or negative.

nitrogenous pesticides: pesticides containing one or more nitrogen atom(s).

oxidize: to combine with oxygen; to take away hydrogen.

p-value: a measure of the partition characteristics of a pesticide between two immiscible organic phases (solvents).

packed columns: hollow tubing ranging in internal diameter from 2-4 mm and in length from a few inches to 50 feet, filled with particles coated with an inviolatile liquid.

partitioning: the process of distributing between two immiscible solvents so that the pesticide will appear in one phase and potential interferences in another, which can then be discarded.

pesticides: toxic chemicals used against insects (insecticides), fungi (fungicides), weeds (herbicides), and other pests.

Pestrak: FDA computerized data base used to track whether pesticides can be analyzed using one of FDA's five routinely used multiresidue methods.

photo-diode array detector: a detector that contains several diodes arranged in series that respond to the characteristic emitted light of the chemical being analyzed.

photo-ionizable functional groups: chemical groups such as halides (e.g., Cl, Br) that can be removed from a larger molecule by the effect of light.

photoconductivity detector: a detector that measures the change in the conductivity of a chemical in solution produced by the decomposition of the chemical by light.

photolyze: the degradation or structural transformation of a chemical by light.

photoreaction: a chemical reaction caused by the reaction of the chemical with light.

polar: that chemical characteristic that favors a chemical's solubility in water.

polyclonal antibodies: heterogeneous antibodies derived from different B lymphocyte cells in the serum of a vertebrate.

ppm: micrograms of chemical per gram of material in which the chemical is found.

preparative chromatography: the use of columns having the capability of separating milligram or larger quantities of chemicals.

pyrolysis: decomposition of chemicals under the influence of high temperatures.

qualitative: of or pertaining to the quality or identity of a substance.

qualitative test: identifies a pesticide residue if it occurs at concentrations above a pre-established level.

quantitative: of or pertaining to the measuring of the quantity of a substance.

relative retention time: the time that a compound is eluted from a chromatographic column expressed relative to that of a standard compound.

resolution: the true separation of two consecutive chromatographic peaks.

retention data: retention volume (volume of a carrier gas required to elute a compound from a column) and retention time (time required to elute a compound from a column).

semiquantitative: intermediate between quantitative and qualitative.

semiquantitative test: identifies a pesticide residue over a pre-established concentration and determines the range of their concentrations.

silica gel: a highly adsorbent gelatinous form of silica.

single residue method: analytical method that detects only one pesticide during an analysis of a sample.

size-exclusion chromatography: see gel chromatography.

solid phase extraction: a technique for concentrating chemicals by absorption and subsequent elution from a liquid phase that is chemically bonded to silica.

solvating power: the ability of a solvent to interact with a solute to form a solution.

solvent: a substance that dissolves another to form a solution.

standard: a chemical, of known concentration and purity, used as a reference substance in analytical work.

Subdivision "O" Guidelines: guidelines provided by the U.S. Environmental Protection Agency which describe the data to be submitted as part of the tolerance-setting process.

supercritical fluid chromatography (SFC): chromatography in which supercritical fluids are used as the mobile phase.

supercritical fluids (SF): fluids that are more dense than gases but not as dense as liquids.

support: the material to which the stationary phase is attached in a chromatographic column.

surveillance samples: for FDA, these are samples of food and feed that have been collected for general monitoring purposes; for FSIS these are meat samples suspected or known to violate pesticide tolerances.

thermionic detectors (NPD and AFID): detectors that measure those elements in a chemical compound that are ionized by heated rubidium (NPD; nitrogen and phosphorus are selectively detected) or by a heated alkali metal (AFID; nitrogen and phosphorus are selectively detected).

tolerance: the maximum legal level of a specific pesticide residue on a specific type of commodity, established by EPA.

Total Diet Study: FDA study that monitors the dietary intake of pesticides in a "market basket" of foods by various age-sex groups in the U.S.

UV absorbance detector: a detector that measures the absorbance of light in the ultraviolet range by chemicals moving through it.

unidentified analytical response (UAR): responses that appear on a chromatogram which do not coincide with standards of the pesticides or pesticide metabolites under investigation.

validating: the process by which one chemist or more test(s) the suitability of a particular method for collecting analytical data.

validation: the verification that a technology or method provides useful analytical data and operates within acceptable performance parameters.

variable wavelength detector: a detector in which a wide range of wavelengths of light can be detected.

violation rate: percentage of samples analyzed that violate tolerances.

volatile: evaporating rapidly.

wide bore columns: a type of capillary column used in gas chromatography that has an internal diameter ranging from 0.53 to 0.75 mm.

Superintendent of Documents Publication Order Form

Order Processing Code:

*6476

Charge your order.
It's easy!

☐ **YES**, please send me the following indicated publications:

Pesticide Residues in Food: Technologies for Detection.
GPO stock number 052-003-01132-8; price $10.00.

1. The total cost of my order is $_____ (International customers please add an additional 25%.) All prices include regular domestic postage and handling and are good through 2/89. After this date, please call Order and Information Desk at 202-783-3238 to verify prices.

Please Type or Print

2.

_____
(Company or personal name)

_____
(Additional address/attention line)

_____
(Street address)

_____
(City, State, ZIP Code)

(_____)_____
(Daytime phone including area code)

3. Please choose method of payment:

☐ Check payable to the Superintendent of Documents

☐ GPO Deposit Account ☐☐☐☐☐☐☐–☐

☐ VISA, CHOICE or MasterCard Account

☐☐☐☐☐☐☐☐☐☐☐☐

☐☐☐☐ (Credit card expiration date) *Thank you for your order!*

_____
(Signature)   10/88

4. Mail To: Superintendent of Documents, Government Printing Office, Washington, D.C. 20402-9325

DO NOT REMOVE
SLIP FROM POCKET